RISK FACTORS IN BREAST CANCER

Edited by Basil A. Stoll

Honorary Consultant Physician to the Radiotherapy and Oncology Departments at St. Thomas' Hospital and Royal Free Hospital, London

VOLUME 2 in the Series

NEW ASPECTS OF BREAST CANCER

A WILLIAM HEINEMANN MEDICAL BOOKS PUBLICATION

DISTRIBUTED BY

YEAR BOOK MEDICAL PUBLISHERS, INC.

35 EAST WACKER DRIVE

CHICAGO

1976

First Published 1976

Distributed in Continental North, South and Central America,
Hawaii, Puerto Rico and The Philippines by
Year Book Medical Publishers, Inc.

by arrangement with William Heinemann Medical Books Ltd.

ISBN 0-8151-8268-6

Library of Congress Catalog Card Number 74-25399

Printed in Great Britain

Preface to Series

In planning a new Series for which both scientists and clinicians will be invited to write, it is hoped to extend the horizons of the very large number of specialists with a major interest in breast cancer. There are, unfortunately, too few meeting grounds in the literature between the scientist engaged in research and the clinician involved in the investigation and management of the patient, and the intention of the Series is to bridge their divergent philosophy and language. Its purpose is to provide the specialist clinician with an authoritative and balanced interpretation of new scientific findings and thinking, and this is to be specifically orientated to a possible application to the clinical problem.

Breast cancer is an obvious choice of topic for such a Series. Its incidence in Western women is increasingly high and its epidemiology, aetiology, diagnosis and life history are currently the subject of very extensive investigations. Moreover, the management of the disease, both early and late, is at the moment in a state of agonizing reappraisal. Each volume will select one particular aspect of breast cancer where recent research has suggested the need for a pressing reorientation of thinking in the clinical field. While the individual experts will each discuss one facet of the problem, it is intended that every volume will be a review of the whole topic and complete in itself.

January 1975 *Basil A. Stoll*

Preface to Volume 2

This volume is intended to discuss the recognition and management of two specific groups of patients. Firstly women with an increased predisposition to the development of breast cancer, and secondly those tumour-bearing patients whose disease carries a relatively poor prognosis.

Recent technical advances in the treatment of breast cancer have not had the impact on the prognosis that had been hoped for, and for the immediate future, the diagnosis of breast cancer at an earlier stage in its development must remain the measure most likely to reduce the mortality of the disease. For this reason, there is a considerable body of opinion which advocates the regular screening of women for the presence of breast cancer, as soon as they enter the age groups at maximum risk. The yield of such a procedure is increased by concentrating on those women who carry a relatively higher predisposition to the tumour. The recognition of these individuals and the earlier diagnosis of their disease is discussed.

In the case of the patient with an established diagnosis of early breast cancer, the symposium aims to define the factors which identify the high risk patient. The biological characteristics of the disease in any individual patient depend on the interplay of tumoral aggressiveness on the one hand with specific host defence factors on the other. As increasing knowledge of these factors becomes available, we are increasingly able to select the most rational treatment for each individual. Even the avoidance of deleterious treatment alone would undoubtedly lead to very marked improvement in the survival rates of breast cancer patients.

January 1976 *Basil A. Stoll*

Contributors

David E. Anderson, Ph.D.
Professor and Acting Head, Department of Biology, University of Texas System Cancer Center, M.D. Anderson Hospital and Tumor Institute, Houston, Texas.

J. E. Devitt, M.D.C.M., M.Sc., F.R.C.S. (Ed.), F.R.C.S.(C)
Director of Continuing Medical Education and Associate Professor of Surgery, University of Ottawa; Consultant in Breast Surgery, Civic Hospital Division, Ottawa Clinic, Ontario Cancer Foundation, Canada.

Santiago Dexeus, M.D., F.I.A.C.
Director of Department of Obstetrics and Gynaecology, Instituto Dexeus, Universidad Autonoma de Barcelona, Spain.

J. A. Dossett, M.D., F.R.C. Path.
Consultant Pathologist, Leeds University Hospitals, St. James's Hospital, Leeds.

Bernard Fisher, M.D.
Professor of Surgery, University of Pittsburgh School of Medicine, Pittsburgh, Pennsylvania.

Edwin R. Fisher, M.D.
Director, Institute of Pathology, Shadyside Hospital, Pittsburgh, Pennsylvania.

H. Steven Greer, M.D., F.R.C. Psych.
Senior Lecturer and Consultant, Department of Psychological Medicine, and Faith Courtauld Unit, King's College Hospital, London, S.E.5.

Remigio M. Gregorio, M.D.
Associate Pathologist, Institute of Pathology, Shadyside Hospital, Pittsburgh, Pennsylvania.

Henry P. Leis, Jr., M.D., F.A.C.S., F.I.C.S. (Hon.)
Clinical Professor of Surgery and Chief of Breast Service, Department of Surgery, New York Medical College, New York City.

Edward F. Lewison, M.D.
Associate Professor of Surgery, The Johns Hopkins University School of Medicine; Chief of Breast Clinic (Emeritus), The Johns Hopkins Hospital, Baltimore, Maryland.

Abraham M. Lilienfeld, M.D., M.P.H., D.Sc.(Hon.)
Professor of Epidemiology, The Johns Hopkins University School of Hygiene and Public Health, Baltimore, Maryland.

H. Miller, M.D., F.R.C.P., F.R.C.Path.
Consultant Chemical Pathologist, Portsmouth and S.E. Hampshire District Pathology Service, St. Mary's Hospital, Portsmouth.

Robert W. Morgan, M.D.
Professor Department of Preventive Medicine and Biostatistics, University of Toronto, Ontario.

James L. Quinn, III, M.D., F.R.C.S. (I)
Professor of Radiology, Associate Chairman and Director of Nuclear Medicine, Northwestern University, McGaw Medical Center, Chicago, Illinois.

Alfio Raciti, M.D.
Chief Surgical Resident, Department of Surgery, New York Medical College, New York City.

Ole Scheike, M.D.
Physician to Radium Center, Finsen Institute and to Frederiksberg Hospital, Copenhagen.

Basil A. Stoll, F.R.C.R.
Honorary Consultant Physician to the Radiotherapy/Oncology Departments, St. Thomas' Hospital and Royal Free Hospital, London.

Philip Strax, M.D.
Associate Clinical Professor of Community Medicine, New York Medical College; Medical Director Guttman Breast Diagnostic Institute, New York; Consultant in Radiology to LaGuardia Hospital, Flushing Hospital, Jewish Memorial Hospital and City Hospital Center at Elmhurst, N.Y.

David P. Thomas, M.D., Dr.P.H.
Associate Professor Department of Epidemiology and International Health, School of Public Health and Community Medicine, University of Washington, Seattle, Washington.

Damodar V. Vakil, B.V.Sc., M.S., Ph.D.
Assistant Professor Department of Preventive Medicine and Biostatistics, University of Toronto, Ontario.

Contents

Section 1
WOMEN AT RISK

1

Familial and Genetic Predisposition

David E. Anderson

That breast cancer may occasionally aggregate in families has been amply demonstrated by numerous observations and studies during the past century. Although a family history has long been accepted as doubling a woman's risk of the disease, there is still doubt as to its etiological significance. Some advocate that familial aggregation represents an inherited tendency to the disease, others that it is the consequence of sharing common customs, dietary habits or other environmental factors. Moreover, breast cancer is sufficiently frequent in the population, at least in westernized cultures, for some familial occurrences to be explained by the phenomenon of chance.

A genetic basis has been clearly established for mammary tumor development in inbred strains of mice. First was the development of high and low mammary tumor strains by inbreeding and selection, which constituted evidence that hereditary factors were influential in the causation of the tumor (see review by Heston, 1973). Second was the evidence from crosses between the inbred strains that provided insight into the nature of the genetic effect. The action of some genes was shown to be localized in the physiology of hormone production by the ovaries; others controlled the response of mammary tissue to hormones; and others, apparently few in number, were responsible for the propagation and transmission of the mammary tumor virus (Heston, 1959; Nandi and Helmich, 1974).

FAMILY STUDIES

The establishment of a genetic basis for breast cancer in women has been much more difficult. The primary difficulty has been the collection of reliable data with which to assess the problem. Evidence of a genetic basis is indicated by certain distribution patterns of the disease in families. These patterns are difficult to identify if family members die of other causes at early ages, or are too young to provide clues as to their susceptibility, or if medical records are not available to document either the presence or absence of breast cancer in deceased family members. Moreover, the disease may be influenced by a number of reproductive and environmental variables, and, as will be discussed later, breast cancer may not be a single disease but a composite of several diseases. Then, too, human beings are characterized by small family sizes, long generation interval, and lack of controlled matings, which are clearly not problems in experimental animals.

Statistical surveys

In spite of these difficulties, an impressive number of genetic investigations of human breast cancer has been undertaken. Generally, one of three basic approaches has been used, i.e., retrospective statistical surveys, comparison of monozygotic and dizygotic twins, and pedigree studies. The retrospective statistical survey involves a comparison of the morbidity and/or mortality rates in the relatives of breast cancer patients with the rates in a control population or those expected from population statistics (see reviews of the method by Woolf, 1955; Anderson, Goodman and Reed, 1958; Clemmesen, 1965).

One of the early studies of this type was conducted by Lane-Claypon (1926), who noted an aggregation of cancer, generally of the same organ, in relatives of patients. Wainwright (1931) and Waaler (1932) added the methodological improvement of evaluating specific types of cancer. They observed a 2- to 4-fold excess of breast cancer in the mothers and sisters of patients over that in comparable control relatives. Excesses were also reported by Wassink (1935) and Martynova (1937). Waaler (1932) made the significant added observation that cancer of the breast, ovary and uterus each had distinct etiologies, while excesses were not observed in relatives of patients with other types of tumors.

The results from some of these early studies have been questioned because of inadequacies in methodology, i.e., lack of comparability between the study and control groups in such factors as age, reproductive or other variables, or completeness of study; questionable controls, lack of validation of the presence or absence of cancer in relatives of patients or controls, or deficiences in analytical procedures. However, the trends observed in the early studies were confirmed and more clearly delineated by later studies using improved methodologies (Jacobsen, 1946; Busk, 1948; Penrose, MacKenzie and Karn, 1948; Woolf, 1955; Anderson, Goodman and Reed, 1958; Tokuhata, 1969).

In one of the most complete and illustrative studies of this type, Macklin (1959) convincingly demonstrated that grandmothers, aunts, mothers and sisters of breast cancer patients manifested a significant 2- to 4-fold excess of breast cancer when compared with women of similar age from the general population or two independent sets of control women. Biased selection and chance were shown not to be involved because the excesses were too large to be adequately explained by either of these factors. She was also able to rule out the possibility of environmental factors as an explanation because increased rates of the disease were found in both paternal and maternal sides of the family and at higher rates than in controls. The genetic effect for breast cancer was enhanced in childless women, thereby demonstrating an interaction between genetic and extrinsic factors.

Excesses of breast cancer in close relatives of patients were also recorded by Bucalossi and Veronesi (1957), Oliver (1958) and Nakano (1967), but not by Chorlton (1966). He found no significant excess of the disease in any category of relative. However, his study was based on only 99 patients and 99 control persons, although 5,042 and 4,753 relatives were involved in the two comparison groups, respectively. The latter numbers indicate a preponderance of distant relatives and a relatively small number of first-degree relatives. The latter group would be of primary importance in a genetic study of a disease such as breast cancer; in more distant relatives the genetic effect would tend to be minimized and would lessen their importance in such a study. The other exception was that of Murphy and Abbey (1959) where an excess of breast cancer was observed in mothers of patients but not in sisters.

It seemingly has not mattered from whence the study has originated, whether in high-risk countries, such as the United States or England, or in moderate-risk countries such as Denmark, Norway or Russia, or in a low-risk country such as Japan; nor has the type of data mattered, whether based on moribidity and/or mortality statistics; nor the type of control, whether in-laws, general population, or some type of cancer or noncancer patients. The studies have consistently indicated approximately a 2- to 3-fold excess of the disease in mothers, sisters and daughters of patients when comparisons were made with women in general (Post, 1966).

This type of result is not indicative of a strong hereditary effect. It is more in keeping with a polygenic mechanism, involving the action of several genes, presumably with small effects and accounting for only a relatively small portion of the total variation in breast cancer. One possible reason for this type of finding is that past survey studies were based on the implicit assumption of a single disease entity. More recent clinical, epidemiologic and genetic evidence points to a heterogeneous disease (Lilienfeld, 1963; de Waard, Halewijn and Huizinga, 1964; von Berndt and Landmann, 1969; Hems, 1970, Anderson 1970a). If the disease were indeed heterogeneous as evidence now strongly suggests, and not homogeneous as previously assumed, then the effect of such an assumption would be to dilute or obscure any measure of a genetic influence.

That the disease may be genetically heterogeneous is suggested by the recent studies of Anderson (1971, 1972, 1974). He found a significantly higher frequency of bilateral breast cancer in patients who had a family history of the neoplasm and whose disease developed in the premenopausal period than that found in familial patients with postmenopausal disease, or in nonfamilial patients of all ages. Moreover, familial patients with bilateral disease had a noticeably earlier average age at diagnosis than unilateral familial patients or nonfamilial patients.

These two characteristics, early age and bilaterality, appeared to have genetic significance because the risk of breast cancer was about twice as high (3.1) in the first-degree relatives of patients with premenopausal disease than in relatives of patients with postmenopausal diagnoses (1.5) when both groups of relatives were compared with control relatives of similar age. It was further observed that bilateral disease in the patient increased the risk to 5.4-fold. When the patient had both premenopausal and bilateral disease, the risk for her relatives increased to 8.8-fold, while relatives of patients with unilateral disease, whether premenopausal or postmenopausal, manifested only 1.2- to 1.8-fold higher risks than control relatives. These results suggested genetic heterogeneity among familial patients and a stronger genetic effect in the premenopausal and/or bilateral group than in the postmenopausal and/or unilateral group of patients.

Even more dramatic differences were found when the familial patients were classified according to type of family history, i.e., who in the family had breast cancer prior to that in the patient (Anderson, 1974). Three general types of familial patterns were observed, where: (1) prior disease involved a second-degree relative of the patient but no other; (2) prior disease involved a sister of the patient and no other; and (3) prior disease involved at least the patient's mother.

The strong genetic effect of premenopausal and/or bilateral disease previously observed was found to be confined to one familial pattern, where prior disease involved the mother of the patient. In such families, the patients' sisters (excluding those who may also have had prior disease) manifested a 30% frequency of breast cancer in the 20 to 39 age group, a frequency 47-fold higher than that in control sisters of similar age. The risks declined to a 6-fold excess for 40- to 59-year-old sisters and were little different from controls in the oldest age group.

In families in which prior disease involved a sister of the patient, the risks for the three age classes averaged about 3-fold in excess of controls. The results for families in which prior disease involved a second-degree relative were little different from controls.

The category of families with affected mothers was concluded to refer to a heritable form of breast cancer where disease susceptibility was transmitted by a mother to a significant fraction of her daughters, such that the daughters had at least a 30% probability of developing their first breast cancer before age 40. The daughters also manifested a significant excess of bilateral cancer, as did the affected mothers. This heritable component appeared to relate to ovarian function in keeping with the proposals of

MacMahon, Cole and Brown (1973) and Lemon (1972), since the frequencies of the disease and risks were highest during the early reproductive period when the ovaries are most active and declined in the period of decreasing ovarian function, and were lowest in the postmenopausal period when the ovaries are largely nonfunctional.

The families in which prior disease occurred only in sisters seemingly referred to another form of heritable cancer with lower risks averaging about 3-fold higher than controls, and in which the disease was usually confined to one breast, was later occurring, and, therefore, was not highly related to ovarian function. De Waard, Halewijn and Huizinga (1964) and Bulbrook, Hayward and Allen (1969) proposed that a predisposition to breast cancer in some families could be operating through adrenocortical hormones.

On the basis of these numerous studies utilizing a variety of survey approaches, a hereditary tendency for breast cancer has been demonstrated much too frequently and consistently to be readily attributed to chance or environmental factors, and, as stated by Clemmesen (1965), it is as real as the hereditary effect found in mice. This should not be construed to mean that all breast cancers involve a transmissable hereditary component. Rather, among breast cancer patients, there will be some fraction, approximately 30% (Knudson, Strong and Anderson, 1973), whose disease will have some type of genetic causation, the same as exists in inbred strains of mice, in which some but not all strains are hereditarily so predisposed. Moreover, the hereditary basis apparently need not be the same in all patients, i.e., it may be genetically heterogeneous, since the risks in the patient's family may vary according to clinical onset of her disease, whether bilateral or unilateral, and type of family history.

Several studies have evaluated the possibility that the hereditary basis for breast cancer susceptibility might extend to other cancers as well, as initially suggested by Martynova (1937), Jacobsen (1946), and Busk (1948). But no evidence favoring this proposal has been found. The results clearly point to an inherited tendency specific for cancer of the breast in the majority of families (Penrose, MacKenzie and Karn, 1948; Smithers, 1948; Wolf, 1955; Anderson, Goodman and Reed, 1958; Macklin, 1959; Tokuhata, 1969; Anderson, 1974). Some apparent exceptions to this finding will be discussed later.

The possibility has also been raised that environmental rather than genetic factors might "run in families", such as the transmission of a virus through the mother's milk from one generation to the next. This possibility takes on added significance in view of the observation of murine B type particles in the milk of 60% of women with family histories of breast cancer and in 5% of women with no family histories (Moore *et al.*, 1971), and the homology observed between the base sequences of RNA molecules from extracts of human breast cancer tissue and the Bittner mouse mammary tumour virus (Axel, Schlom and Spiegelman, 1972). The homology was observed in 66% of 29 human breast tumors and in 29% of 17 tumors in a more recent study by Vaidya *et al.* (1974). The significance of the occurrence of particles in the milk of women with and without family histories of the disease has been diminished, since no evidence of a difference was detectable in a later study by Sarkar and Moore (1972).

If a virus were transmitted through the milk, higher frequencies of the disease would be expected in the maternal than in the paternal side of the family. Comparisons have been made of the disease occurrence in paternal and maternal grandmothers of patients, paternal and maternal aunts and sisters of patients whose paternal or maternal grandmothers and/or aunts had breast cancer. No differences have been found (Macklin, 1959; Anderson, Goodman and Reed, 1958; Chorlton, 1966; Anderson, 1974). These findings thus provide no support for the transmission of a virus through the milk of the mother. They do not, however, negate the possibility of a virus in human breast cancer, but if one is involved, it must be ubiquitous or be integrated into the DNA of the host, whether male or female.

Huebner and Todaro (1969) have proposed that all normal cells of animals possess genes (oncogenes) which when expressed, release the cells from the constraints which regulate normal growth. These cells also possess virogenes, the genetic information required to specify an RNA virus. The expression of oncogenes and virogenes to produce tumor and/or viruses was assumed to be under the genetic control of the cell but could also be influenced by physical and chemical carcinogens. Bentvelzen *et al.* (1972) postulated a similar mechanism in mice: that all cells contain the information necessary for mammary tumor virus production, which is normally repressed, but under appropriate genetic, hormonal or other conditions could be activated to form virus and tumor.

At present, the only evidence that a virus could possibly be involved in human breast cancer rests on the homology between the RNA of human breast cancer tissue and the murine mammary tumor virus, and on the actual existence of the virus in mammary cancer development in mice. But even in the mouse, the virus is not necessarily sufficient for tumor induction but requires the action of one or two specific genes interacting with other necessary genetic factors, including those of the histocompatibility system (Walford, Smith and Waters, 1971; Heston, 1973; Nandi and Helmich, 1974). Consequently, the question of viruses in human breast cancer is still unresolved; their possible existence does not conflict with any proposed genetic hypotheses.

Twin studies

Comparison of the concordance rates for breast cancer in monozygotic and dizygotic twins has high theoretical importance for providing insight into the importance of genetic versus nongenetic factors in breast cancer. Unfortunately, such studies, primarily because of the difficulty in generating sufficient numbers of unselected twins with and without breast cancer, have added little new information to that provided by statistical surveys. These studies have, however, clearly indicated much closer correlation of ages at diagnosis in monozygotic than in dizygotic twins (Munford and Linder, 1936; Macklin, 1940; Gorer, 1938; Heizer and Lewison, 1964). Clinical studies although based on selected material, have also pointed to a high degree of similarity in the clinical course of the disease in pairs of monozygotic twins (Macklin, 1940; Heizer and Lewison, 1964).

Using the twin data summarized by Knudson, Strong and Anderson (1973), the concordance rate of breast cancer is about 28% in monozygotic twins and 12% in dizygotic twins, a 2-fold excess similar to that observed with the survey approach. These rates yield a heritability estimate of 18%, suggesting that genetic factors play a relatively small role among all breast cancers. But the estimate is subject to large error owing to the relatively small number of twin pairs in the comparison; moreover, twin studies are subject to many of the same potential errors as retrospective statistical surveys, namely, errors stemming from lack of comparability between the two types of twins and selection of twins because of their likeness. There is also the problem of knowing for certain, in the absence of blood groups or other genetic markers, whether the twins are indeed monozygotic and dizygotic. And, similar to statistical surveys, twin studies have been based on the assumption of a single homogeneous disease, which could reduce or minimize any estimate of a genetic effect.

Pedigree studies

The approach of evaluating single families or pedigrees for breast cancer has been widely used and has a longer history than either the survey or twin approaches. Although it bypasses the need for controls, it may be criticized on the grounds that the resulting data are biased. The families frequently come to the attention of an investigator and are reported because they contain an impressive array of patients and so could contain an unrealistic excess of multiple cases. Pedigrees become genetically more meaningful when they are not selected, and the familial aggregation becomes evident by continued study. They become still more meaningful when the relatives resemble one another in the age at which they develop the disease and the clinical behavior of the disease. A highly variable disease picture among distantly related individuals is suggestive of chance phenomena. The pedigree method has the distinct advantage of avoiding the problem of heterogeneity and providing data amenable to tests of specific genetic hypotheses, i.e. segregation ratios, linkage relationships, and other basic questions of genetic and clinical interest that cannot be attempted or adequately answered with either survey or twin data.

Several pedigrees have been reported in which a genetic basis cannot be readily dismissed. The most meaningful one was initially published by Gardner and Stephens (1950) and then up-dated by Stephens, Gardner and Woolf (1958). Breast cancer occurred in direct descent through three generations in 13 individuals (one male), and benign breast tumors occurred in 11 others. The death rate from breast cancer was about 1 in 4 for ages over 30, well in excess of the expected rate for the same ages in the general population, clearly dismissing the possibility of chance. Significantly, the affected individuals were not randomly distributed throughout the kindred, as might be expected with chance, but were confined to specific branches of the pedigree, a finding compatible with genetic segregation. All new cases of breast cancer developing between the initial study in 1949 and the later study in 1957 were confined to the same branches as the original cases.

The age at diagnosis was relatively early, averaging about 45 years, and the course of the disease in the four branches was surprisingly parallel. The benign tumors were primarily fibrocystic in type and occurred in the same branches of the pedigree as the breast cancer cases, suggesting some association. The women with breast cancer lived in widely separated points of the United States and Canada, so it was unlikely that they were exposed to the same diet or other environmental factors. The distribution of breast cancer in this kindred was interpreted as agreeing with a dominant mode of inheritance, with almost complete penetrance in females and almost complete lack of penetrance in males. Similar to this pedigree are several smaller pedigrees, probably selected to some extent (Handley, 1938; family S of Papadrianos, Haagensen and Cooley, 1967; Smith, 1968; Cady, 1970; and Dmytryk, 1971); also similar are the high-risk families with affected mothers and early onset reported by Anderson (1974).

Another large pedigree was described by Woolf and Gardner (1951). It contained 1137 individuals, but all breast cancers were confined to only one of the 10 branches of this large pedigree. In this branch, the neoplasm occurred in three generations in 8 of 35 women over age 35, all descendents of one afflicted woman. Neither of her two sisters was affected and only three cases of cancer (uterus, kidney and breast sarcoma) occurred among the 775 descendents of her nine brothers and two sisters. Yet, seven of 9 of her direct descendents died from breast cancer, which was well in excess of the expected mortality rate of 1 of 33 for ages over 35 years. As concluded by the authors, it is doubtful that such a concentration could have occurred by chance. No environmental factors could be found for this occurrence, particularly as the descendents of the progenitor were raised in the same rural community as the unaffected descendents of her brothers and sisters. The authors concluded that the distribution of cases in this family was best explained by an inherited tendency to breast cancer.

This pedigree bears similarities to those described by Smithers (1948) and family Z of Papadrianos, Haagensen and Cooley (1967), but it differs from the one initially reported by Gardner and Stephens (1950) because the age at diagnosis was later, averaging 58 years of age compared with 45 years. It also included only one benign breast tumor occurrence, an adenofibroma, while 11 cases of fibrocystic disease were observed in the other. Although the numbers are small, the course of the disease may also have differed, since 7 out of 8 women died from the disease in the pedigree of Woolf and Gardner (1951), compared with a ratio of 1 in 4 in the pedigree of Gardner and Stephens (1950).

Further evidence of genetic heterogeneity is provided by the pedigrees reported by Li and Fraumeni (1969 a,b); Bottomley, Trainer and Condit (1971); and Lynch *et al.* (1973). They described an entity characterized by an early and multiple type of breast cancer occurring in association with lukemia, brain tumor, sarcoma, and/or carcinomas of the lung, pancreas, and skin in the same families. The most frequently associated tumors were breast cancer, acute leukemia, and sarcoma, which occurred in the pedigrees at higher than expected frequencies. These tumor occurrences also tended to be confined to specific branches of the pedigrees and appeared to conform to a dominant mode of inheritance. Anderson (1974) observed 8 such families among 234 breast cancer families. Wood and Darling (1943) described a family which appears to refer to this entity, as does one of the three families (his Fig. 2) reported by Oliver (1958). The other of his families (Fig. 3) is interesting because it could refer to still another hereditary form of breast cancer, namely, one associated with adenocarcinoma of the colon and rectum, stomach and uterus, so-called hereditary adenocarcinomatosis (Anderson, 1970b). At least one of the families reported by Mersheimer and Dursi (1971) seems to refer to this association (their Family 1).

Hermann (1972), Lynch *et al.* (1972) and Lunch, Krush and Guirgis (1973) have also commented on this association in breast cancer families, and Schoenberg, Greenberg and Eisenberg (1969) have described the association in breast cancer patients in general. This association was observed in 14 of 234 breast cancer families reported by Anderson (1974). The latter study also suggested another less frequent association involving breast cancer and ovarian cancer. This association was previously observed in 3 of 34 families by Lynch and Krush (1971) and may be possibly involved in one of the families reported by Mersheimer and Dursi (1971). The association has also been discussed by Schoenberg, Greenberg and Eisenberg (1969) and Schottenfeld and Berg (1971).

Smaller pedigrees more difficult to interpret have been reported by Kobb (1968), Kerr and Ross (1967), George (1973), and Saikkonen and Sääf (1973). They are not presented in sufficient detail to determine the age at onset of breast cancer or if other neoplasms occurred in the families at higher than expected frequencies. Broca and Lugol described a large family in 1866 in which breast cancer developed in 10 women distributed in direct descent through three generations (presented by Jacobsen, 1946; Lynch *et al.*, 1972). Four other women had hepatic cancer, which could represent either another primary or metastatic breast cancer. Whether this family was involved by a metastarizing type of breast cancer and/or one of the forms involving an associated neoplasms(s) cannot be ascertained from the available data.

Several interesting observations emerge from the pedigree studies. An impressive number of relatives may demonstrate the disease, including males, such as the male described by Gardner and Stephens (1950) and the two males by Papadrianos, Haagensen and Cooley (1967). Males may also transmit the disease. Chance as well as environmental contributions can be excluded as an explanation of the multiple occurrences in the large and most meaningful pedigrees. Affected family members may have fairly similar ages at onset, some pedigrees being characterized by relatively young average ages and others by older ages.

Some pedigrees involve associated neoplasms and others do not. Another interesting observation is that the tumor type and clinical course of the disease are sometimes highly similar in affected members of the same pedigree. A significant observation is that frequency of bilateral occurrences is often higher than that generally encountered (Smith, 1968; Cady, 1970; Dmytryk, 1971; Anderson, 1970a, 1974), a feature which would be expected with genetic causation (Knudson, Strong and Anderson, 1973).

The pedigree approach has thus provided convincing evidence of a hereditary basis for breast cancer and, furthermore, that the hereditary and clinical characteristics may well differ among pedigrees, pointing again to genetic heterogeneity. The data as they now exist suggest at least one and perhaps two dominantly inherited site-specific types, one with early onset and other with later onset. But whether these refer to the same or to different genetic defects is not known at present.

A minimum of three other dominantly inherited disorders also appear to exist, such as the one involving the association of breast cancer, leukemia and sarcoma; another, the association of breast, colon, stomach and uterine cancer; and another, the association of breast and ovarian cancer. A more recessive type of pattern is suggested by the low-risk families with affected sisters reported by Anderson (1974) and the families described by Oliver (1958), Kobb (1968), George (1973) and Saikkonen and Sääf (1973). These may or may not refer to the same genetic defect.

The high rate of breast cancer in the Parsi community of Bombay has been attributed to their high level of inbreeding (Moore *et al.*, 1971), which, if true, could suggest a recessively inherited type of breast cancer in that community. Although 49% of the cancers in Parsi females involve the breast (Paymaster and Gangadharan, 1970), their incidence of 34.8 per 100,000 is not far removed from the 39.0 per 100,000 in Norway, and is lower than the 46.9 per 100,000 in England and Wales (Jussawala *et al.*, 1970), populations with lower levels of inbreeding. Japanese also manifest a higher inbreeding rate than other populations, yet they have one of the lowest incidence rates of breast cancer, 27.5 to 31.8 per 100,000 (Doll, 1972).

At face value, these comparisons suggest the lack of consanguinity effect in Parsis, but actually they provide no evidence for or against such an effect. They fail to take into consideration possible differences in gene frequency among the populations as well as the occurrence of dominantly inherited breast cancers. Moreover, such comparisons could be influenced by extraneous environmental factors, which could seriously compromise any genetic inferences. Evidence of consanguinity will have to come from a special investigation within a community, such as the Parsis, or some other specified population, in which the gene frequency and other variables are relatively constant or can be controlled and in which different degrees of consanguinity can be directly related to breast cancer incidence.

GEOGRAPHIC DIFFERENCES

Post (1966) proposed an interesting hypothesis to explain the wide population differences in mortality rates from breast cancer, based on the evidence pointing to genetic factors for lactation and for breast cancer and assuming these two sets of factors to be related. He proposed that in prehistorical and early historical Caucasian populations, and only in Caucasian populations, the widespread use of artificial infant food and animal milk may have permitted the survival of children whose mothers had genetic factors for hypolactation. In non-Caucasian populations, in the absence of animal milk, such children would have died.

This relaxed selection of genetic factors for hypolactation might have led to the high breast cancer rates in these populations today, while selection against these factors would have resulted in low frequencies of hypolactation genes and thus low breast cancer rates in non-Caucasian populations. Although this proposal was consistent with the epidemiologic features of the disease at that time, more recent evidence indicates that lactation in high- and low-risk populations has little or no effect on breast cancer risk (MacMahon, Cole and Brown, 1973).

Dietary factors and their effect on hormone synthesis and metabolism are now considered to be prime suspects for explaining population differences in breast cancer rates (see reviews by de Waard, 1969; MacMahon, Cole and Brown, 1973). These differences are clearly not the consequence of geography, race, or ethnic background *per se*, because white populations generally have a high incidence whether they reside in the United States, Canada, New Zealand, Australia or Israel. This is also indicated by Japanese immigrants to the United States or Hawaii, whose incidence rates become higher than those of women in Japan, and higher in the second generation Nisei than in the first generation Issei (Haenszel and Kurihara, 1968). Indeed, the 1969–71 rates of Japanese–American women in the San Francisco Bay area now closely approximate the rate of white women for the 35- to 45-year age interval, but still fall below the rates for whites in the postmenopausal period, although they are higher than the postmenopausal rates in Japan or Japanese–Hawaiians (Buell, 1973).

The rates in Polish immigrants to the United States have also rapidly approached the United States rates up to age 55 years. This is true to a lesser extent for older ages but the rates are still higher for older Polish immigrants than those prevailing at older ages in Poland (Staszewski and Haenszel, 1965). The increase in incidence rates among Polish migrants has been more rapid than that in Japanese migrants, which has been attributed to their having had earlier exposure to and adopting a more western-type culture than Japanese migrants.

A similar effect is also evident among descendents of Chinese in Hawaii, whose incidence rates now closely approach those of Caucasian women. Blacks in the United States have almost the same rates as whites (Doll, 1972). Among Jewish populations in Israel, those born in Europe and America have markedly higher risks than Asian or African-born Jews, while Yemenite immigrants maintain low incidence (Steinitz and Costin, 1972; Seidman, 1971; Bertini *et al.*, 1971).

Had the incidence rates of immigrants to westernized cultures remained closer to those of their native countries, rather than increasing, this would have pointed to a genetic effect (Haenszel and Kurihara, 1958; Buell and Dunn, 1965). But the tendency of the rates to ever more closely approach the westernized rates is indicative of an important environmental influence (MacMahon, Cole and Brown, 1973). The possibility of some genetic effect should not be totally discounted because a genetic effect has been demonstrated in various countries, regardless of whether risk is high, low or moderate, and the shape of the age-incidence curves notably in the postmenopausal period is still different between migrants and native born and between Caucasians and non-Caucasians.

Moreover, differences in tumor type and survival persist between Caucasians and non-Caucasians (Wynder *et al.*, 1963; Morrison *et al.*, 1972). The low-risk Japanese have higher frequencies of intraductal, medullary, and colloid tumors than high-risk Caucasians. Anderson (1974) also noted high frequencies of these tumor types in his low-risk Caucasian families, while those at high risk manifested high frequencies of ductal carcinomas and adenocarcinomas. However, no one tumor type has been implicated in the various families exhibiting aggregations of the disease. Further studies utilizing more refined pathologic classifications will be required to assess the relation between histologic type and etiology (MacMahon, Cole and Brown, 1973).

GENETIC MARKERS

Genetic studies of inbred strains of mice have identified specific genes that are associated with mammary cancer, namely, the gene for brown (br), dwarf (dw), obese (ob), lethal yellow (A^y) and viable yellow (A^{vy}), as well as alleles at the histocompatibility-2 (H-2) locus. The affect of these genes on suceptibility is primarily through a direct or pleiotropic effect on susceptibility, not through linkage with primary susceptibility genes (Heston, 1973). Identification of individual gene effects in human breast cancer would have important practical relevance toward identification of high-risk individuals, if the degree of association were strong. Furthermore, such evidence would provide added support to a genetic or hereditary basis for familial-occurring breast cancer and would serve to distinguish between clinically similar but genetically different forms of the disease.

An association between blood type A and breast cancer was suggested by Rai *et al.* (1970). Vogel (1970) also observed a slight (1.08) excess of type A to type O, similar to the 1.06 excess noted by Anderson (1971). Although the excess in Vogel's study was statistically significant, it is still too small to be of practical utility. Moreover, Aird *et al.* (1954), Buckwalter *et al.* (1956), Damon (1960), Torti (1963) and Newell *et al.* (1974) found no association between breast cancer and the ABO blood group system. Lee (1971) and Badellino *et al.* (1973) have related the response and survival rates from oophorectomy to the ABO blood groups, but the numbers of patients have been small.

The Boston Collaborative Drug Surveillance Programme (1971) found an excess of the ss blood type in two populations of breast cancer patients compared with controls, the excess being larger in patients with diagnoses before age 50 than after this age. This association, whether diagnosis was early or late, was not confirmed by Anderson (1971) nor by the study of Morosini *et al.* (1972), using data from England and Finland.

No associations have been detected for the Rh, MN and Duffy blood groups, nor for haptoglobin, phosphoglucomutase 1, or acid phosphatase markers (Anderson, 1971).

In mice, certain alleles at the histocompatibility-2 locus, such as H-2 a, d, f, k and m, have been shown to enhance susceptibility to mammary tumors (up to 89 per cent) compared with the H-2b allele (14 per cent), according to Walford, Smith and Waters (1971). The human counterpart of this complex polymorphic genetic system (HL-A) has also been related to breast cancer, but with equivocal results. Patel *et al.* (1972) typed 123 controls and 52 breast cancer patients for thirteen HL-A antigens. Only one,

HL-A7 and haplotypes bearing this antigen, was significantly increased in the patients. This finding was not corroborated by the larger study of Takasugi *et al.* (1973), nor by Martz and Benacerraf (1973), nor Cordon and James (1973).

These recent studies of HL-A specificities suffer from the same deficiency as many studies, that is, the possible pooling of etiologically different but histopathologically or clinically similar entities into one heterogeneous category (Walford, Smith and Waters, 1971). An association may well exist between some HL-A specificity and a given type of breast cancer, which will simply not be detected when other types that are not associated obfuscate the issue. This effect is illustrated by a study of prolactin where no association with general breast cancer was detected (Kwa *et al.*, 1974; Wilson *et al.,* 1974), but an association was detected when high-risk families were evaluated separately (Kwa *et al.,* 1974).

A somewhat similar situation was observed in relating the ABO blood group system to familial breast cancer (Anderson, 1971). No association was detected for combined cases except a slight excess of A, but a significant excess of type O was observed when the patients were grouped into those with premenopausal diagnoses and in whom the genetic effect was strongest, while patients with postmenopausal diagnoses and a weak genetic effect manifested no excess of type O but an excess of type A. The effect of heterogeneity is also indicated by the genetic studies which indicated 2- to 3-fold risks for relatives of patients, but which increased to 9-fold or 47-fold when the patients were classified into more homogeneous groupings. Future studies of HL-A or other genetic markers, to be more meaningful, should attempt to avoid the problem of heterogeneity.

Matsunaga (1962) demonstrated that cerumen (ear wax) was a polymorphic genetic trait determined by a simple genetic mechanism, the wet form of wax being dominant to the dry. Races were observed to vary widely in their frequencies of the two alleles. Petrakis (1971) related the frequency of the wet allele to mortality rates in 9 countries or population groups and to breast cancer frequency ratios in 15 countries or population groups. The correlations were large and positive, suggesting that breast cancer mortality and frequency increased with an increase in frequency of the wet allele. The suggestion was made that the genetic mechanism for cerumen had a pleiotropic effect on the apocrine system (cerumenous, mammary, axillary sweat glands) and possibly other systems, which in turn affected susceptibility to breast cancer. A subsequent study of Chinese patients in Hong Kong by Ing, Petrakis and Ho (1973) indicated no important differences in the frequency of the dry allele among patients with breast cancer, other malignancies, thyrotoxicosis or controls. This study did not support the hypothesis of a genetic apocrine factor in susceptibility to breast cancer.

No concerted effort has been made to compare anthropometrics in breast cancer patients and controls. Damon (1960) evaluated the height, weight, height $^3\surd$ weight index, somatotype, dysplasia and gynandromorphy and other variables in various types of patients. Those with breast cancer were found to be shorter, heavier, more stockily built, more endomorphic (fat) and less mesomorphic (bone and muscle) then aged-matched normal women, but to a lesser extent than uterine cancer patients. Brinkley, Carpenter and Haybittle (1971) concluded that women with breast cancer had a larger biacromial-biiliac ratio for a given sitting height than normal women, i.e., they were more masculine, while Ravnihar, MacMahon and Lindtner (1971) noted that breast cancer patients in Slovenia were taller and heavier than controls. Anthropometrics, which could be strongly influenced by environmental factors, appear to be of little use in identifying women in the general population who are at an increased risk for breast cancer.

CONCLUSION

The one clear fact emerging from etiological studies of breast cancer is its complexity. This complexity is evident in the different clinical and morphological forms of the disease and their characteristic rates of development, age at onset, responses to endocrine therapy and survival rates; the clinical and epidemiologic evidence of differences in the development of the disease in the premenopausal and postmenopausal periods; differences in shape of the age incidence curves among various populations; the variety of etiologic hypotheses, involving hormones, viruses, genes and nutritional and exogenous agents that have been proposed or implicated in the disease, no one of which is sufficient in itself to explain all of its vagaries; and the present evidence of genetic heterogeneity.

Genetic heterogeneity implies different etiological mechanisms, and if the heritable forms comprise 30% of all breast cancer cases, then the remaining 70% would also appear to involve several mechanisms and not merely one. But the major effort in most etiological studies, whether epidemiological, viral, genetic, immunologic or hormonal, is to explain the disease on the basis of a single, unifying hypothesis. More progress would seem to be possible in understanding not only the disease but its etiological mechanisms if the concept of heterogeneity rather than that of homogeneity were more widely adopted.

Understanding the underlying mechanisms has relevance to disease control through early detection or perhaps ultimately through prevention. But, even without awareness of the specific metabolic pathways that may be involved, awareness of certain attributes could lead to identification of high-risk groups and thence to screening, early detection, and treatment. On the basis of the present summary, one high-risk group would be women with a family history of the neoplasm, in which the disease appears to have a genetic basis and in which risks could range from a 2-fold to a 47-fold excess compared with women without family histories. Aside from their clinical interest, the various categories of genetically high-risk women would also be a fruitful and homogeneous source of experimental material for etiological studies, namely, relating estrogen, 16 alpha hydroxylase, and adrenocortical steroid patterns to breast cancer risk. HL-A studies would be of further interest because of the possible involvement of a virus(es), an area which should also be related to inherited susceptibility.

Acknowledgement

The original work cited in this report was supported in part by CA05831 and GM 19513, C-1, from the National Institutes of Health.

REFERENCES

Aird, I., Bentall, H. H., Mehigan, J. A. and Roberts, J. (1954): The blood groups in relation to peptic ulceration and carcinoma of colon, rectum, breast and bronchus. *Br. Med. J.*, **2**, 315.

Anderson, D. E. (1970a): Genetic considerations in breast cancer. In *Breast Cancer: Early and Late*, p. 27, Year Book Medical Publishers, Chicago.

Anderson, D. E. (1970b): Genetic varieties of neoplasia. In *Genetic Concepts and Neoplasia*, p. 85, The Williams and Wilkins Co., Baltimore.

Anderson, D. E. (1971): Some characteristics of familial breast cancer. *Cancer*, **28**, 1500.

Anderson, D. E. (1972): A genetic study of human breast cancer. *J. Natl. Cancer Inst.*, **48**, 1029.

Anderson, D. E. (1974): Genetic study of breast cancer: Identification of a high risk group. *Cancer*, **34**, 1090.

Anderson, V. E., Goodman, H. O. and Reed, S. (1958): In *Variables Related to Human Breast Cancer*, University of Minnesota Press, Minneapolis.

Axel, R., Schlom, J. and Spiegelman, S. (1972): Presence in human breast cancer of RNA homologous to mouse mammary tumour virus RNA. *Nature*, **235**, 32.

Badellino, F., Santoro, L., Lesca, F., Panazzolo, A. and Bianco, R. (1973): Risultati in 125 ovariectomie per cancro mammario, con particolare riguardo al la risposta in relazione al gruppo sanguigno. *Cancro*, **26**, 45.

Bentvelzen, P., Daams, J. H., Hageman, P., Calafal, J. and Timmermans, A. (1972): Interactions between viral and genetic factors in the origin of mammary tumors in mice. *J. Natl. Cancer Inst.*, **48**, 1089.

Bertini, B., Ber, A., Posener, L. and Zelikson-Singer, S. (1971): Ethnic and constitutional differences and their relation to breast diseases in Israel: Educational and socio-economic status. *Br. J. Cancer*, **25**, 428.

Boston Collaborative Drug Surveillance Programme (1971): Relation between breast cancer and S blood-antigen system. *Lancet*, **I, 301.**

Bottomley, R. H., Trainer, A. L. and Condit, P. T. (1971): Chromosome studies in a "cancer family". *Cancer,* **28**, 519.

Brinkley, D., Carpenter, R. and Haybittle, J. (1971): An anthropometric study of women with cancer. *Br. J. Prev. Soc. Med.,* **25**, 65.

Bucalossi, P. and Veronesi, U. (1957): Some observations on cancer of the breast in mothers and daughters. *Br. J. Cancer,* **11**, 337.

Buckwalter, J. A., Wohlwend, E. B., Colter, D. C., Tidrick, R. T. and Knowler, L. A. (1956): ABO blood groups and disease. *J.A.M.A.*, **162,** 1210.

Buell, P. (1973): Changing incidence of breast cancer in Japanese–American women. *J. Natl. Cancer Inst.,* **51**, 1479.

Buell, P. and Dunn, J. E., Jr. (1965): Cancer mortality among Japanese Issei and Nisei of California. *Cancer,* **18**, 656.

Bulbrook, R. D., Hayward, J. L. and Allen, D. S. (1969); Further observations on steroid excretion and subsequent breast cancer in Guernsey. In *Hormonal Aspects on the Epidemiology of Human Breast Cancer,* p. 163; De Bussy, J. H. (Ed.) Amsterdam (as cited in *Lancet 2*, 1035, 1969).

Busk, T. (1948): Some observations on heredity in breast cancer and leukemia. *Ann. Eugen.,* **14**, 213.

Cady, B. (1970): Familial bilateral cancer of the breast. *Ann. Surg.,* **172,** 264.

Chorlton, S. H. (1966): Breast cancer in families. In *New South Wales State Cancer Council Publication No. 13*, p. 6, Australasian Publishing Co., Sydney.

Clemmesen, J. (1965): Statistical studies in the aetiology of malignant neoplasms. I. Review and results. *Acta. Path. Microbiol.,* **174,** 1.

Cordon, A. L. and James, D. C. O. (1973): HL-A and carcinoma of the breast. *Lancet,* **2**, 565.

Damon, A. (1960): Host factors in cancer of the breast and uterine cervix and corpus. *J. Natl. Cancer Inst.,* **24,** 483.

de Waard, F. (1969): The epidemiology of breast cancer: Review and prospects. *Int. J. Cancer,* **4,** 577.

de Waard, F., Baanders-van Halewign, E. A. and Huzinga, J. (1964). The bimodal age distribution of patients with mammary carcinoma: Evidence for the existence of two types of human breast cancer. *Cancer,* **17,** 141.

Dmytryk, E. T. (1971): Familial breast carcinoma. *J.A.M.A.,* **216,** 1350.

Doll, R. (1972): Cancer in five continents. *Proc. R. Soc. Med.,* **65,** 49.

Gardner, E. J. and Stephens, F. E. (1950): Breast cancer in one family group. *Am. J. Hum. Genet.,* **2,** 30.

George, W. D. (1973): Two sisters with breast cancer. *Proc. R. Soc. Med.,* **66,** 15.

Gorer, P. A. (1938): The genetic interpretation of studies on cancer in twins. *Ann. Eugen.,* **8,** 219.

Haenszel, W. and Kurihara, M. (1968): Studies of Japanese migrants. I. Mortality from cancer and other disease among Japanese in the United States. *J. Natl. Cancer Inst.,* **40,** 43.

Handley, W. S. (1938): Chronic mastitis and breast cancer: A family history of five sisters. *Br. Med. J.,* **2,** 113.

Heizer, W. D. and Lewison, E. F. (1964): Concordant disease in identical twins. *J.A.M.A.,* **188,** 217.

Hems, G. (1970): Epidemiological characteristics of breast cancer in middle and late age. *Br. J. Cancer,* **24,** 226.

Hermann, J. B. (1972): Breast cancer and associated extramammary malignant neoplasms. *Am. J. Surg.,* **124,** 620.

Heston, W. E. (1973): Genetics of mammary cancer. In *Methods in Cancer Research, Vol. 7,* p. 115, Academic Press, New York.

Heston, W. E. (1959): Site of gene action and carcinogenesis. In *Genetics and Cancer,* p. 226, University of Texas Press, Austin.

Huebner, R. J. and Todaro, G. J. (1969): Oncogenes of RNA tumor virsues as determinants of cancer. *Proc. Natl. Acad. Sci. USA,* **64,** 1087.

Ing, R., Petrakis, N. L. and Ho, H. C. (1973): Evidence against association between wet cerumen and breast cancer. *Lancet,* **1,** 31.

Jacobsen, O. (1946): Heredity in Breast Cancer: *A Genetic and Clinical Study of Two Hundred Probands,* H. K. Lewis, London.

Jussawala, D. J., Deshpande, V. A., Haenszel, W. and Natekar, M. V. (1970): Differences observed in the site incidence of cancer between the Parsi community and the total population of Greater Bombay: A critical appraisal. *Br. J. Cancer,* **24,** 56.

Kerr, I. F. and Ross, R. M. (1967): Breast cancer and heredity. *Lancet,* **1,** 1332.

Knudson, A. G., Jr, Strong, L. C. and Anderson, D. E. (1973): Heredity and cancer in man. *Prog. Med. Genet.,* **9,** 113.

Kobb, H. J. (1968): Carcinoma of the breast and schizophrenia in two sisters: A case report. *J. Med. Soc. N.J.,* **65,** 354.

Kwa, H. G., Engelsman, E., De Jong-Bakker, M. and Cleton, F. J. (1974): Plasma-prolactin in human breast cancer. *Lancet,* **1,** 433.

Lane-Claypon, J. E. (1926): A further report on cancer of the breast, with special reference to its associated antecedent conditions. In *Rep. Min. Health No. 32,* H. M. Stationery Office, London.

Lee, Y. N. (1971): The ABO blood groups and results of therapeutic oophorectomy for advanced carcinoma of the breast. *Surg. Gynecol.*

Obstet., **132,** 871.

Lemon, H. M. (1972): Genetic predisposition to carcinoma of the breast: Multiple human genotypes for estrogen 16 alpha hydroxylase activity in Caucasians. *J. Surg. Oncol.,* **4,** 255.

Li, F. P. and Fraumeni, J. F., Jr. (1969a): Soft-tissue sarcomas, breast cancer and other neoplasms. A familial syndrome? *Ann. Intern. Med.,* **71,** 747.

Li, F. P. and Fraumeni, J. F., Jr. (1969b): Rhabdomyosarcoma in children: Epidemiologic study and identification of a familial cancer syndrome. *J. Natl. Cancer Inst.,* **43,** 1365.

Lilienfeld, A. M. (1963): The epidemiology of breast cancer. *Cancer Res.,* **23,** 1503.

Lynch, H. T. and Krush, A. J. (1971): Carcinoma of the breast and ovary in three families. *Surg. Gynecol. Obstet.,* **133,** 644.

Lynch, H. T., Krush, A. J. and Guirgis, H. (1973): Genetic factors in families with combined gastrointestinal and breast cancer. *Am. J. Gastroenterol.,* **59,** 31.

Lynch, H. T., Krush, A. J., Harlan, W. I. and Sharp, E. A. (1973): Association of soft tissue sarcoma, leukemia, and brain tumors in families affected with breast cancer. *Am. Surg.,* **39,** 199.

Lynch, H. T., Krush, A. J., Lemon, H. M., Kaplan, A. R., Condit, P. T. and Bottomley, R. H. (1972): Tumor variation in families with breast cancer. *J.A.M.A.,* **222,** 1631.

Macklin, M. T. (1940): An analysis of tumors in monozygous and dizygous twins: With a report of fifteen unpublished cases. *J. Hered.,* **31,** 277.

Macklin, M. T. (1959): Comparison of the number of breast cancer deaths observed in relatives of breast-cancer patients, and the number expected on the basis of mortality rates. *J. Natl. Cancer Inst.,* **22,** 927.

MacMahon, B., Cole, P. and Brown, J. (1973): Etiology of human breast cancer: A review. *J. Natl Cancer Inst.,* **50,** 21.

Martynova, R. P. (1937): Studies in the genetics of human neoplasms. Cancer of the breast, based upon 201 family histories. *Am. J. Cancer,* **29,** 530.

Martz, E. and Benacerraf, B. (1973): Lack of association between carcinoma of the breast and HL-A specificities. *Tissue Antigens,* **3,** 30.

Matsunaga, E. (1962): The dimorphism in human normal cerumen. *Ann. Hum. Genet.,* **25,** 273.

Mersheimer, W. L. and Dursi, J. F. (1971): Familial cancer susceptibility. *Rev. Surg.,* **28,** 316.

Moore, D. H., Charney, J. C., Kramarsky, B., Lasfargues, E. Y., Sarker, N. H., Brennan, M. J., Burrows, J. H., Sirsat, S. M., Paymaster, J. C. and Vaidya, A. B. (1971): Search for a human breast cancer virus. *Nature,* **229,** 611.

Morosini, P., Lee, E. G., Jones, M. N., Vessey, M. P., Heinonen, O. P., Nevanlinna, H. R. and Svinhufvud, U. L. M. (1972): Breast cancer and the S blood group system. *Lancet,* **1,** 411.

Morrison, A. S., Low, C. R., MacMahon, B. Warram, J. H., Jr. and Yuasa, S. (1972): Survival of breast cancer patients related to incidence risk factors. *Int. J. Cancer,* **9,** 470.

Munford, S. A. and Linder, H. (1936): Carcinoma of the breast in homologous twins. *Am. J. Cancer,* **28, 393.**

Murphy, D. P. and Abbey, H. (1959): *Cancer in Families: A Study of the Relatives of 200 Breast Cancer Probands,* Harvard University Press, Cambridge.

Nakano, K. (1967): Genetical studies of malignant tumor. I. Genetical studies on breast cancer. *Kumamoto Med. J.,* **20,** 112.

Nandi, S. and Helmich, C. (1974): Transmission of the mammary tumor virus by the GR mouse strain. II. Genetic studies. *J. Natl. Cancer Inst.,* **52,** 1567.

Newell, G. R., Gordon, J. E., Monlezun, A. P. and Horwitz, J. S. (1974): ABO blood groups and cancer. *J. Natl. Cancer Instit.,* **52,** 1425.

Oliver, C. P. (1958): Studies on human cancer families. *Ann. N.Y. Acad. Sci.,* **71,** 1198.

Papadrianos, E., Haagensen, C. D. and Cooley, E. (1967): Cancer of the breast as a familial disease. *Ann. Surg.,* **165,** 10.

Patel, R., Habal, M. B., Wilson, R. E., Birtch, A. G. and Moore, F. D. (1972): Histocompatibility (HL-A) antigens and cancer of the breast. Association with antigen HL-A7. *Am. J. Surg.,* **124,** 31.

Paymaster, J. C. and Gangadharan, P. (1970): Cancer in the Parsi community of Bombay. *Int. J. Cancer,* **5,** 426.

Penrose, L. S., MacKenzie, H. J. and Karn, M. N. (1948): A genetical study of human mammary cancer. *Ann. Eugen.,* **14,** 234.

Petrakis, N. L. (1971): Cerumen genetics and human breast cancer. *Science,* **173,** 347.

Post, R. H. (1966): Breast cancer, lactation, and genetics. *Eugen, Quart.,* **13,** 1.

Rai, S., Saronwala, K. C., Mittal, P. K. and Arora, S. (1970): ABO blood group distribution in carcinoma breast. *Indian J. Cancer,* **7,** 135.

Ravnihar, B., MacMahon, B. and Lindtner, J. (1971): Epidemiologic features of breast cancer in Slovenia, 1965–67. *Eur. J. Cancer,* **7,** 295.

Saikkonen, J. and Sääf, J. (1973): Familial occurrence of breast cancer. *Lancet,* **2,** 626.

Sarkar, N. and Moore, D. (1972): On the possibility of a human breast cancer virus. *Nature,* **236,** 103.

Schoenberg, B., Greenberg, R. A. and Eisenberg, H. (1969): Occurrence of certain multiple primary cancers in females. *J. Natl. Cancer Inst.,* **43,** 15.

Schottenfeld, D. and Berg, J. (1971): Incidence of multiple primary cancers. IV. Cancers of the female breast and genital organs. *J. Natl. Cancer Inst.,* **36,** 161.

Seidman, H. (1971): Cancer mortality in New York City for country-of-birth, religious, and socioeconomic groups. *Environ. Res.,* **4,** 390.

Smith, B. C. (1968): Bilateral carcinoma of the breast in living mother and daughter: A report of cases. *Arch. Surg.,* **97,** 590.

Smithers, D. W. (1948): Family histories of 459 patients with cancer of the breast. *Br. J. Cancer,* **2,** 163.

Staszewski, J. and Haenszel, W. M. (1965): Cancer mortality among the Polish-born in the United States. *J. Natl. Cancer Inst.,* **35,** 291.

Steinitz, R. and Costin, C. (1972): Investigation on the epidemiological significance of detailed cancer data—Preliminary results. *Recent Results Cancer Res.,* **39,** 7.

Stephens, F. E., Gardner, E. J. and Woolf, C. M. (1958): A recheck of Kindred 107, which has shown a high frequency of breast cancer. *Cancer,* **11,** 967.

Takasugi, M., Terasaki, P. I., Henderson, B., Mickey, M. R., Menck, H. and Thompson, R. W. (1973): HL-A antigens in solid tumors. *Cancer Res.,* **33,** 648.

Tokuhata, G. K. (1969): Morbidity and mortality among offspring of breast cancer mothers. *Am. J. Epidemiol.,* **89,** 129.

Torti, R. A. (1963): ABO blood groups and Rh antigens in patients with carcinoma of the breast. *Med. Times,* **91,** 1167.

Vaidya, A. B., Black, M. M., Dion, A. S. and Moore, D. H. (1974): Homology between human breast tumour RNA and mouse mammary tumour virus genome. *Nature,* **249,** 565.

Vogel, F. (1970): ABO blood groups and disease. *Am. J. Hum. Genet.,* **22,** 464.

von Berndt, H. and Landmann, R. (1969): Zwei epidemiologische typen des mammakarzinoms. *Arch. Geschwulstforsch.,* **33,** 157.

Waaler, G. H. M. (1932): Ueber die Erblichkeit des Krebses. Shrifter Utgitt av det Norske Videnskaps-Akademie i Oslo, I. Mat. – Nature. Klasse, 2 (abstract by M. Greenwood). *Cancer Rev.,* **7,** 464.

Wainwright, J. M. (1931): A comparison of conditions associated with breast cancer in Great Britain and America. *Am. J. Cancer,* **15,** 2610.

Walford, R. L., Smith, G. S. and Waters, H. (1971): Histocompatibility systems and disease states with particular reference to cancer. *Transplant. Rev.,* **7,** 78.

Wassink, W. F. (1935): Cancer et hérédité. *Genetica,* **17,** 103.

Wilson, R. G., Buchan, R., Roberts, M. M., Forrest, A. P. M., Boyns, A. R., Cole, E. N. and Griffiths, K. (1974): Plasma prolactin and breast cancer. *Cancer,* **33,** 1325.

Wood, D. A. and Darling, H. H. (1943): A cancer family manifesting multiple occurrences of bilateral carcinoma of the breast. *Cancer Res.,* **3,** 509.

Wolf, C. M. (1955): Investigations on genetic aspects of carcinoma of the stomach and breast. *Univ. Calif. Publ. Public Health,* **2,** 265.

Woolf, C. M. and Gardner, E. J. (1951): The familial distribution of breast cancer in a Utah kindred. *Cancer,* **4,** 515.

Wynder, E. L., Kajitani, T., Kuno, J., Lucas, J. C., Jr., de Palo, A. and Farrow, J. (1963): A comparison of survival rates between American and Japanese patients with breast cancer. *Surg. Gynecol. Obstet.,* **117,** 196.

2

Geographic, Reproductive and Sociobiological Factors

David B. Thomas and Abraham M. Lilienfeld

INTRODUCTION

Most primary malignant tumors of the breast are carcinomas that arise from mammary tissues. In this chapter, the terms "breast cancer" and "mammary carcinoma" will be used interchangeably and refer only to these tumors. Rare breast tumors that arise from the skin, connective tissue, or adipose tissue, and metastatic tumors of the breast, will not be discussed.

Breast cancer is primarily a disease of women. In the United States, for example, breast cancer death rates are approximately 100 times higher for women than men (Lilienfeld, Levin and Kessler, 1972). This chapter deals primarily with cancer of the female breast, with a section specifically devoted to cancer of the male breast at the end of the chapter.

In industrialized western nations, where breast cancer occurs with the highest frequency, it is the most common neoplasm in women. Based on data from the New York cancer registry, it has been estimated that 6.9% of newly born girls, or about 1 in 14, develop breast cancer during their lifetime (Seidman, 1972). Figure 1 shows that both incidence and mortality rates of breast cancer in the United States increase markedly with age between the usual ages of menarche and menopause. The rate continues to increase with age in older women, but the rate of change is less for women in their post-reproductive years (Lilienfeld *et al.*, 1972). In addition, Fig. 1 shows that for breast cancer, mortality rates in the United States (although lower than incidence rates) accurately reflect the same relationship of age to disease occurrence as do incidence rates. This suggests that studies of breast cancer based on mortality statistics, if interpreted with caution, may provide valid information regarding the epidemiology of breast cancer.

However, the general limitations of both mortality and morbidity data are widely recognized, and have been systematically discussed (Lilienfeld, Pedersen and Dowd, 1967). These must consistently be kept in mind in interpreting data presented in this chapter, in which geographic, reproduc-

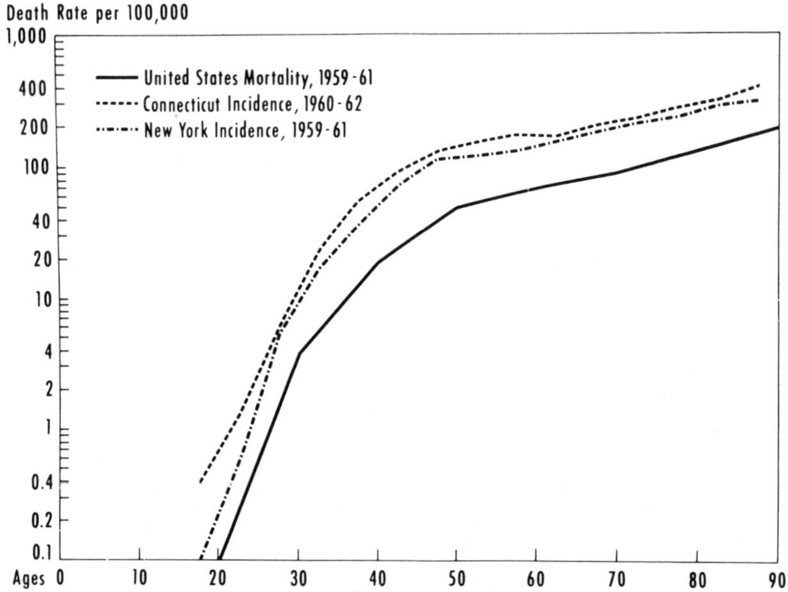

Fig. 1 Death rates for malignant neoplasms of the breast for United States, 1959–61, and incidence rates for Connecticut, 1960–62, and New York State (exclusive of New York City), 1959–61, by age for white females (from Lilienfeld *et al.*, 1972).

tive and sociobiological factors will be reviewed in separate sections. An attempt will also be made to speculate on possible interrelationships between these factors, and the mechanisms by which they may operate to alter the risk of breast cancer.

GEOGRAPHIC FACTORS

Geographic factors that may influence the occurrence of breast cancer have been studied by investigating: (1) variations in mortality and morbidity rates due to breast cancer between different countries; (2) differences between regions within countries, although only limited data for the latter are available; and (3) differences in individuals who have migrated from one country or area to another.

Differences between countries

As shown in Fig. 2, breast cancer death rates vary markedly from one country to another (Seidman, 1972). Rates tend to be high in the developed countries with populations of predominantly European descent, and low in

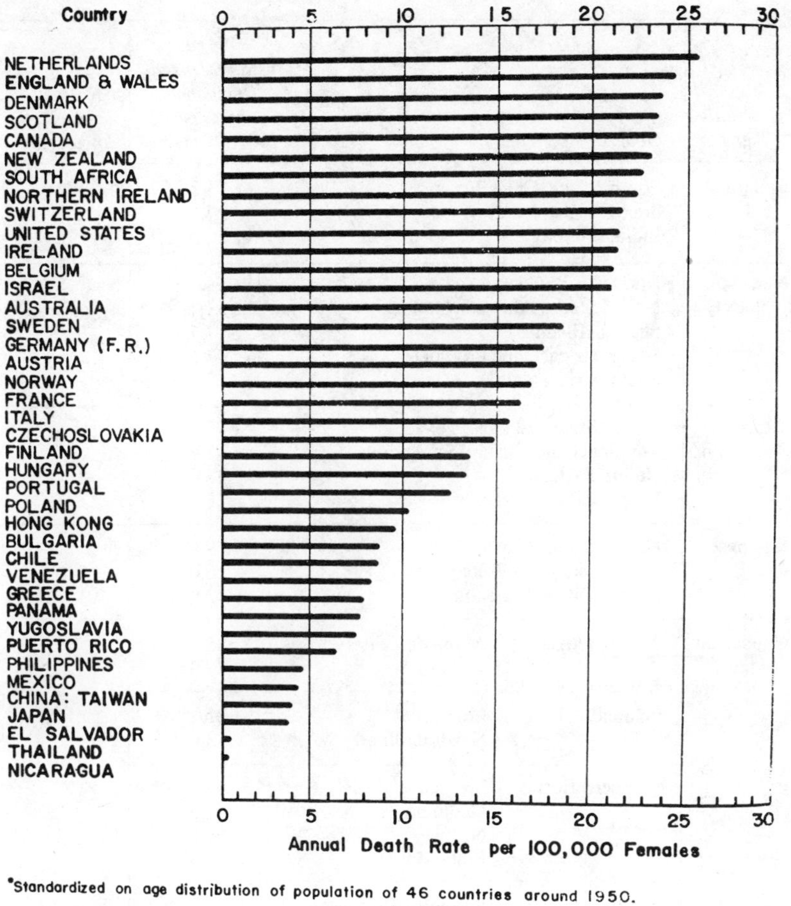

Fig. 2 Age standardized female breast cancer death rates* for various countries, 1964–65. (From Seidman, 1972).

less developed countries, and in those with non-Caucasian populations. The considerable variation in rates among countries in the first category suggests that racial factors are not solely responsible for the observed differences, and the low rates for Japan suggest that economic and industrial development *per se* is not responsible.

These observations are consistent with reported incidence rates of breast cancer for ethnic groups and geographic areas shown in Table 1 (Doll, Muir and Waterman, 1970). Native Japanese show the lowest incidence rates. For each of the five racial/ethnic groups represented, there is

Table 1 Age-standardized Incidence Rates of Breast Cancer by Ethnic Group and Geographic Area (from Doll *et al.*, 1970)

Racial/ ethnic group	*Geographic area*		**Age standardized incidence rates per 100,000 women*	*Ratio of highest to lowest rate*
Indian (colored)	South Africa, Cape Province		35.3	
	South Africa, Natal		27.1	1.26
	India, Bombay		28.0	
Negro (black)	Rhodesia, Bulawayo		54.1	
	United States, Alameda County		53.1	
	Nigeria, Ibadan		17.7	3.38
	South Africa, Cape Province		17.6	
	South Africa, Natal		16.0	
Latin American	United States, El Paso, Texas		42.2	
	Jamaica, Kingston and St. Andrew		47.8	
	Columbia, Cali		37.0	1.68
	Puerto Rico		28.3	
Japanese	United States, Hawaii		29.6	
	Japan, Okayama Prefecture		16.0	2.13
	Japan, Miyagi Prefecture		13.9	
Caucasian (white)	†United States	Alameda County	85.4	
		Nevada	77.3	
	†Canada	Manitoba	83.1	
		Newfoundland	53.0	
	Northern Europe	Sweden	67.5	
		Denmark	62.5	
		Norway	56.2	
		Finland	39.9	
	†United Kingdom	England, Birmingham region	69.5	4.17
		Scotland	57.3	
	Eastern Europe	†Hungary, Miskolc	33.5	
		Hungary, County Szaboles-Szatmar	22.6	
		†Poland, Warsaw City	38.5	
		Poland, 4 rural areas	20.5	
		Romania, Banat region	34.0	
		Yugoslavia, Slovenia	30.5	

* Standardized to a European population.

† Regions within these countries for which rates are shown include only those with the highest and lowest available rates.

considerable variation in incidence by geographic area, suggesting that environmental, not racial factors are responsible for these differences.

Mortality rates from breast cancer have changed with time, but not uniformly in all countries. This is shown in Table 2 for 24 countries for which reasonably valid breast cancer death rates are available for the period 1950–51 to 1964–65 (Seidman, 1972). In general, rates have increased in most countries with low and intermediate rates in 1950–51, with the striking exception of Japan, where the rates were lowest at that time. Although overall rates in Japan have continued to decline, this trend has only occurred in older women; breast cancer mortality rates in women under age 55 years showed no appreciable change from 1947 to 1962 (Segi, Kurihara and Matsuyama, 1965).

Japan is the only country with a non-European population represented in the table. In countries where death rates were above 20 per 100,000 women in 1950–51, the rates have tended to vary less in magnitude, and inconsistently from one country to another. It seems reasonable to conclude that during the past three decades the mortality rates in most predominantly European populations, if initially low, have increased and, if initially high, have remained relatively stable. The increasing rates in the countries with initially low mortality rates may at least in part be due to improvements in diagnosis, registration and reporting of the cause of death.

The United States (with high breast cancer mortality rates) is one country where the mortality rates have been stable from 1930 to at least 1959–61 (Lilienfeld *et al.*, 1972). Based on data from the State of Connecticut, it has been suggested that this unchanging mortality rate is due to the combined effect of an increasing incidence and a decreasing case-fatality

Table 2 Distribution of 24 Countries by Breast Cancer Death Rates in 1950–51 and Temporal Trend between 1950–51 and 1964–65 (from Seidman, 1972).

Death rate in 1950–51 per 100,000 females	*Number of countries*	
	Total	*With increased death rate by 1964–65*
0–4	1*	0
5–9	2	2
10–14	5	5
15–19	6	5
20–24	10	6
Total	24	18

*Japan

ratio (Cutler, Christine and Barclay, 1971). Although this is supported by data from the Canadian province of Saskatchewan (Cutler *et al.*, 1971), the incidence of breast cancer has not increased in all areas of North America. In New York state, for example, the incidence declined in the years from 1941 to 1960 (Lilienfeld *et al.*, 1972).

These differences in time trends of incidence between areas, as well as the reported changes in incidence, may at least in part, be a result of differences and improvements in diagnosis and registration. These factors will have to be evaluated before one can definitely conclude that the

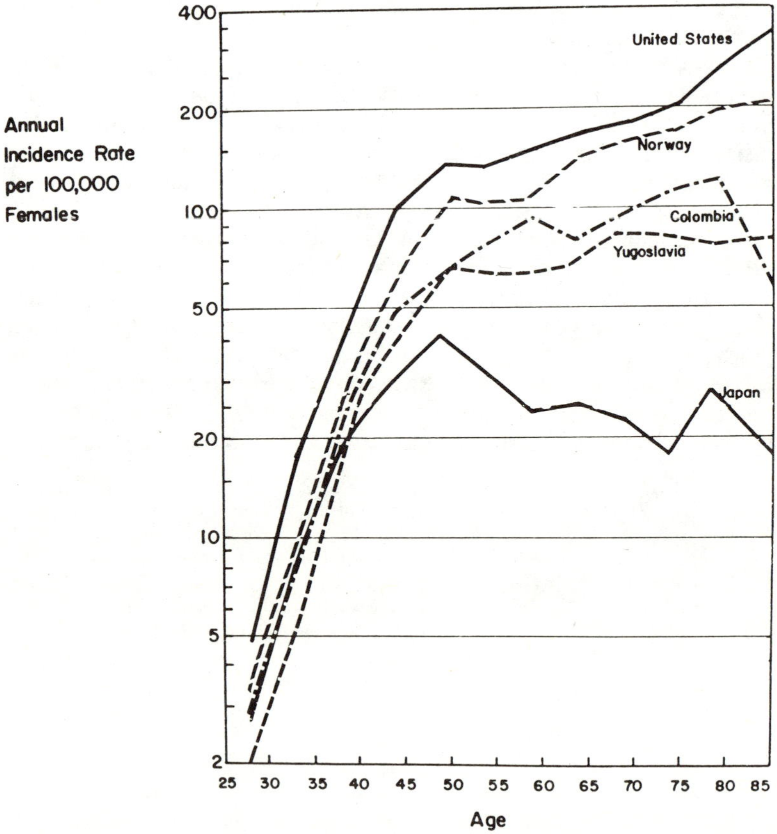

Fig. 3 Female breast cancer incidence rates by age for five countries, periods around 1965 (from Seidman, 1972).

Note: Colombia (Cali), 1962–66; Japan (averages of Miyagi Prefecture, 1962–64 and Okayama Prefecture, 1966); Norway, 1964–66; United States, 1966–68; Yugoslavia (Slovenia), 1961–65.

observed changes in incidence are real. If they are real, they support the notion that environmental rather than genetic factors play a major role in influencing the occurrence of breast cancer. In spite of the limitations of mortality and incidence statistics, this inference is probably a reasonable one, particularly if one considers the expected stability of rates during this time period that would result if genetic factors were predominant.

Environmental factors that may be responsible for the geographic differences in breast cancer rates appear to have a greater effect on the occurrence of the disease in post-menopausal than pre-menopausal women. As shown in Fig. 3, the slope of the curves of incidence rates during the reproductive years is similar in countries with high and low overall rates, but the diminution in the slope of the curves at menopause is more marked for countries with low rates. In Japan, the death rates actually decline with age after the usual age of menopause.

In addition, qualitative differences have been noted in the breast tumors that occur in high and low risk countries. Breast tumors in women in Tokyo were found to differ histologically from breast tumors in women in Boston. In Tokyo, tumors were more frequently of the medullary type, with circumscribed margins and a higher degree of cellular reaction than in Boston (MacMahon *et al.*, 1972a). Such qualitative differences tend to support the contention that the observed quantitative differences are real, and suggest that different etiologic factors may be operative in different areas.

Table 3 Incidence of Breast Cancer in Urban and Rural Areas of Three European Countries (from Doll *et al.*, 1970).

	Area		**Age standardized incidence rate per 100,000 women*		
Country	*Urban*	*Rural*	*Urban*	*Rural*	*Ratio of urban to rural rates*
Norway	Total urban	Total rural	63.2	50.4	1.25
Poland	Warsaw City	4 rural areas	38.5	20.5	1.22
Hungary	Miskolc	County Szaboles-Szatmar	33.5	22.6	1.48

The incidence of breast cancer tends to be higher in urban than rural areas. However, differences in the degree of urbanization do not explain the variability in breast cancer incidence among countries, as demonstrated in Table 3 (Doll *et al.*, 1970). The higher rates for Norway than Poland or Hungary are seen for both urban and rural populations of these countries. Also, the ratios of urban to rural rates, which are fairly similar for all three countries, tend to be lower than the ratios of high to low rates for the various ethnic groups shown in Table 1.

Studies of immigrants

Further evidence for environmental factors being primarily responsible for geographic differences in breast cancer rates has been obtained from studies of immigrants. In Table 4, the breast cancer death rates for 13 countries of origin are listed in order of increasing breast cancer death rates (Lilienfeld *et al.*, 1972). The first 11 countries have rates that are lower than for the United States white population (22.3 per 100,000), but the rates are higher for the migrants from all these 11 countries than for

Table 4 Age Adjusted Breast Cancer Death Rates per 100,000 Females for Migrants in Urban and Rural Counties in the United States and from Selected Countries, 1956–61, and for Residents of These Countries of Origin, 1960 (from Lilienfeld *et al.*, 1972).

		Migrants		
Country of origin	*Country of origin*	**Total in U.S.*	*Metropolitan counties (urban)*	*Non-metropolitan counties (rural)*
Mexico	4.0	13.4	14.4	10.4
Poland	7.1	20.3	20.8	14.5
Yugoslavia	7.3	15.5	16.0	12.1
Hungary	12.5	23.0	23.5	20.1
Czechoslovakia	13.9	21.9	21.8	24.9
Finland	14.1	20.3	19.5	25.7
Italy	15.0	19.5	20.0	14.6
Austria	16.9	25.5	26.5	17.5
Norway	17.4	18.6	18.6	19.0
Sweden	20.3	21.7	20.8	26.0
Ireland	20.7	33.1	32.5	38.3
Canada	24.2	27.3	28.2	24.4
United Kindom	24.4	22.2	22.6	20.1

*U.S. white rates = 22.3

their respective country of origin. Rates for 8 of these 11 migrant groups are intermediate between those in the country of origin and the rates for the United States whites. Three of these 11 migrant groups actually have higher rates than the United States whites, although appreciably so only for the Irish immigrants, a group for which the validity of cancer mortality statistics has been questioned (Lilienfeld *et al.*, 1972).*

Migrants from one of the two countries with higher breast cancer rates than the United States whites have rates that are similar to the United

* The data for both the Irish and Canadian immigrants are questionable because rates for 14 out of 15 different types of cancer in the Irish, and for 11 out of 15 in the Canadians, are higher for the migrants than in either the country of origin or the United States. This may reflect differences in death certification or underenumeration of the migrants in the census.

States whites (United Kingdom), whereas migrants from the other high risk country (Canada), are shown to have even higher rates than resident Canadians, but the validity of this observation has also been questioned (see Footnote p. 32). The general pattern for migrants is that they tend to develop breast cancer at a rate more comparable to that of the country of adoption than to the country of origin.

Although many immigrants to the United States came from rural areas and settled in cities, the change in their rates cannot be explained simply by the move from an urban to a rural environment. In all but one category (Italians in rural areas), the death rates among immigrants from all of the first 11 countries in Table 4 to both urban and rural areas of the United States are higher than in the respective country of origin.

Exclusive of Mexico, the only country in Table 4 with a predominantly non-European population, there is no relationship between death rates in the country of origin, and rates among immigrants from the country. This observation, too, is not compatible with a genetic basis for the geographic differences in rates. The lower rates for Mexicans can be explained by differences in culture as adequately as by differences in genetic makeup. Unlike migrants from Europe and Canada, Mexicans in the United States tend more strongly to adhere to cultural patterns that are similar to those of the country of origin.

This is also true for United States residents of Chinese and Japanese descent, and more detailed studies of the latter have provided additional information regarding breast cancer. Both Polish and Japanese migrants came to the United States primarily during the last two decades of the 19th and the first three decades of the 20th century, and both came from rural areas of countries that have lower breast cancer rates than the United States (Buell, 1973). By 1950, breast cancer mortality rates among Polish immigrants had nearly reached the level for United States white women

Table 5 Average Annual Breast Cancer Death Rates (per 100,000 women) for Japanese and White Women in California During Two Time Periods (from Buell, 1973).

	Japanese					
	Issei (Immigrants)		*Nisei (Second generation)*		*Whites*	
	1956–62	*1968–72*	*1956–62*	*1968–72*	*1959–61*	*1969–71*
Number of deaths	14	7	11	33	6024	7990
Age adjusted death rate*	7.4	11.5	14.6	22.8	45.7	48.4

*For women from 35 to 64 years of age.

(Staszewski and Haenszel, 1965); rates among Japanese immigrants although higher than in Japan, had not reached the level for United States white women even by the early 1970s (Buell, 1973).

Table 5 shows that breast cancer rates have been increasing for both the Issei and Nisei (Buell, 1973) suggesting that longer exposure to a western environment may be a factor, although the number of deaths available for analysis is small. The higher rates for the latter than the former suggest that more prolonged exposure to a western culture, beginning at an early age, increases the rise of breast cancer more than exposure later in life. Unlike the Polish migrants, but similar to the Mexicans and Chinese, the Japanese in the United States tend to maintain the cultural patterns of their native country, which are distinct from those of the white residents of the United States. Some factor inherent in non-western cultures that is maintained by descendents of migrants from such cultures thus appears to offer a degree of protection against breast cancer.

This factor is at least partially specific for breast cancer. Rates in Japanese migrants from some other forms of cancer that occur less frequently in Japan than in the United States, such as cancer of the colon and pancreas, more rapidly approached United States white rates with the passage of time than did rates of breast cancer (Buell and Dunn, 1965).

An explanation of the geographic differences in rates of breast cancer would undoubtedly provide valuable information regarding the etiology of this disease. For this reason, attempts have been made to correlate rates of breast cancer in various geographic areas with other characteristics of these areas. This is a valid approach, but it can also lead to biologically implausible correlations, and great care must be taken in interpreting the results of such studies. For example, breast cancer death rates in various regions of Norway, Sweden and Great Britain have been directly correlated with mean annual temperature, and inversely correlated with latitude (Lea, 1965). It seems unlikely, however, that latitude or temperature *per se* alter the risk of breast cancer, because many eastern European countries of lower latitude (see Table 1) have lower incidence rates than either of the three countries studied.

A more biologically plausible correlation has been noted between breast cancer mortality and morbidity rates in 22 countries and mean annual amounts of sugar and fats consumed per capita (Hems, 1970). This observation is later discussed in the section that deals with sociobiological characteristics.

Although studies of the characteristics of high and low risk countries, or other definable areas or groups of individuals, have limitations because of the danger of inferring fallacious correlations, they have provided hypotheses upon which to plan more detailed investigations. Moreover, it should be emphasized that any acceptable etiological hypotheses must explain the observed geographic variation in the occurrence of breast cancer.

REPRODUCTIVE FACTORS

Marital status

As early as 1713 it was recognized that nuns have more breast cancer than lay women (Ramazzini, 1713), and this observation has been well documented in subsequent studies (Fraumeni *et al.*, 1969; Wagoner, Chiazze and Lloyd, 1967). Single women are at higher risk of breast cancer than married women. This has been observed in such diverse regions of the world as Australia (Lancaster, 1951), India (Paymaster and Gangadharan, 1972a; Wynder, Bross and Hirayama, 1960), Israel (Stewart *et al.*, 1966), the United States (Lilienfeld, 1956; Shapiro, Strax and Venet, 1968), and Japan (Wynder *et al.*, 1960), as well as in an international collaborative study conducted in seven cities of North and South America, Europe and Asia (MacMahon *et al.*, 1970).

The excess risk in single women tends to be confined to women in their post-menopausal years (Lilienfeld, 1956; Paymaster *et al.*, 1972a; Lancaster, 1951; Wagoner *et al.*, 1967; Fraumeni *et al.*, 1969). As described below, artificial menopause reduces the risk of post-menopausal breast cancer, and it has been shown that at least part of the excess risk in single women is due to their less frequently having artificial menopause than married women (Lilienfeld, 1956). This explanation, however, cannot account for the excess risk among nuns prior to the advent of modern surgery.

Data from the international collaborative study suggest that much of the excess risk in unmarried women can be explained by the fact that most single women are nulliparous, and have not been subjected to the apparent protective effect of an early pregnancy (MacMahon *et al.*, 1970), a phenomenon discussed below. This collaborative study also shows that the observed inverse relationship between age at first marriage and risk of breast cancer can be explained by the correlation between the ages of first marriage and first confinement. The absence of a relationship between age at first marriage and breast cancer has subsequently been confirmed by an independent study (Lilienfeld *et al.*, 1975).

Childbearing

Married women who have never been pregnant are at a higher risk of breast cancer than married women who have borne children (Lancaster, 1951; Paymaster and Gangadharan, 1972b; Levin *et al.*, 1964). As shown in Table 6, three independent groups of investigators have shown that this is due to the low risk experienced by women with an early first birth, and that the risk of breast cancer increases with age at first birth (MacMahon *et al.*, 1970; Henderson, Powell and Rosario, 1974; Lilienfeld *et al.*, 1975).

Table 6 Relative Risks[1] of Breast Cancer for Parous Women by Age at First Birth and Interval from First Marriage to First Birth

Age at first birth	*Study (and age of cases)*								
	[2]*International study*[5] *(all ages)*	[3]*Los Angeles County* *(<65)*	[4]*Three Buffalo Studies*						
				(>40)		(>40)		(<40)	
			Time in years from first marriage to first birth						
			Total	⩽2	>2	⩽2	>2	⩽2	>2
<20	0.26–0.81	0.66	0.34	0.30	—	0.40	—	0.57	—
20–24	0.49–0.74	0.95	0.62	0.60	0.72	0.66	0.77	1.26	1.93
25–29	0.37–0.94	1.36	0.79	0.76	0.82	1.08	1.14	1.20	3.27
30–34 35+	0.73–1.12 1.06–1.75	1.57 2.25	0.71 1.07	} 0.86	0.77	1.22	1.45	2.75	—

[1]Risks relative to 1.00 for nulliparous women.
[2]From MacMahon *et al.*, 1970.
[3]From Henderson *et al.*, 1974
[4]From Lilienfeld *et al.*, 1975.
[5]Range of relative risks for 7 centers.

Women who first have a child when in their 30s actually tend to be at higher risk of breast cancer than nulliparous women.

The relationship between early first birth and reduced risk of breast cancer could be due to either a direct protective effect of an early first birth, or due to a third factor which both reduces fertility (and hence delays pregnancy), and increases the risk of breast cancer. Table 6 shows that the reduced risk associated with an early first pregnancy is evident for those whose first birth occurred less than two years after marriage, as well as for those who first gave birth more than two years after marriage. This suggests that an early first birth *per se*, and not lowered fertility, reduces the risk of breast cancer. This interpretation is supported by the observation that only full-term births are associated with an altered risk; there is no relationship between breast cancer and a history of spontaneous abortions (MacMahon, Cole and Brown, 1973; Paymaster *et al.*, 1972a; Wynder *et al.*, 1960).

On the other hand, Table 6 also shows that, with but one exception (the women over 29 in the first Buffalo study), for each age at first birth the relative risk is greater for those whose first birth was after rather than before two years subsequent to marriage. This is supportive evidence for the hypothesis that there is a third factor that both reduces fertility and increases the risk of breast cancer, except for the fact that the differences are not large relative to the age at first birth effect.

Thus, the presently available evidence suggests that an early first birth *per se* does confer a degree of protection against breast cancer. But the suggestion that ovulatory failure predisposes to the development of breast cancer and also to late or no pregnancies (Grattarola, 1964; Swain, Bulbrook and Hayward, 1974; Sherman and Korenman, 1974) appears to have some degree of support and although it is relatively weak, it should be further investigated.

The protective effect associated with an early first pregnancy may last for decades, but appears to diminish with aging. Protection was not noted in women over age 55 in India (Paymaster *et al.*, 1972a), in women over 65 in the international collaborative study (MacMahon *et al.*, 1970), and in women over 45 in a small study conducted in a defined United States population (Craig, Comstock and Geiser, 1974). Because the geographic differences are greatest for post-menopausal women, and because the association between age at first birth and breast cancer is evident both in countries with high and low rates of breast cancer (MacMahon *et al.*, 1970), differences in the age at first pregnancy cannot explain the international mortality differences.

Births other than the first do not appear to appreciably alter the risk of breast cancer although a second birth occurring below age 25 may exert a small additional protective effect (MacMahon *et al.*, 1970).

An inverse relationship between risk of breast cancer and number of pregnancies has been reported by many investigators (Bucalossi and Veronesi, 1959; Kaplan and Acheson, 1966; Stewart *et al.*, 1966; Shapiro *et al.*, 1968; Paymaster *et al.*, 1972a). However, two independent investigations have now shown that, when the relationship between number of pregnancies and age at first birth is taken into account, then little or no association between breast cancer and number of pregnancies is evident (Wynder *et al.*, 1960; MacMahon *et al.*, 1970).

Breast feeding

Compared to women in the United States and Britain, women in Japan and India more frequently breast feed their children and do this for a longer period of time, so that the mean number of months during which a woman lactates is longer for Japanese and Indian women than for American and British women (Wynder *et al.*, 1960). This observation is compatible with the hypothesis that lactation provides a degree of protection against breast cancer. Because lactation suppresses ovarian function and, as discussed below, oophorectomy reduces the risk of breast cancer, this hypothesis is biologically reasonable.

The relationship between risk of breast cancer and breast feeding was studied in women from the United States, Britain, India and Japan (Wynder *et al.*, 1960). A strong inverse relationship between breast cancer and lifetime total months of lactation was observed in the Japanese and Indian women, but this relationship was weak in British women and nonexistent in American women, both of whom tend to lactate for shorter periods than the Asians. Duration of lactation was noted to be correlated with such factors as age at first birth and parity, although the investigators did not analyse their data to take this into account. These observations nonetheless suggest that prolonged lactation may protect against breast cancer. This conclusion is compatible with the results of a study in Buffalo, New York, that showed that lactation for more than 17 months, but not for shorter periods, may be protective (Levin *et al.*, 1964).

Despite these early observations, more recent evidence does not support the concept that lactation is protective. Breast feeding has declined in the United States in recent decades (Meyer, 1968), but breast cancer rates have remained relatively stable; and the differences in breast cancer rates in Japan and the United States are as great for men as for women (Doll *et al.*, 1970). More importantly, the international collaborative study (MacMahon *et al.*, 1970) showed no consistent relationship between breast cancer at any age and either any length of breast feeding or prolonged lactation. This study not only looked at this problem in high, intermediate, and low risk populations, but in the United States using two differently selected control groups. More recently, a study in a defined United States population has shown a positive relationship between history of lactation and breast cancer in women over age 45, but not in younger women (Craig *et al.*, 1974).

One may conclude that there is probably no protective effect of lactation against breast cancer. If there is, it is small, confined to women who breast feed for a prolonged period of time, and does not explain the marked international differences in breast cancer rates.

A number of virologic studies have provided evidence that an RNA tumor virus, with properties similar to those of the mouse mammary tumor virus, may be related to the genesis of breast cancer in women (Schlom and Spiegelman, 1974; Moore, 1974). The suspect virus particles have been identified in breast milk from both normal women and women with breast cancer. An association between having been breast fed and developing breast cancer would thus support the hypothesis that a viral agent responsible for breast cancer is transmitted in human milk.

However, only evidence contrary to this hypothesis is available. Case-control studies have shown that women with breast cancer and normal controls do not differ in their history of having been breast fed (Bucalossi *et al.*, 1959; Wynder *et al.*, 1960; Henderson *et al.*, 1974). Prospective studies have shown that the incidence of breast cancer is the same among women who were and were not breast fed. This is true for the daughters of predominantly normal women (Morgan, Vakil and Chipman, 1974), as well as for the daughters of women with benign and malignant breast disease (Tokuhata, 1969). It can safely be concluded that having been breast fed as an infant does not alter one's risk of breast cancer.

Menstrual activity

Data from Buffalo, New York (Lilienfeld, 1956; Levin *et al.*, 1964) and India (Paymaster *et al.*, 1972b) have shown no relationship between age at menarche and risk of breast cancer. Other studies have indicated that the mean age at menarche is slightly younger for women with breast cancer than for unaffected individuals, although the observed differences in age at menarche between cases and controls have tended to be small (Bucalossi *et al.*, 1959; Wynder *et al.*, 1960; Henderson *et al.*, 1974; Kaplan *et al.*, 1966).

Two studies have shown a clear inverse relationship between age at menarche and risk of breast cancer (MacMahon and Cole, 1972b; Shapiro *et al.*, 1968), although in one, the international collaborative study, this was not noted consistently in all seven centers. Early menarche appears to have a greater influence on the risk of breast cancer in women under 45 than in older women (Staszewski, 1971). The facts currently available regarding age at menarche and breast cancer are thus inconclusive. If early menarche influences the risk of breast cancer, its role is probably a minor one compared to other factors.

A more striking relationship is seen between risk of breast cancer and age at either natural or artificial menopause. With few exceptions (Lilienfeld, 1956), most investigators have noted that post-menopausal women with breast cancer went through menopause at a later age than normal women (Leven *et al.*, 1964; Paymaster *et al.*, 1972b; Wynder *et al.*, 1960; Bucalossi *et al.*, 1959; Henderson *et al.*, 1974); and three studies (MacMahon *et al.*, 1972b; Shapiro *et al.*, 1968; Trichopoulos, MacMahon and Cole, 1972) have shown a direct relationship between age at natural menopause and risk of breast cancer.

Table 7 shows results from one study indicating that the risk in women with natural menopause under age 45 is only 73% that of women having menopause between the ages of 45 and 54. This study (Trichopoulas *et al.*, 1972) showed an apparent protective effect of an early menopause for post-menopausal women of all ages. Women in their 70s who had an early menopause appeared to benefit as much as younger women and conversely, the increased risk that resulted from a late menopause was greater for older than younger women. These data suggest a long term effect of ovarian or pituitary function on the risk of breast cancer and that breast cancer in both older and relatively younger women is influenced by ovarian or other endocrine activity.

Table 7 Relative Risk of Breast Cancer in Women with Natural Menopause and Menopause due to Oophorectomy at Various Ages (from Trichopoulos *et al.*, 1972).

Age at menopause	*Relative risks**	
	Natural menopause	*Artificial menopause*
>35	0.73 (>35–44)	0.36
35–39		0.68
40–44		0.65
45–49	0.93	0.73
50–54	1.07	0.98 (50–55+)
55+	1.48	

*Risks relative to 1.00 for women having natural menopause between 45 and 54 years of age.

A number of studies have shown a lower frequency of artificial menopause among breast cancer cases than comparable controls (Bucalossi *et al.*, 1959; Paymaster *et al.*, 1972a; Kaplan *et al.*, 1966; Levin *et al.*, 1964; Lilienfeld, 1956, Hirayama and Wynder, 1962; Trichopoulos *et al.*, 1972), and that the mean age at which artificial menopause was induced was older for cases than controls (Levin *et al.*, 1964; Lilienfeld, 1956). Artificial menopause thus appears to be protective, but only if ovarian function is disrupted; hysterectomy without oophorectomy does not alter the risk (Hirayama *et al.*, 1962; Feinleib, 1968). The degree of protection is greater for women with bilateral oophorectomy than for those with unilateral oophorectomy or menopause induced by pelvic radiation (Hirayama *et al.*, 1962; Feinleib, 1968). Presumably some women in the later group retain partial ovarian function, as do those from whom only one ovary is removed.

Similar to natural menopause, the degree of protection afforded by oophorectomy is also inversely related to the age at cessation of menstruation (Table 7). Two independent groups of investigators (Hirayama *et al.*, 1962; Feinleib *et al.*, 1968) have estimated that women who have had an oophorectomy by about age 40 have approximately a 75% reduction in their risk of breast cancer, a finding roughly in agreement with the data in Table 7. This table also shows that, for any age at menopause, the degree of protection is about the same for artificial and natural menopause. As with natural menopause, the protective effect of oophorectomy is considered to be a long-term one. It has been estimated to last at least 30 years (Trichopoulas *et al.*, 1972), and data from the international collaborative study shows that the degree of protection actually increases with the passage of time following oophorectomy. A reduction in breast cancer risk has also been noted in spayed female dogs, and the amount of reduction is inversely related to the age of the dog at surgery (Schneider, Dorn and Taylor, 1969).

Support for the idea that pre-menopausal oophorectomy protects against breast cancer is also provided by the observation that women who have had both ovaries removed have histologic evidence of severe large-duct hyperplasia in their breasts less frequently than do women whose ovaries are intact (Swerdlow and Humphrey, 1964).

As stated previously, the greater frequency of induced menopause in married than single women has been shown to account for at least part of the lower rates of post-menopausal breast cancer in married than single women in New York State (Lilienfeld, 1956). It must be realized, however, that castration prior to the usual age of menopause is relatively rare in many parts of the world, and therefore the impact of this procedure on the overall risk of breast cancer in many populations must be small. In spite of this fact, studies of the relationship of artificial as well as natural menopause to breast cancer have provided important information regarding mammary carcinogenesis. It can be concluded from such studies that premature disruption of ovarian function, whether by artificial means or not, provides a degree of protection against breast cancer that lasts for decades.

A relationship between an increase in the total lifetime years of menstrual activity and a higher risk of breast cancer has been reported (Bucalossi *et al.*, 1959; Levin *et al.*, 1964; Shapiro *et al.*, 1968). Length of menstrual activity is a function of age at menarche, age at menopause, and duration of time spent in a pregnant or lactating state. Because parity and lactation do not appear to be correlated with breast cancer, and because the association between breast cancer and age at menarche is weak at best, the age at menopause probably is the primary component of this relationship.

The relationship between breast cancer and a number of other aspects of menstrual activity has been investigated. No association has been found between risk of this disease and menstrual irregularity (Shapiro *et al.*, 1968; Paymaster *et al.*, 1972a), length of cycle (Wynder *et al.*, 1960), pain during menstruation (Wynder *et al.*, 1960), or strength or duration of flow each month (Wynder *et al.*, 1960). Most studies have shown no association between risk of breast cancer and a prior history of swelling or tenderness of the breasts during menstruation (Wynder *et al.*, 1960; Shapiro *et al.*, 1968), but at least one study has shown such an association (Kaplan *et al.*, 1966). Breast size has not been found to be related to breast cancer risk (Wynder *et al.*, 1960).

SOCIOBIOLOGICAL FACTORS

In this section, the only strictly social factor discussed is that of socioeconomic status, but as will be indicated, this factor must act through some biological mechanism. In fact several of the reproductive factors previously discussed can be regarded as being socially determined. In addition, however, there are several non-reproductive factors that have been shown to be related to breast cancer, which have both social and biological relationships such as diet and obesity, the use of reserpine, and exposure to ionizing radiation. These will be discussed in this section.

Socioeconomic status

Breast cancer occurs more frequently in women of higher than lower socioeconomic status, as measured in the United States by educational level (Lilienfeld *et al.*, 1972; Wynder *et al.*, 1960; Shapiro *et al.*, 1968) and income (Zippin and Petrakis, 1971) and in the United Kingdom by social class (Campbell, 1972). In western India, the relatively more prosperous Parsis have more breast cancer and less uterine cancer than Hindus, Muslims, Christians and Jews (Paymaster *et al.*, 1972a).

Like geographic comparisons, relationships between breast cancer and various indices of socioeconomic status provide little specific etiologic information regarding mammary carcinoma. Such indices are statistically related to breast cancer only because they are also associated with one or more reproductive or other factor of more direct etiologic importance. For example, the relationship between breast cancer and education has been accounted for by the fact that education is related to marital status and parity (Shapiro *et al.*, 1968; Wynder *et al.*, 1960), as well as to age at first pregnancy (Wynder *et al.*, 1960); and, compared to women of other Indian communities, the high risk Parsis tend to marry less frequently, marry and have their first child at a later age, and also have fewer children (Paymaster *et al.*, 1972a). The main value in identifying socioeconomic variables associated with breast cancer is that such variables can aid in defining groups of women at high risk of breast cancer who could be studied in the search for etiological factors and who should receive high priority in case finding programs.

Diet and obesity

Breast cancer rates in a number of countries have been correlated with mean annual per capita consumption of sugar, proteins and fats (Hems, 1970; Drasar and Irving, 1973). Like international differences in rates of breast cancer, these correlations are especially evident for breast cancer in post-menopausal women. Both "good" nutrition in general, and high fat diets in particular, have been hypothesized to account for the international differences in rates of breast cancer as well as for differences between socioeconomic groups within countries.

High levels of nutrition in general could result in an increased risk of breast cancer both by producing obesity and/or lowering the age at menarche. Evidence for the latter mechanism include the observation that the age of menarche is delayed by protein-calorie malnutrition, and tends to occur earlier in better nourished western industrialized countries and relatively high socioeconomic groups (with high rates of breast cancer) than in more poorly nourished and underdeveloped countries and lower socioeconomic groups (with lower rates of breast cancer) (Johnston, 1974). Also, in some European countries the mean age at menarche decreased from age 17 in 1830 to age 13 in 1960, a time during which nutrition generally improved (Johnston, 1974). During at least the latter portion of this time period, there was an apparent increase in rates of breast cancer (Table 2) (Seidman, 1972).

Breast cancer cases have been observed to be obese more frequently than normal controls (Wynder *et al.*, 1960; Wynder, 1967). One study showed this only for post-menopausal breast cancer patients (DeWaard, Baanders-van Halewijn and Huizinga, 1964), a relationship that has been confirmed by a prospective study (DeWaard and Baanders-van Halewijn, 1974). Furthermore, in normal post-menopausal women, it was shown that evidence of endogenous estrogens, as determined by the cytologic appearance of cells seen in urinary sediment, was directly related to body weight (DeWaard and Baanders-van Halewijn, 1969a). It is now known that after the menopause, estrogens are produced by conversion of androstenedione, which is produced by the adrenal cortex, to estrone; a conversion that takes place primarily in adipose tissue, and more readily in obese women (Kirschner, 1974).

Based on these and other considerations, DeWaard (1969b) has hypothesized that dietary excesses lead to obesity, which in turn increases the production of estrogens that enhance the development of breast cancer. This hypothesis is attractive in that it is consistent with international and socioeconomic differences in the occurrence of post-menopausal breast cancer, and with the associated differences in dietary habits. It is also consistent with the observation that delayed menopause, with its accompanying prolongation of the period of production of ovarian estrogens, is associated with an increased risk of breast cancer. Both indicate the importance of endogenous estrogens in the genesis of post-menopausal breast cancer. To test this hypothesis, a prospective study designed to relate the incidence of breast cancer to the presence of post-menopausal estrogen activity is currently being conducted (DeWaard, 1969b).

Induction of obesity as the intermediate mechanism by which overnutrition increases the risk of breast cancer is not incompatible with the hypothesis that early menarche is the mechanism. Either both may be operative, or the association between dietary induced early menarche and breast cancer may be an indirect reflection of the association of early menarche with obesity (Johnston, 1974).

The Japanese are one group of people who are generally well nourished but have a low rate of breast cancer. But the Japanese diet tends to be low in fat content, and a high fat diet has been shown to enhance breast tumor formation in rats given the carcinogen 7,12-dimethylbenz(a)anthracene (DMBA) (Carroll, Gammal and Plunkett, 1968). These observations suggest that fat rich diets specifically enhance the risk of breast cancer.

Two mechanisms for this action have been proposed. One, based on rat experiments (Chan and Cohen, 1974), is that the increased risk may result from an alteration in levels of circulating prolactin. The other (Hill, Goddard and Williams, 1971) is based on observations in humans and experiments with bacteria in vitro, and is particularly attractive because it is consistent with the hypothesis that endogenous estrogens alter the risk of breast cancer. It has been noted that a high fat diet increases the amount of biliary steroids (cholesterol and bile-salt degradation products) in feces, and also renders the intra-intestinal environment more favorable to the growth of anerobic lecithinase-negative clostridia. In vitro, these organisms can produce estrone, estradiol, and 17-methoxy-estradiol from cholesterone, a bacterial metabolite of cholesterol that is present in human feces. This suggests that dietary fat may influence the development of breast cancer by affecting the production of these hormones in the gut and thereby altering their levels in the body.

A prospective study reported a higher risk of breast cancer with increased height (DeWaard *et al.*, 1974), which is not surprising because good nutrition both enhances ultimate height and may be related to breast cancer development. The mechanism by which height *per se* could directly influence breast cancer is unclear. An analogous indirect association probably accounts for the relationship between impaired glucose tolerance and hypertension, and breast cancer, that was reported from one case-control study (DeWaard *et al.*, 1964). These two factors were not related to the presence of endogenous estrogens as detected from cytologic smears of urinary sediment (DeWaard, 1969b), and an independent prospective study showed no relationship between blood pressure and the subsequent development of breast cancer (Garfinkel and Hammond, 1974).

Reserpine

Although hypertension probably does not alter the risk of breast cancer, treatment of this condition with the rauwolfia alkaloid, reserpine, may. Three case-control studies have reported a 2.0 to 3.5-fold increased risk of breast cancer among users of reserpine (Boston Collaborative Drug Surveillance Program, 1974; Armstrong, Stevens and Doll, 1974; Heinonen *et al.*, 1974). Since these three studies employed somewhat different study designs, and were conducted in different countries by different investigators, the consistency of the results suggests that they are not spurious, even though the methods used in each individual study have been criticized on methodological grounds.

Reserpine could theoretically alter the risk of breast cancer in at least three possible ways: (1) by stimulation of prolactin production, which can lead to galactorrhea in humans; in rodents, stimulation of prolactin by reserpine enhanced the growth of mammary tumors that were induced by DMBA (Welsch and Meites, 1970); (2) by immunologic suppression, since reserpine suppresses delayed hypersensitivity, which may influence breast tumor growth and metastasis (Cazenave *et al.*, 1974; Black 1973); and (3) by serving as a precursor of a chemical carcinogen and metabolites of reserpine are chemically similar to some compounds known to induce nasal squamous-cell carcinoma in rats, as well as to others that may have caused mammary and hepatic tumors in mice (Schoental, 1974). Reserpine is excreted in human milk (O'Brien, 1974).

Although it cannot be stated with certainty that reserpine can cause breast cancer in women, the possibility exists. Additional epidemiologic studies to answer this questions are currently underway.

Ionizing radiation

The evidence is overwhelming that ionizing radiation can cause breast cancer. Studies of women who received multiple fluoroscopies during artificial pneumothorax treatment of tuberculosis (MacKenzie, 1965; Myrden and Hiltz, 1969; Cook, Dent and Hewitt, 1974) and of women who were treated with x-rays for acute post-partum mastitis (Mettler *et al.*, 1969) have shown that these irradiated women have an increased risk of breast cancer. The breast cancer nearly always occurred on the same side that received the radiation. These tumors also tended to occur on the inner aspects of the breast, in contrast to tumors in unirradiated women that occur more frequently in the outer regions. In addition, a study of breast cancer among survivors of the atomic bomb explosions at Hiroshima and Nagasaki (Wanebo *et al.*, 1968) also demonstrates a striking dose-response relationship; the risk of breast cancer increased with the degree of exposure to radiation. Estimates from these data (Wanebo *et al.*, 1968; MacKenzie, 1965) suggest that the dose of radiation which doubles breast cancer is between 20 and 46 rads and evidence is lacking for a threshold dose below which ionizing radiation does not alter the risk of breast cancer (Tamplin and Gofman, 1970).

It must be realized, however, that few women are now subjected to amounts of radiation comparable to those received in these studies. Such exposure can therefore account for only a small proportion of all breast cancer cases. The carcinogenic potential of radiation received from chest x-rays and mammography has not been evaluated. This potential will ultimately have to be compared to the benefits of these diagnostic aids.

BREAST CANCER IN MALES

Although a separate chapter of this book is devoted to the high risk male patient, a brief summary of the similarities and differences in the epidemiologic features of male and female breast cancer is presented here because such contrasts provide information regarding the etiology of mammary carcinomas that is not apparent from independent considerations of breast cancer in the two sexes.

Like female rates, mortality rates of breast cancer in males increase with age. Furthermore, the change in the rate of increase with age, although not as great as in females, is also noted in males (Schottenfeld and Lilienfeld, 1963a). This suggests that endocrine changes at menopause may not totally account for the age trend in women.

Married men have lower rates of breast cancer than single, divorced, or widowed men, as is true for women. However, the rates for widowed or divorced men are higher than for single men, whereas the opposite is true for women (Schottenfeld and Lilienfeld, 1963a). This suggests that the reasons for the variation in rates by marital status are different for men and women, and is consistent with the hypothesis that early first pregnancy and premature artificial menopause are the important etiologically-related factors in females. Obviously these cannot be operative in males. One theoretical mechanism that could account for the marital difference in males is that divorced and widowed males are known to have a higher frequency of alcoholic liver cirrhosis than married men. Pathological changes in the liver impair the excretion of endogenous estrogens, resulting in gynecomastia, and as noted later, gynecomastia has been related to male breast cancer.

The same international and ethnic differences in male rates of breast cancer have been noted as in females. Rates for both sexes are low in Japan and Finland, and higher for Jews than Christians in New York City (Schottenfeld and Lilienfeld, 1963a). This suggests that the environmental factors responsible for the difference in rates of (predominantly post-menopausal) breast cancer in females may also be of importance in males.

Evidence has been presented that implicates hormonal factors in the etiology of female breast cancer. Although of a different nature than for females, studies have also implicated hormones in the genesis of male breast cancer. Compared to controls, male breast cancer patients were shown to have more frequently a prior history of orchitis, orchietomy, treatment with hormones (thyroid, cortisone, testosterone, or stilbesterol), and gynecomastia (Schottenfeld and Lilienfeld, 1963b). Male transvestites treated with high doses of estrogens to stimulate mammary growth have developed breast cancer (Symmers, 1968). Men with Klinefelter's syndrome have both testicular disorders and gynecomastia and estimates indicate that such men have a risk of breast cancer that is about one fifth that of women, representing about twenty times the normal male rate (Scheike, Visfeldt and Petersen, 1973). It has been suggested that the relatively high percentage of all breast cancer cases that are males in Egypt (2.3 to 9.5%) refleccts the high prevalence of liver damage due to bilharziasis (El-Gazayerli and Abdel-Aziz, 1964). The relationship of male breast cancer to alcoholic cirrhosis in western countries is unknown and should be studied.

As has been discussed in the previous chapter, female relatives of women with breast cancer more frequently develop breast cancer than do relatives of unafflicted controls. A similar finding has been reported for the male relatives of men with breast cancer (Schottenfeld and Lilenfeld, 1963b). This indicates that the factor responsible for familial aggregation of breast cancer is not a sex-linked inherited trait, and is not solely transmitted transplacentally or by breast feeding.

Ionizing radiation also increases the risk of male as well as female breast cancer (Schottenfeld and Lilienfeld, 1963b).

CONCLUSION

The epidemiologic characteristics of female breast cancer suggest that: (1) environmental factors are of etiologic importance; (2) endogenous hormones play a causative role; and (3) different factors may be responsible for the development of breast cancer in the pre- and post-menopausal years. Evidence that environmental factors are important include the marked variability in incidence by geographic area and socioeconomic status, the fact that migrants tend to develop breast cancer at rates comparable to those of the population in their country of adoption, and the observation that this tendency is related to the degree of acculturation and duration of residence in the adopted country.

The importance of endocrine factors in the genesis of breast cancer is suggested by the differences in the rates of increase of breast cancer with age in the pre- and post-menopausal years. In addition, hormonal influence in pre-menopausal breast cancer is suggested by its inverse relationship with age at menarche and its direct association with early age at birth of first child. The latter factor is the more important; it also influences risk of post-menopausal breast cancer, although to a lesser extent. Breast cancer risk after menopause is also related inversely to age at natural or artificial cessation of ovarian function, and directly to obesity.

International differences in breast cancer rates cannot be explained by differences in childbearing practices or age at menopause, and are greater for post- than pre-menopausal women. Dietary factors have been hypothesized to explain these differences. Better nutrition lowers the age at menarche, which is weakly related to the risk of pre-menopausal breast cancer, and might explain the small geographic variability in the frequency of early breast cancer.

The larger geographic differences in post-menopausal disease rates may be due to differences in the frequency of obesity and/or the fat content of the diet. Obesity enhances peripheral conversion of androstenedione of adrenal origin to estrogens, and a high fat diet may enhance the conversion of bile salts to estrogens in the gut. These estrogens may then enhance the risk of post-menopausal breast cancer in a manner similar to ovarian estrogens in women with late menopause. They may also alter breast cancer risk for decades by inducing hormonal patterns early in life that are similar or analogous to those that are thought to be induced by an early pregnancy. Specific endocrinologic abnormalities that may be etiologically related to breast cancer are discussed in a subsequent chapter.

Acknowledgements

This work was partially supported by grant numbers 5 PO1 CA 11489 06 and 5 RO1 CA 14031 03 from the National Cancer Institute. Dr. Lilienfeld is a recipient of Research Career Award number K 06 GM 13901 from the National Institute of General Medical Sciences.

REFERENCES

Armstrong, B., Stevens, N. and Doll, R. (1974): Restrospective study of the association between use of rauwolfia derivatives and breast cancer in women. *Lancet,* **2,** 672.

Black, M. M. (1973): Human breast cancer. A model for cancer immunology. *Israel J. Med. Sci.,* **9,** 284.

Boston Collaborative Drug Surveillance Program (1974): Reserpine and breast cancer. *Lancet,* **2,** 669.

Bucalossi, P. and Veronesi, U. (1959): Researches on the etiological factors in human breast cancer. *Acta Union Internationale Contre le Cancer* **15,** 1056.

Buell, P. and Dunn, J. E., Jr. (1965): Cancer mortality among Japanese Issei and Nisei of California. *Cancer,* **18,** 656.

Buell, P. (1973): Changing incidence of breast cancer in Japanese–American women. *J. Natl. Cancer Inst.,* **51,** 1479.

Campbell, H. (1972): A review of studies of breast cancer in human populations excluding endocrine studies. *Proc. Royal Soc. Med.,* **65,** 641.

Carroll, K. K., Gammal, E. B. and Plunkett, E. R. (1968): Dietary fat and mammary cancer. *Canad. Med. Ass. J.,* **98,** 590.

Cazenave, J., Reimers, H., Perey, D. Y. E., *et al.* (1974): Rauwolfia derivatives and breast cancer. *Lancet,* **2,** 1571.

Chan, P. and Cohen, L. A. (1974): Effect of dietary fat, antiestrogen, and antiprolactin on the development of mammary tumor in rats. *J. Natl. Cancer Inst.,* **52,** 25.

Cook, D. C., Dent, O. Hewitt, D. (1974): Breast cancer following multiple chest fluoroscopy: The Ontario experience. *Canad. Med. Ass. J.,* **111,** 406.

Craig, T. J., Comstock, G. W. and Geiser, P. B. (1974): Epidemiologic comparison of breast cancer patients with early and late onset of malignancy and general population controls. *J. Natl. Cancer Inst.,* **53,** 1577.

Cutler, S. J., Christine, B. and Barclay, T. H. C. (1971): Increasing incidence and decreasing mortality rates for breast cancer. *Cancer,* **28,** 1376.

DeWaard, F., Baanders-van Halewijn, E. A. and Huizinga, J. (1964): The bimodal age distribution of patients with mammary carcinoma. Evidence for the existence of 2 types of human breast cancer. *Cancer,* **17,** 141.

DeWaard, F. and Baanders-von Halewijn, E. A. (1969a): Cross-sectional data on estrogenic smears in a post-menopausal population. *Cytologica,* **13,** 675.

DeWaard, F. (1969b): The epidemiology of breast cancer; review and prospects. *Int. J. Cancer,* **4,** 577.

DeWaard, F. and Baanders-van Halewijn, E. A. (1974): A prospective study in general practice on breast-cancer risk in post-menopausal women. *Int. J. Cancer,* **14,** 153.

Doll, R., Muir, C. S. and Waterhouse, J. A. H. (Eds.) (1970): *Cancer incidence in five continents, Volume II.* Springer-Verlag, Berlin–Heidelberg–New York.

Drasar, B. S. and Irving, D. (1973): Environmental factors and cancer of the colon and breast. *Brit. J. Cancer,* **27,** 167.

El-Gazayerli, M. M. and Abdel-Aziz, A. S. (1964): On bilharziasis and male breast cancer in Egypt: a preliminary report and review of the literature. *Brit. J. Cancer,* **17,** 566.

Feinleib, M. (1968): Breast cancer and artificial menopause: a cohort study. *J. Natl. Cancer Inst.,* **41,** 315.

Fraumeni, J. F., Lloyd, J. W., Smith, E. M. *et al.* (1969): Cancer mortality among nuns: role of marital status in etiology of neoplastic disease in women. *J. Natl. Cancer Inst.,* **42,** 455.

Garfinkel, L. and Hammond, E. C. (1974): Breast cancer and hypertension. *Lancet,* **2,** 1381.

Grattarola, R. (1964): The premenstrual endometrial pattern of women with breast cancer. *Cancer,* **17,** 1119.

Heinonen, O. P., Shapiro, S., Tuominen, L. *et al.* (1974): Reserpine use in relation to breast cancer. *Lancet,* **2,** 675.

Hems, G. (1970): Epidemiological characteristics of breast cancer in middle and late age. *Brit. J. Cancer,* **24,** 226.

Henderson, B. E., Powell, D., Rosario, I. *et al.* (1974): An epidemiologic study of breast cancer. *J. Natl. Cancer Inst.,* **53,** 609.

Hill, M. J., Goddard, P. and Williams, R. E. O. (1971): Gut bacteria and aetiology of cancer of the breast. *Lancet,* **2,** 472.

Hirayama, T. and Wynder, E. L. (1962): A study of the epidemiology of cancer of the breast. II. The influence of hysterectomy. *Cancer,* **15,** 28.

Johnston, F. E. (1974): Control of age at menarche. *Human Biology,* **46,** 159.

Kaplan, S. D. and Acheson, R. M. (1966): A single etiological hypothesis for breast cancer? *J. Chron. Dis.,* **19,** 1221.

Kirschner, M. (1974): Relation of endocrine functions to epidemiological characteristics of breast cancer. *Presented at* Breast Cancer Task Force "Report to the Profession" Meeting. September 30, 1974. National Institutes of Health, Bethesda, Maryland, U.S.A.

Lancaster, H. O. (1951): The mortality in Australia from cancers peculiar to the female. *Med. J. Australia,* 1.

Lea, A. J. (1965): New observations of distribution of neoplasms of female breast in certain European countries. *Brit. Med. J.,* **1,** 488.

Levin, M. L., Sheehe, P. R., Graham, S. *et al.* (1964): Lactation and menstrual function as related to cancer of the breast. *Amer. J. Publ. Hlth.,* **54,** 580.

Lilienfeld, A. M. (1956): The relationship of cancer of the female breast to artificial menopause and marital status. *Cancer,* **9,** 927.

Lilienfeld, A. M., Pedersen, E. and Dowd, J. E. (1967): *Cancer Epidemiology: Methods of Study,* Chapter 3, The Johns Hopkins Press, Baltimore.

Lilienfeld, A. M., Levin, M. L. and Kessler, I. I. (1972): *Cancer in the United States,* Harvard University Press, Cambridge.

Lilienfeld, A. M., Coombs, J., Bross, I. D. J. *et al.* (1975): Marital and reproductive experience in a community-wide epidemiological study of breast cancer. The Johns Hopkins Medical Journal (in press).

MacKenzie, I. (1965): Breast cancer following multiple fluoroscopies. *Brit. J. Cancer,* **19,** 1.

MacMahon, B., Lin, T. M., Lowe, C. R. *et al.* (1970): Lactation and cancer of the breast. A summary of an international study. *Bull. Wld. Hlth. Org.,* **42,** 185.

MacMahon, B., Morrison, A. S., Ackerman, L. V. *et al.* (1972a): Histologic characteristics of breast cancer in Boston and Tokyo. *Int. J. Cancer,* **11,** 338.

MacMahon, B. and Cole, P. (1972b): The ovarian etiology of human breast cancer. *In* Recent results in Cancer Research: current problems in the epidemiology of cancer and lymphomas. Grundman, E. and Tulinius, H. (Eds.). Springer-Verlag, New York.

MacMahon, B., Cole, P. and Brown, J. (1973): Etiology of human breast cancer: a review. *J. Natl. Cancer Inst.,* **50,** 21.

Mettler, F. A., Jr., Hempelmann, L. H., Dutton, A. M. *et al.* (1969): Breast neoplasms in women treated with x-rays for acute post-partum mastitis. A pilot study. *J. Natl. Cancer Inst.,* **43,** 803.

Meyer, M. F. (1968): Breast feeding in the United States. Report of a 1966 national survey with comparable 1946 and 1956 data. *Clin. Pediat.,* **7,** 708.

Moore, D. H. (1974): Evidence in favor of the existence of human breast cancer virus. *Cancer Research,* **34,** 2322.

Morgan, R. W., Vakil, D. V. and Chipman, M. L. (1974): Breast feeding, family history, and breast disease. *Amer. J. Epidemiol.,* **99,** 117.

Myrden, J. A. and Hitlz, J. E. (1969): Breast cancer following multiple fluoroscopies during artificial pneumothorax treatment of pulmonary tuberculosis. *Canad. Med. Ass. J.,* **100,** 1032.

O'Brien, T. E. (1974): Excretion of drugs in human milk. *Amer. J. Hosp. Pharm.,* **31,** 844.

Paymaster, J. C. and Gangadharan, P. (1972a): Some observations on the epidemiology of cancer of the breast in women of western India. *Int. J. Cancer,* **10,** 443.

Paymaster, J. C. and Gangadharan, P. (1972b): Epidemiology of breast cancer in India. *J. Natl. Cancer Inst.,* **48,** 1021.

Ramazzini, B. (1713): Diseases of workers. The Latin text of 1713, translated by W. C. Wright, New York, Hafner, 1964, 191.

Scheike, O., Visfeldt, J. and Petersen, B. (1973): Male breast cancer. 3. Breast carcinoma in association with the Klinefelter's syndrome. *Acta Path. Microbiol. Scand., Section A.,* **81,** 352.

Schlom, J. and Spiegelman, S. (1974): Breast cancer: molecular basis for a viral etiology. *New York State J. Med.,* **74,** 1373.

Schneider, R., Dorn, C. R. and Taylor, D. O. N. (1969): Factors influencing canine mammary cancer development and post-surgical survival. *J. Natl. Cancer Inst.,* **43,** 1249.

Schoental, R. (1974): Are rauwolfia alkaloids carcinogenic? *Lancet,* **2,** 1571.

Schottenfeld, D. and Lilienfeld, A. M. (1963a): Some epidemiological features of breast cancer among males. *J. Chron. Dis.,* **16,** 71.

Schottenfeld, D. and Lilienfeld, A. M. (1963b): Some observations on the epidemiology of breast cancer among males. *Amer. J. Publ. Hlth,* **53,** 890.

Segi, M., Kurihara, M. and Matsuyama, T. (1965): Cancer mortality in Japan (1899–1962). Dept. Public Health. Tohoku Univ. School of Medicine, Sendai, Japan.

Seidman, H. (1972): *Cancer of the Breast: Statistical and Epidemiological Data,* American Cancer Society.

Shapiro, S., Strax, P., Venet, L. *et al.* (1968): The search for risk factors in breast cancer. *Amer. J. Publ. Hlth.,* **58,** 820.

Sherman, B. M. and Korenman, S. G. (1974): A pathophysiological interpretation of human breast cancer epidemiology. *Cancer,* **33,** 1306.

Staszewski, J. and Haenszel, W. (1965): Cancer mortality among the Polish-born in the United States. *J. Natl. Cancer Inst.,* **35,** 291.

Staszewski, J. (1971): Age and menarche and breast cancer. *J. Natl. Cancer Inst.,* **47,** 935.

Stewart, H. L., Dunham, L. J., Casper, J. *et al.* (1966): Epidemiology of cancers of uterine cervix and corpus, breast and ovary in Israel and New York City. *J. Natl. Cancer Inst.,* **37,** 1.

Swain, M. C., Bulbrook, R. D. and Hayward, J. L. (1974): Ovulatory failure in a normal population and in patients with breast cancer. *J. Obst. Gyn. Brit. Commonwealth,* **81,** 640.

Swerdlow, M. and Humphrey, L. J. (1964): The relationship of breast disease to gynecologic disease. *Cancer,* **17,** 1165.

Symmers, W. S. (1968): Carcinoma of the breast in transsexual individuals after surgical and hormonal interference with the primary and secondary sex characteristics. *Brit. Med. J.,* **2,** 82.

Tamplin, A. R. and Gofman, J. W. (1970): Radiation-induction of human breast cancer. Testimony presented at hearings of the joint committee on atomic energy. 91st Congress of the United States, January 28, 1970.

Tokuhata, G. K. (1969): Morbidity and mortality among offspring of breast cancer mothers. *Amer. J. Epidemiol.,* **89,** 139.

Trichopoulos, D., MacMahon, B. and Cole, P. (1972): Menopause and breast cancer. *J. Natl. Cancer Inst.,* **48,** 605.

Wagoner, J. K., Chiazze, L. and Lloyd, J. W. (1967): Cancer of the breast at menopausal ages. *Cancer,* **20,** 354.

Wanebo, G. K., Johnson, K. G., Sato, K. *et al.* (1968): Breast cancer after exposure to the atomic bombings of Hiroshima and Nagasaki. *New Eng. J. Med.,* **279,** 667.

Welsch, C. W. and Meites, J. (1970): Effects of reserpine on development of 7,12-dimethylbenzanthracene induced mammary tumors. *Experientia,* **26,** 1133.

Wynder, E. L., Bross, I. J. and Hirayama, T. (1960): A study of the epidemiology of cancer of the breast. *Cancer,* **13,** 559.

Wynder, E. W. (1969): Identification of women at high risk for breast cancer. *Cancer,* **24,** 1235.

Zippin, C. and Petrakis, N. L. (1971): Identification of high risk groups in breast cancer. *Cancer,* **28,** 1385.

3

Malignant Potential of Breast Lesions

J. A. Dossett

INTRODUCTION

The diagnosis of infiltrating breast cancer depends on histological evidence of abnormal epithelial cells no longer confined by their natural boundaries but infiltrating the surrounding tissues. Except in relatively uncommon instances, the diagnosis causes little disagreement between different histologists. Such unanimity is however not found in the diagnosis of lesions likely to lead to infiltrating cancer. Here abnormal cells must be recognized while they are still confined by their natural boundaries. Alternatively, a lesion must be recognized which leads to cancer in a high proportion of cases.

In cancerous breasts, the lesion we find most closely connected with infiltration is a proliferation of epithelial cells within pre-existing boundaries. In our series, over 90% of infiltrating cancers show evidence of neoplastic proliferative lesions still within their natural boundaries, either within or in direct continuity with the infiltrating cancer. Both the infiltrating and the non-infiltrating cells show similar cytological features. Multiple cancers are sometimes found in the same breast segment, arising from a common intraduct neoplastic lesion.

The conclusion is inescapable that whether or not there are other precancerous conditions, the majority of breast cancers arise from pre-existing, non-infiltrating, neoplastic proliferating cells. The histological evidence is very strong, yet most surgeons of experience will confirm that infiltrating cancer is not a common sequel when patients in whom biopsy has shown a non-invasive lesion, are followed over a number of years. This has led to doubt and contention which is perhaps best illustrated by the statement of Willis (1953): "any competent pathologist who has examined a considerable number of surgically removed breasts will find it difficult to remain patient with those surgeons who deny the precancerous potentialities of cystic hyperplasia."

It is not difficult to find reasons for this discrepancy. In the first place the nomenclature of simple breast conditions is confused. Different pathologists give different names to the same condition or include differing conditions under the same name. For example chronic mastitis and fibrocystic disease are still widely used all-embracing terms but interpreted differently in different centres. Cystic hyperplasia is used to refer to cystic disease with no proliferative component, and also to cystic disease with epithelial proliferation, occurring in the same breast as distinct though not necessarily unrelated conditions. There is even confusion as to what constitutes normal or abnormal breast structure and for example, normal involutional changes are frequently classed as pathological disorders. It is not surprising therefore that studies of precancerous lesions are not strictly comparable and yield different statistical results.

This is not the place to embark upon a detailed nomenclature. Here we shall use the terminology of Bonser, Dossett and Jull (1960), revised by Dossett, Herlinger and Shucksmith (1974) to exclude eponyms and words which in a restricted situation are given a special meaning. As far as is possible words will be used only in their general pathological sense.

EARLY STUDIES

Allowing for differences in terminology, follow-up studies would be expected to have shown a clear relationship between certain benign lesions and infiltrating cancer, yet conflicting conclusions have been reached. The earlier workers dealt mainly with small numbers of patients and correspondingly small numbers developed cancer. When larger numbers of cases were reported, guesses were made as to the expected frequency of cancer, and no comparison was made with the actual incidence in women of corresponding ages. The almost uniform conclusion that no relationship existed between "cystic disease" and cancer, therefore had no factual basis.

The first adequate study was by Warren (1940). He first tried to ascertain the morbidity rate for breast cancer in the Massachusetts area. In this state, there was no cancer register and the morbidity rate could be calculated only from the death rate, making allowance for cancer cures and undiagnosed cases. In order to avoid biasing the figure in favour of a causal relationship Warren accepted twice the death rate as the morbidity rate although a factor of 1.5 would have been more than adequate.

Overall, 35 cancers occurred in 1044 individuals with "cystic disease" followed from 5 to 21 years, representing a total exposure of 9393 risk years. This gives a figure of 0.37 per 100 as a corrected annual breast cancer rate in this series contrasted with an average breast cancer morbidity rate of 0.058 per 100 for the Massachusetts female population of 1930.

When age specific rates were used, the breast cancer rate was 4.5 times greater in the biopsy series than for the normal female population. Below the age of 50 the rate was 11.7 times greater than normal. Over the age of 50 it was only 2.5 times greater. This excess risk has persisted in this group of patients diagnosed between 1915 and 1955. This is shown in a recent follow-up 30 to 40 years after the diagnosis of benign disease (Warren, Monson and MacMahon, 1973).

Thus Warren has shown conclusively that cancer arose more frequently in a breast where biopsy had proved the pre-existence of certain pathological lesions, than it did in the general population of women of similar ages. His figures do not, however, tell us just how much greater is the risk. Neither do they tell us which lesions are likely to be the most dangerous. Warren divided his cases into the following groups: chronic mastitis, chronic cystic mastitis, adenocystoma and adenofibroma. These subdivisions are too imprecise to permit assessment of the malignant potential of individual breast lesions.

Similar remarks apply to the subsequent studies of Lewison and Lyons (1953) and Clagett, Plimpton and Rood (1944). They respectively found a cancer rate 2.6 and 5 times greater in women with pre-existing breast disease than in the general population. The former authors were not able to support Warren's findings of higher incidence below the age of 50, as all their cases of cancer arose after the menopause (average age 54 years).

Some indication of the malignant potential of specific types of breast lesion can be obtained from comparing cancerous and noncancerous breasts for the frequency of certain benign lesions in each group. Bonser *et al.* (1960) divided their cases into: cystic disease, which comprised lobular degeneration cysts, tension cysts and lobular sclerosis; epithelial proliferation in the sense used in this chapter; and cystic disease and epithelial proliferation occurring together which was referred to as cystic hyperplasia at that time. For comparison they used the normal series of Frantz *et al.* (1951) who had subdivided breast lesions in a similar manner.

The incidence of these benign lesions in "normal" compared with cancerous breasts was:

1 to 1.7 for cystic disease
1 to 3.3 for proliferative lesions
1 to 3.8 for cystic disease and proliferative lesions occurring together

More detailed analysis is required to tell us precisely the chances of any given lesion becoming malignant but the above findings indicate that proliferative lesions, with or without cystic disease, require particularly close attention.

There is no standard way of reporting proliferative breast lesions and because of the diversity of type, extent and situation, it is unlikely that any simple acceptable method will emerge. However it is essential that every report should indicate concisely

1. The degree of differentiation of the lesion
2. Its anatomical site
3. The absence of infiltration or its presence and degree.

PROLIFERATIVE LESIONS

By neoplastic epithelial proliferation we refer to an increase in the number of cells within a a pre-existing breast structure, the cells being confined by their basement membranes. All epithelial structures in the breast may show such a change although some are affected more frequently than others. Ducts, terminal ducts and acini may be involved. Abnormal structures such as cysts or rarely the clefts in a fibroadenoma may also show evidence of these lesions. Even the cells in an area of lobular sclerosis may take on neoplastic properties terminating in infiltrating cancer.

The multiplication of cells may be no more than a heaping up of epithelium in a portion of the duct wall, or perhaps in a lobule the acini will appear solid and slightly distended. On the other hand ducts can be distended to very large dimensions and acini reach such a size that they can be distinguished from distended ducts only by the absence of elastic tissue in their walls. The cellular masses may be well differentiated with an acinar or cribriform pattern or may present as a solid core of undifferentiated cells.

Individual cells may be small, regular and pale staining, differing only slightly from normal ducts and acinar cells in the surrounding breast. In such cases, pathologists often diagnose simple epithelial proliferation although cells of this regular type are known to constitute a proportion of infiltrating breast cancers. In other cases the cells are irregular and hyperchromatic and then intraduct cancer is readily diagnosed. Mitotic figures may be absent, scanty or abundant.

The pathologist assesses these protean manifestations using similar criteria to those he would use for non-infiltrating neoplastic lesions elsewhere in the body, e.g. rectal polypi, bladder papillomata or carcinoma *in situ* of the cervix uteri. In effect he grades the lesions into those with low and those with high malignant potential, and advises the surgeon accordingly.

GRADING OF PROLIFERATIVE LESIONS

If any planned large scale study is to give the additional information we need on the malignant potential of the proliferative lesion, grading, using a method such as that of Bloom and Richardson (1957), will be essential.

Bloom graded infiltrating breast cancers according to: structural differentiation of the tumour as shown by tubular arrangement of the cells; variation in size, shape and staining quality of the nuclei; frequency of hyperchromatism and mitotic figures. Points are given in each category so that finally three grades emerge ranging from low (Grade I) to high (Grade III). The duration of survival was found to be $2\frac{1}{2}$ to 3 times greater in Grade I than in Grade III.

Clearly it could not be expected that such grading applied to non-infiltrating lesions would be reflected in survival but its use could be to assess the potential for infiltration. Grade I lesions would be expected to infiltrate infrequently whilst Grade III lesions would suggest a constant source of danger. Therefore a prospective study would have to be restricted to patients with Grade I and II lesions, for it would be considered unethical by many surgeons not to proceed to mastectomy in Grade III cases.

The following observations illustrate the relative dangers. We have followed up large numbers of Grade I lesions and in only one case has metastasis occurred when infiltration has not been apparent. Here a biopsy was undertaken for a small proliferative lesions distending a terminal duct and related acini. There was a well differentiated cribriform pattern with pale regular cells and no mitotic activity. The woman returned three years later with bone secondaries. Adrenalectomy revealed secondary deposits in the adrenal glands of similar pattern to the intraduct lesion of the original biopsy. At autopsy nine months later no residual breast lesion was found and no other source of primary growth could be demonstrated.

Grade III lesions are less predictable. Particularly dangerous are the Grade III comedo cancers with huge masses of bizarre cells stuffing and distending ducts and acini in which there is central necrosis and calcification. Secondary deposits are sometimes found in axillary nodes even when serial sections fail to reveal a point of infiltration. Seven per cent (8 of 115 consecutive cases) showed this phenomenon. Clearly biopsy alone must be regarded as insufficient treatment for this particular lesion.

STATISTICAL CONSIDERATIONS

Other considerations in addition to grading require to be taken into account in planning a large scale study of the proliferative lesion. The extent of the tumour and its situation in the duct acinar system will be considered later. But first the number of women that would need to be followed up, the possible outcome and the limitations of this method of approach must be considered. We shall calculate the number of women with and without proliferative lesions which would be expected to yield 100 cancers if followed over a five year period. These numbers and times are taken for convenience to give a measure of the size and effort required in such an investigation.

Campbell (1968) calculated that of women reaching the age of 40, 3% will die from breast cancer and a further 2% will contract cancer but die from other causes. In all, 5% of women over the age of 40 years will develop breast cancer. Assuming an expectancy of 30 more years of life, i.e. an average life span of 70 years, 100 breast cancers will be expected to develop from 12,000 unselected women over each 5 year period. We have already indicated that over 90% of cancers can be seen to develop from pre-existing non-invasive proliferative lesions, whilst in about 10% the origin of the cancer cannot be determined. Therefore 100 breast cancers showing contained neoplastic lesions within or in direct continuity with the infiltrating cancer would be expected from 13,200 unselected women over a 5 year period.

Frantz *et al.* (1951) in a study of breasts of women coming to autopsy with no previous history of breast disease, found proliferative lesions in 17% of women of this age group. It follows that if women with proliferative lesions are selected by biopsy, 2,244 of these women will be required to produce 100 cancers in 5 years, a cancer incidence of 4.5% or 0.89% per annum. This is much higher than the incidence of 0.37% per annum arrived at by Warren (1940). He would have required 5,400 cases to produce 100 cancers in 5 years.

This difference is expected, for our calculations relate to the tissue removed at biopsy in contrast to those of Warren which relate to the tissue remaining after biopsy. Warren could make no allowances for the tissue removed which presumably included the most severely affected portion of the breast. In many of his cases mastectomy had been undertaken so that only half the tissue at risk remained and Warren was estimating the malignant potential of the field with the lesion removed. This information is of more value to the surgeon managing the patient than a knowledge of the malignant potential of the tissue removed if the biopsy has eradicated the entire local lesion. Where the biopsy is inadequate however, the converse is true and it is important to know both the malignant potential of the lesion removed and that of the field change in the remaining breast tissue.

From these arguments it will be apparent that follow-up studies are unsuitable for the assessment of the malignant potential of individual breast lesions; this information can be obtained only by indirect methods. Unfortunately there is insufficient information available so far to compare the malignant potential of individual proliferative lesions. The most that can be done is to give a very rough estimate of the malignant potential in the two large groups into which most pathologists separate their cases.

These are intraduct proliferation, a term commonly used when the pathologist does not wish to alarm the surgeon, and intraduct cancer which is used when he considers the surgeon should take further action. For this purpose, proliferative lesions can be divided into two equal groups, one of high grade and one of low grade. If the not unreasonable assumption be made that 90% of infiltrating tumours will develop in the high grade group, it can be calculated that in the low grade group 11,220 women would be required to produce 100 cancers in 5 years, an incidence of 0.18% per annum. This figure is only slightly in excess of that for women in the general population where the cancer incidence as calculated here is 0.16% for women over 40 years of age per annum. This slight increased risk of cancer developing would not justify any surgical procedure additional to biopsy.

In the high grade group however, 1,246 women would be expected to produce 100 infiltrating cancers in 5 years, an incidence of 1.6% per annum. Here the risk is high indeed and the surgeon would need to be very sure that the entire local lesion had been removed if he decides not to proceed to mastectomy.

ANATOMICAL SITE OF PROLIFERATIVE LESIONS

Terminal duct and intralobular proliferation

Intraduct proliferative lesions most commonly affect the terminal ducts at the point where the elastic mantle surrounding the duct disappears and the duct joins the lobule. This has been elegantly shown in whole breast studies using a quantitative, three-dimensional, thick-section method, confirming the results with conventional histology (Wellings and Jensen, 1973). Their findings are supported by a study of very early infiltrating cancers in our material where two types of infiltration are apparent at this site; one associated with proliferation of elastic tissue; the other associated with acinar unfolding and distension.

In the former type there is tremendous hyperplasia of the elastic network of the terminal ducts as the cancer cells penetrate the duct wall so that dense masses of finely fibrillar elastic tissue result. This is visible as pale pink areas with ordinary Haematoxylin and Eosin staining with sparse surviving cancer cells detectable in the elastic masses. The proliferating intraduct lesion and surrounding elastica form the nidus on which the contracted (scirrhous) cancer is based (Shucksmith and Dossett, 1965; Dossett, 1968).

The prognostic implications of this early elastic cancer are important. In the absence of infiltrating cancer elsewhere in the breast, metastasis at this stage has not been observed in our material. Furthermore, because the lesion is localized to a very small section of the duct its complete removal with the biopsy is assured. Hence we do not advise mastectomy for this lesion, and in a follow-up of over 100 cases in the last 8 years there has been no recurrence. It would seem therefore that excision biopsy is adequate treatment although our total numbers and the length of follow-up are insufficient to assess the effect of field change in the breast. When cancer cells appear beyond the hyperplastic elastic zone, the above considerations do not apply and lymph node metastases have been found even with the smallest infiltrating tumours.

The second method of spread, i.e. into the lobule, follows the pattern described by Wellings and Jensen who find a process of "progressive lobular and ductular distension and unfolding with concomitant coalescence of ductular lumens converting the lobular structure into large ovoid and circular profiles". An examination of their material leaves no doubt that the various types of intralobular carcinoma are produced in this way.

A particular variety of *in situ* lobular carcinoma of the breast was described by Muir (1941) and Foote and Stewart (1941) as "lobular carcinoma *in situ*". This is sometimes called "small cell carcinoma", for the cells are small, fairly regular and darkly staining, and are crowded together within the distended lobule in undifferentiated masses. When infiltration occurs there is a tendency for the cells to lose cohesion and infiltrate diffusely in the tissue spaces as individual cells or very small groups of cells. Cancers which spread in this manner are highly malignant and it has been shown by Ashikari *et al.* (1973) among others that this cancer carries a worse than average prognosis. Because of this most authors recommend mastectomy as curative for "lobular carcinoma *in situ*". However Gordans and Klopp (1973) report on 19 patients with non-infiltrating "lobular carcinoma" who refused mastectomy. Only two developed carcinoma in the ipsilateral breast 3 and 6 years after biopsy. At mastectomy axillary nodes were negative and both patients were alive and well 8 and 11 years later. They conclude that the good results suggest a careful follow-up as a valid alternative to simple mastectomy for this variety of intralobular cancer.

Clearly, as with the early contracted cancers, biopsy may eradicate the entire lesion and the problem becomes one of field change in the remaining breast tissue. Even so the tendency to infiltrate is higher than with other intralobular proliferations and this may be due to several factors acting together. Thus the absence of any elastic barrier in the lobule to impede infiltration may be a factor. Furthermore a dedifferentiated type of intralobular cancer has been selected for study and with better differentiated varieties it is likely that subsequent infiltration would be less of a hazard. Further study might be directed to an estimation of the bulk of the initial lesion in relation to prognosis and to evidence of multifocal lesions as shown in a step series through the biopsy.

Intraduct proliferations

Intraduct proliferations are far less frequent than those affecting terminal ducts and acini. They may be confined to a short length of the duct and distend the duct to such dimensions that a palpable tumour results. Typical of this is the multiradicular papilloma which is usually found in the larger ducts. The tumour is well differentiated and although infiltrating cancers can be seen to arise from this lesion, excision biopsy is curative in the non-infiltrating cases we have encountered.

When extensive areas of the duct system are involved the situation is more dangerous. Multifocal cancers are found in 8 to 10% of the cancerous breasts and although some of these arise from independent lesions a large number originate from a single involved duct system. Breakout usually occurs at the weak points in the system where the elastica is deficient, i.e. from lobules secondarily involved or from the junction of terminal ducts and acini. A typical cancer of this type is the comedo cancer described earlier in this chapter. The treatment of choice for extensive duct lesions must be mastectomy. Mammography may be of value in gauging the extent of an intraduct cancer in those cases where calcification is a feature.

Neoplastic lesions of nipple sinuses and intraepidermal spread

In the male breast the nipple sinuses account for almost all the glandular epithelium. A few rudimentary ducts may lie beneath the nipple and it is from these that gynaecomastia can develop. Primary neoplastic lesions of the male breast are therefore predominantly of sinusoidal origin. Neoplastic lesions arising in sinuses or the tubules of the rudimentary duct system beneath will present as a lump centrally placed under the nipple and are frequently accompanied by a sanguineous discharge. This facilitates early diagnosis before infiltration occurs.

Secondary carcinoma of the male breast is more common than primary cancer. It presents as a tumour eccentrically placed beneath the nipple and is not accompanied by bleeding from the nipple ducts. Carcinoma has been reported in breasts affected with gynaecomastia but this has not been observed in our material.

In the female breast the nipple sinuses account for only a small percentage of the total breast epithelium and consequently the incidence of primary neoplastic lesions of the sinuses is low. It is more usual for the sinuses to show secondary involvement from neoplastic cells growing up from the main ducts beneath the nipple. In either event, as in the male breast, bleeding from the nipple ducts is not uncommon and infiltration from lesions of the sinuses is rarely seen.

When a nipple is ulcerated and destroyed by cancer a large tumour arising deeper in the breast is usually responsible. Intrasinusoidal neoplastic lesions may involve the terminal galactophores and spread into the epidermis of the nipple to produce Paget's disease. This method of spread indicates a high malignant potential, for in about half the cases an infiltrating cancer will already be present deeper in the breast at the time of the initial diagnosis of Paget's disease. The infiltrating tumour may arise from a duct proliferation continuous with the intraepidermal and sinusoidal lesions, or from a discontinuous multifocal lesion. Nevertheless, where operation has been refused, cases are reported where twenty years have elapsed between the first appearance of a lesion in the nipple and the development of infiltrating cancer. A detailed study of histogenesis of Paget's disease was made by Bonser *et al.* (1960).

PROLIFERATIVE LESIONS IN PATHOLOGICAL CONDITIONS

Cystic disease and cancer

Cystic disease of the breast carries an increased risk of cancer even when unassociated with proliferative lesions, and cancer has been observed to develop directly from pink metaplastic epithelium by many competent observers. However, it is generally accepted that the risk is too small to warrant excisional procedures and aspiration of cysts is undertaken in most clinics. Those cases where the metaplastic pink epithelium forms papillary projections into the cyst lumen appear to carry no greater risk than those where the epithelium is of simple columnar type. However, it has been shown (Bonser *et al.*, 1960) that tension cysts may result either from kinking of a terminal duct supplying a lobular degeneration cyst in the course of breast involution, or from a proliferative lesion blocking the terminal duct. Hence, follow-up after aspiration is essential and mammography may be of help in detecting certain duct lesions.

Cancer may develop from a cyst wall or result from a proliferative lesion within the terminal duct growing into a cyst. Carcinoma of either type tends to carry a relatively good prognosis; the cancer tends to grow freely into the cyst lumen rather than infiltrate deeply into the cyst wall. In many cases the cancer is purely intracystic with no infiltrating component. Cytology of aspirated cyst contents is usually sufficient for diagnosis but a cyst which cannot be completely aspirated must be subjected to biopsy.

Lobular sclerosis

Lobular sclerosis is an abnormal form of lobular involution allied to cystic disease. It results when fibrosis occurs in the involuting lobule with fusion of the basement membranes and newly formed intralobular collagenous tissue. We do not subscribe to the view that lobular sclerosis (sclerosing adenosis) is a myoepithelial hyperplasia. The fibrosis distorts the tubules and acini and produces the characteristic picture with a superficial resemblance to infiltrating cancer, but the cytological appearances are not those of neoplasia and there is no true infiltration.

Although there is general agreement that this lesion is not precancerous, sometimes the cells do undergo neoplastic transformation becoming large and hyperchromatic with a degree of nuclear irregularity. When such changes are pronounced the underlying lobular origin may become difficult to recognise. In the event of carcinomatous change all traces of the structure of origin will soon be obliterated. Further study is required to determine the frequency of neoplasia in lobular sclerosis and the chances of malignant progression.

Fibroadenoma and cystosarcoma

Fibroadenomata result from hyperplasia of single lobules or aggregates of lobules. The process commences as an overgrowth of loose intralobular connective tissue into which lobular epithelium grows to form cysts and tubules. Further overgrowth of loose connective tissue invaginates the cysts to produce clefts and crevices. Finally growth ceases and the loose connective tissue becomes dense and collagenous.

In the early stages of development the hyperplastic epithelium will appear active and may be three or four layers deep but these minor proliferations do not progress to cancer. In old quiescent tumours neoplastic epithelial changes are sometimes seen but infiltration of the dense collagenous stroma is an excessive rarity. Sometimes a fibroadenoma abutting onto a cancer will share similar neoplastic epithelium in its crevices with that in ducts within the infiltrating tumour. In such cases the infiltrating cancer will have originated from structures outside the fibrous tumour. It can be concluded that neoplasia within a fibroadenoma is of limited significance.

Carcino-sarcoma is a rare tumour in which neoplastic change has occurred in the epithelial component of a cysto-sarcoma. The two elements, fibrous and epithelial, metastasize separately as fibrosarcoma and carcinoma.

Duct ectasia

Duct ectasia is initially an inflammation of the wall of a larger duct which results in damage to the myoepithelial and elastic layers so allowing the duct to passively dilate. The subepithelial lymphatic plexus of the duct wall is obliterated by the inflammation and ensuing fibrosis, reabsorption of secretions is disturbed and they accumulate to form an inspissated mass. Stagnation of secretions has been invoked as a possible carcinogenic factor but if this were true intraduct neoplasia and carcinoma would be expected more frequently in duct ectasia than in normal ducts. This is not so since in our material proliferative lesions and infiltrating cancer show no increased incidence in duct ectasia. We have not analysed the types of cancer related to dilated ducts. Whether or not infiltration is modified by the damage and fibrosis in the duct wall must be a subject for further study.

CONCLUSION

Our knowledge of the malignant potential of individual breast lesions and of the likelihood of cancer developing in the remaining breast tissue after biopsy is at the best fragmentary. In most cases treatment depends on local policy and individual bias. Over the last twenty years pathologists have tended to advocate a less radical approach, and improvement in diagnostic facilities has given the surgeon more confidence to engage in follow-up studies.

However, small scale studies are valueless and large scale studies take a vast amount of time and organisation. Nonetheless such studies must be embarked upon for a more rational approach to be realized. The advent of the computor should reduce the labour involved but in order to obtain a sufficient number of cases, and to reduce the work to manageable proportions, several centres would need to be involved with a panel of pathologists to unify nomenclature. A study of this type is urgently needed.

BIBLIOGRAPHY

Ashikari, R., Huvos, A. G., Urban, J. A. and Robbins, G. F. (1973): Infiltrating lobular carcinoma of the breast. *Cancer,* **31,** 110.

Bloom, H. J. G. and Richardson, W. W. (1957): Histological grading and prognosis in breast cancer. A study of 1,409 cases of which 359 have been followed for 15 years. *Brit. J. Cancer,* **11,** 359.

Bonser, G. M., Dossett, J. A. and Jull, J. W. (1960): Human and experimental breast cancer. Pitman Medical Publishing Co. London.

Campbell, H. (1968): Prognostic factors in breast cancer: Proceedings of the first Tenovus symposium. Ed. Forrest, A. P. M. and Kunkler, P. D. Livingstone, Edinburgh.

Clagett, O. T., Plimpton, N. C. and Root, G. T. (1944): Lesions of the breast, the relationship of benign lesions to carcinoma. *Surgery.* **15,** 413.

Dossett, J. A. (1968): Prognostic factors in breast cancer: Proceedings of the first Tenovus symposium. Ed. Forrest, A. P. M. and Kunkler, P. B. Livingstone, Edinburgh.

Dossett, J. A., Herlinger, H. and Shucksmith, H. S. (1975): A simplified nomenclature of breast disorders: histological and radiological aspects. (In press.)

Foote, F. W. Jr. and Stewart, F. W. (1941): Lobular carcinoma in situ. *Amer. J. Path.,* **17,** 491.

Frantz, V. K., Pickren, J. W., Melcher, G. W. and Auchincloss, H. Jr. (1951): Incidence of chronic cystic disease in so-called "normal breasts. *Cancer (Philad),* **4,** 762.

Giordano, J. M. and Klopp, C. T. (1973): Lobular carcinoma in situ: Incidence and treatment. *Cancer,* **31,** 105.

Lewison, E. F. and Lyons, J. G. (1953): Relationship between benign breast disease and cancer. *Arch. Surg.,* **66,** 94.

Muir, R. (1941): The Evolution of carcinoma of the mamma. *J. Path & Bact.,* **52,** 155.

Shucksmith, H. S. and Dossett, J. A. (1965): Pseudolipoma of the breast: a mask for cancer. *Brit. Med. J.*, **2**, 1459.

Warren, S. (1940): The relation of "chronic mastitis" to carcinoma of the breast. *Surg. Gynec. Obstet.*, **71**, 257.

Warren, S., Monson, R., MacMahon, B. *et al.* (1973): Long-term follow-up of patients with benign cystic mastopathy. Quoted in Etiology of Human Breast Cancer: A Review *J. Natl. Cancer Inst.*, **50**, 21–42, 1973.

Wellings, S. R. and Jensen, H. M. (1973): On the origin and progression of ductal carcinoma in the human breast. *J. Natl. Cancer Inst.*, **50**, 1111.

Willis, R. A. (1953): Pathology of tumours, 2nd Ed. Butterworth: London.

4

Role of Exogenous Estrogens

Edward F. Lewison

The exact effect of exogenous estrogens on the incidence of breast cancer must await improved knowledge and ability to determine more precisely the endocrine regulation of the cells of breast tissue. A time-dose relationship is probably most important. The influence of estrogen, progesterone, androgen and corticoid receptors inside the cell, and prolactin, growth hormone and insulin receptors on the cell surface, are exceedingly complex but certainly most important in determining the incidence and control of breast cancer. These hormones can be either promoters of breast cancer or etiologic agents.

Estrogens have been clearly shown by Lyons, Li and Johnson (1958) to act directly on normal breast tissue cells to promote growth and differentiation. Estrogen also stimulates the release of pituitary prolactin which in turn affects the mammary cells. Estrogens cannot support the growth of experimental mammary cancers in the absence of the pituitary gland, but prolactin has been shown by Pearson *et al.* (1969) and others to be able to support the growth of mammary tumors in the absence of both the ovaries and the adrenals.

Our knowledge of the mode of action of hormones has progressed remarkably during the past few years. Steroid hormones are now known to regulate gene activity and the very earliest changes resulting from the activity of even minute amounts of steroid hormone can now be detected. To fully understand the mechanism of steroid activity we must however know the biochemical process whereby information is transferred from the hormone-receptor complex to the nucleus.

The breast and other target organs are known to possess the ability to bind selectively certain circulating hormones such as 17β-estradiol. Breast tumor cells can bind this estrogen at specific receptor sites within the cell, and they also have the enzymatic ability to convert circulating steroids to metabolites of greater or lesser physiological activity.

Clinical evidence clearly indicates that the breast is an estrogen-sensitive target organ. In 1923, Doisey and Allen demonstrated that even crude ovarian extracts were remarkably potent growth stimulants for the epithelium of both the breast and the female genital tract. The dawn of breast development in the female begins at the menarche – the onset of hormonal activity in women. The importance of endogenous estrogens in the development of breast cancer is suggested by the fact that the disease never occurs in the female prior to this time of estrogenic awakening.

Gynecomastia can be caused by hormonal stimulation in men receiving exogenous estrogens therapeutically. Enlargement of the male breast occurs in men with estrogen-producing tumors and in men taking drugs which physiologically resemble estrogens, such as digitalis. Therefore, it seems clear that exogenous estrogens can affect the growth of breast tissue and may be important either directly or indirectly in the development of breast cancer.

Breast cancer has been noted occasionally in men taking estrogens therapeutically and in factory workers exposed to the manufacture of synthetic Stilbestrol. Symmers (1968) recently reported the tragedy of two male transvestites both of whom developed and died of breast cancer after long-term exogenous estrogen treatment. A child taking her mother's birth control pills by mistake has been described as developing breast cancer at a very early age.

A three-and-a-half year old girl developed breast enlargement and other signs of sexual precocity and was found to have been using small but regular doses of estrogen-containing face cream. She developed deeply pigmented nipples and marked bilateral breast enlargement. In premenopausal women, the growth of an existing breast cancer can be exacerbated by low-dose long-term exogenous estrogen stimulation.

During the past thirty years exogenous estrogens were occasionally recommended by obstetricians for pregnant women whose pregnancy was considered to be at risk because of irregular bleeding or previous pregnancy loss. Adenocarcinomas of the vagina are presently developing in some of these young women whose mothers received diethylstilbestrol during their pregnancy. This 20 or 30 year time lag, a prolonged latent period, is indeed quite characteristic of most human carcinogens, and the "time-bomb" represented by this exogenous estrogen has assumed major importance at the present time.

In our modern society, the birth control pill has become an important and convenient method of family planning. It is usually an estrogen–progestagen combination and is currently being taken by millions of women throughout the world. It is the exogenous hormone most widely used at the present time.

Estrogenic hormones used by women in the perimenopausal period are perhaps the next most common exogenous hormone prescribed and the long-term use of these hormones may be of importance in the incidence of breast cancer. These estrogenic hormones are usually prescribed for specific therapeutic replacement purposes at the menopause but may be taken by many women in the false hope of retaining their youthfulness.

Exogenous estrogen may be given by mouth, by injection or in a hormone – containing cream or suppository. Certain drugs also have estrogen-like physiologic properties as do some factors present in our diet. Boyland (1967) has noted that more than a hundred different species of plants contain estrogenic substances, some of which are eaten in our daily diet and others are eaten by domestic farm animals which we ultimately consume as meat. The biologic activity of these estrogenic food-stuffs is, of course, dependent upon many factors the most important of which is the liver. Gut bacteria can produce estrogens from biliary steroids but the actual amount produced and absorbed in vivo is unknown (Hill, Goddard and Williams, 1971).

Does prudence suggest that women with a "high-risk" predisposition to breast cancer and women with known mastopathy avoid the stimulation of long-term estrogen therapy? Several recent epidemiologic studies (Arthes, Sartwell and Lewison, 1967) have explored this relationship between estrogens, the pill and breast cancer. These investigations include our own Johns Hopkins series of 283 cases with carefully matched controls (Arthes *et al.*, 1974), the Boston Drug Survey (1973), the retrospective study of Vessey, Doll and Sutton (1972), the report of Leis (1970), and Burch, Byrd and Vaughn (1974) and finally the most recent interim report of the Royal College of General Practitioners (1974). In all of these surveys there appeared to be *no* convincing clinical evidence to support a significant association between the taking of exogenous estrogens or the pill and the incidence of breast cancer.

In my opinion, however, before these negative conclusions can be accepted as final it will be necessary to study many times more subjects and to wait for a much longer period of time. I would consider the clinical dangers of breast cancer in "high risk" patients to contraindicate the prolonged use of the pill or estrogens but we must await the passage of time before a final reckoning of the risks involved in the long-term use of exogenous estrogens.

REFERENCES

Arthes, F. G., Sartwell, P. E. and Lewison, E. F. (1967): The pill, estrogens and the breast. Epidemiologic aspects. *Cancer,* **28,** 1391.

Arthes, F. G., Sartwell, P. E., Lewison, E. F. and Tonascia, J. (1974): Breast cancer, estrogens and the pill. Presented at the XI International Cancer Congress, Florence, Italy.

Boston Collaborative Drug Surveillance Programme (1973): Oral contraceptives and venous thromboembolic disease surgically confirmed gall-bladder disease, and breast tumors. *Lancet,* **1,** 1399.

Boyland, E. (1967): Natural oestrogens and the safe level of oestrogen intake. *Tumori,* **53,** 19.

Burch, J. C., Byrd, B. F. and Vaughn, W. K. (1974): The effects of long-term estrogen on hysterectomized women. *Am. J. Obst. Gyn.,* **118,** 778.

Doisey, E. A. and Allen, E. (1923): Ovarian hormone; preliminary report on its localisation, extraction and partial purification, and action in test animals. *JAMA,* **81,** 819.

Hill, M. J., Goddard, P. and Williams, R. E. O. (1971): Gut bacteria and aetiology of cancer of the breast. *Lancet,* **2,** 472.

Leis, H. P. (1970): The pill and the breast. *New York State J. Med.,* **70,** 2911.

Lyons, W. R., Li, C. H. and Johnson, R. E. (1958): Recent Progress. *Hormone Research,* **14,** 219.

Pearson, O. H., Llerena, O., Llerena, L., Molina, A. and Butler, T. (1969): *Tran. Ass. Amer. Physicians,* **82,** 225.

Royal College of General Practitioners (1974): Oral contraceptives and health: an interim report. Pitman Medical, London: p. 98.

Symmers, W. S. (1968): Carcinoma of breast in trans-sexual individuals after surgical and hormonal interference with primary and secondary sex characteristics. *Brit. Med. J.,* **2,** 82.

Vessey, M. P., Doll, R. and Sutton, P. M. (1972): Oral contraceptives and breast neoplasia: a retrospective study. *Brit. Med. J.,* **3,** 719.

5

Psychological Correlates of Breast Cancer

H. Steven Greer

The following report is a review of the psychological investigation of a consecutive series of 160 women who were admitted to hospital for biopsy of a lump in the breast (Greer and Morris, 1975). Significant differences were looked for between those whose lumps were subsequently reported positive for cancer, and those who showed benign disease. The patients were compared with respect to four major factors – their history of psychiatric disorders, their social adjustment, their reaction to stress and the extent to which they suppressed anger and other feelings.

INTRODUCTORY

The notion that psychological disorders and stressful life experiences may influence the development and course of cancer is by no means new. In the 18th and 19th centuries a number of eminent clinicians including Guy (1759), Paget (1870) and Snow (1893) argued that depression and antecedent life stresses played a part in the aetiology of cancer (Le Shan and Worthington, 1956). The most consistently reported psycho-social antecedent of cancer has been loss of a major emotional relationship (Le Shan, 1959). Yet a subsequent carefully controlled investigation of this hypothesis failed to demonstrate any significant association between breast cancer and either recent or childhood loss (Muslin, Gyarfas and Pieper, 1966).

In a later British study, Coppen and Metcalfe (1963) reported a statistical association between breast cancer and extraversion. Their findings were based on comparisons between women with breast cancer and patients without cancer who were suffering from "various gynaecological and surgical conditions". Unfortunately, the diagnoses of the latter patients and the stage of breast cancer in the experimental group were not specified, nor did the authors state whether testing was conducted before or after surgery. These omissions make it difficult to interpret Coppen and Metcalfe's findings. It is likely that the emotional state of the breast cancer patients and controls was dissimilar at the time of testing, and this variable may influence the test scores (Kissen, 1964).

In contrast to the generally inadequate studies in this field are the rigorous standards adopted by Kissen in his work on lung cancer patients. Using structured clinical interviews and psychological tests of known reliability and validity, he repeatedly found that lung cancer patients differed significantly from controls with non-cancerous lung diseases in having a personality pattern characterised by "a restricted outlet for emotional discharge" (Kissen, 1963; Kissen, Brown and Kissen, 1969). Kissen's findings, of which only the briefest mention has been made here, raise some fundamental questions concerning the contributory role of personality factors in the aetiology of lung cancer.

INVESTIGATION

A consecutive series of 160 patients was studied psychologically. At the subsequent operation, 69 of these women were found to have breast cancer and 91 benign breast disease; the latter women comprised the control group. The cancer and control groups were closely similar in terms of marital state and social class. Cancer patients were, however, significantly older than controls.

Subjects were interviewed, using a structured psychiatric interview schedule, and given psychological tests on the day before operation. Care was taken to ensure that the interviewers had no knowledge of the provisional diagnosis. In almost all cases, husbands or close relatives were interviewed separately to verify the patients' accounts.

The patients were submitted to psychiatric investigation with respect to four factors – their history of psychiatric disorders, their degree of social adjustment, their reaction to stress and the extent to which they suppressed or expressed anger and other feelings.

1. Psychiatric disorders

During the five years before the first appearance of the breast lump, almost exactly the same proportion of cancer patients (35%) as controls (36%), suffered from depressive illnesses for which they had received medical treatment, in most cases as outpatients. Other psychiatric illnesses during this period were reported by 9% of cancer patients and 6% of controls. The severity of depression just before admission to hospital was assessed quantitatively by means of Hamilton's (1967) Rating Scale on which scores range from 0 (no depressive symptoms whatever) to 50. Of the total, 93% of cancer patients and 95% of controls had scores from 0–15.

Each patient was given the Mill Hill Test of Verbal Intelligence (Raven, 1958), the Eysenck Personality Inventory (*E.P.I.*) Form A (Eysenck and

Eysenck, 1964) and the Caine and Foulds (1967) Hostility and Direction of Hostility Questionnaire (*H.D.H.Q.*).

There were no significant differences between cancer patients and controls in the following respects:

(i) verbal intelligence (Raven's Mill Hill Test)

(ii) hostility and direction of hostility as measured by the *H.D.H.Q.* (Caine and Foulds, 1967)

(iii) extraversion (*E*) and neuroticism (*N*) scores on the *E.P.I.* (Eysenck and Eysenck, 1964). These are personality dimensions as outlined in the Manual of the E.P.I. (op. cit.); briefly, the term extraversion describes the behaviour of a person who is sociable, outgoing, merry and craving excitement, whereas neuroticism is akin to emotional instability.

Table 1 Eysenck Personality Inventory Mean Scores (from Greer and Morris, 1975)

	Patient Group (Cancer n = 65) (Control n = 90)	*Mean Scores and S.D.*	*t-value*	*Significance*
'E' Score	Cancer	10.68 ± 3.98		
(Extraversion)	Control	11.48 ± 3.60	−1.31	N.S.
'N' Score	Cancer	11.29 ± 5.48		
(Neuroticism)	Control	10.74 ± 4.82	0.66	N.S.
'L' Score	Cancer	4.42 ± 2.04		
(Lie)	Control	4.43 ± 1.85	−0.06	N.S.

2. Social adjustment

Measurements of social adjustment were based on rating scales devised for this purpose, the criteria for each point on the scales being clearly specified. Women in the cancer and control groups were found to be similar in terms of their scores on the rating scales for marital, other interpersonal and sexual relations, as well as for work satisfaction and leisure activities.

3. Reaction to stress

Just over one third of patients habitually reacted to life stresses, as defined below, by denying these whenever possible but the remaining patients appeared to be able to face up to stress realistically. The use of denial as a means of coping with stress was not related to diagnosis since this occurred in similar proportions of cancer patients (38%) and controls (32%). Denial was, however, significantly correlated with delay in seeking treatment after the breast lump first appeared. This result, together with other factors which are related to such delay, has been reported separately (Greer, 1974).

Stress was recorded where any event occurred or situation existed – irrespective of its nature – which the patient reported as having caused her severe and prolonged emotional distress. Consequently, the present results are based on the patients' reported experiences, corroborated by the husband or a close relative, and not on any arbitrary judgement by us as to what kinds of events are stressful. Stress was then classified according to its nature (e.g. loss of a loved person, interpersonal conflict) and when it had occurred.

Cancer patients and controls reported similar amounts and types of stress within the previous five years, and, indeed, during their whole lives. In the case of the loss of a major emotional relationship, we found that 18% of cancer patients and 16% of controls had experienced such a loss in the previous five years.

4. Release of emotions

Patients were assessed according to the degree to which they suppressed or expressed (i) anger and (ii) other feelings. *Extreme supressors* were so named if they had never, or not more than twice during their adult lives, openly shown anger, and had always or nearly always concealed or "bottled up" their other feelings. *Extreme expressors*, on the other hand, were those individuals who had a history of frequent temper outbursts, and never or very rarely concealed other feelings. Where a patient's emotional release fell between these extremes, it was termed *apparently normal.* Highly significant differences were found between the cancer patients and controls both in the expression of anger (Table 2) as well as of other feelings (Table 3).

Extreme suppression of anger and of other feelings occurred in a significantly higher proportion of cancer patients than controls. Extreme expressors of anger, though in much smaller numbers, were also found significantly more often among the cancer patients than among controls. Our clinical ratings of release of emotions were discovered to be significantly related to measures on the psychological tests mention earlier. Thus anger was correlated with Acting out Hostility scores on the

Table 2 Release of Emotions: Anger (from Greer and Morris, 1975)

	Cancer Patients	*Control Patients*	*Significance*
Extreme Suppressors	33 (47.8)	14 (15.4%)	$p < 0.0001$
Apparently Normal	20 (29%)	66 (72.5%)	$p < 0.0001$
Extreme Expressors	14 (20.3%)	9 (9.9%)	$p < 0.02$
Uncertain	2 (2.9%)	2 (2.2%)	—
Total	69 (100%)	91 (100%)	

Table 3 Release of Emotions: Feelings Other than Anger (from Greer and Morris, 1975)

	Cancer Patients	*Control Patients*	*Significance*
Extreme Suppressors	36 (52.2%)	27 (29.7%)	p <0.0002
Apparently Normal	20 (29%)	54 (59.3%)	p <0.0001
Extreme Expressors	12 (17.4%)	10 (11%)	N.S.
Uncertain	1 (1.4%)	0 —	—

H.D.H.Q. ($r = 0.412$, $p < 0.001$) and also with extraversion scores on the E.P.I. ($r = 0.142$, $p < 0.04$). Expression of feelings other than anger was correlated with extraversion scores ($r = 0.211$, $p < 0.005$).

In other words, individuals rated as extreme suppressors of anger had low Acting-Out Hostility scores, whereas extreme expressors had high scores. High extraversion scores were associated with extreme expression of anger and of other feelings. These results are in the expected direction and provide some indirect support for the validity of the clinical assessments.

Age *per se* was found to be correlated not only with diagnosis but also with suppression of anger and of other feelings. Consequently, it was necessary to compare release of emotions among cancer patients and controls in different age groups, viz: under 40, 40–49, 50 and over. Since this procedure reduces the numbers in each category, extreme suppression and extreme expression was combined in a single category termed *abnormal* release of anger or other feelings.

The correlation, described above, between abnormal release of anger and the diagnosis of cancer, holds good in each age group, although in patients over 50 it just fails to reach statistical significance (Table 4). In the

Table 4 Abnormal Release of Anger by Diagnosis in Separate Age groups (from Greer and Morris, 1975)

Age Group	*Cancer Patients*	*Control Patients*	*Significance*
Under 40	60% (3/5)	16% (4/25)	p <0.0001
40–49	72% (13/18)	22% (10/46)	p <0.0001
50+	67% (31/46)	45% (9/20)	p <0.06>0.05

Table 5 Abnormal Release of Other Feelings by Diagnosis in Separate Age Groups (from Greer and Morris, 1975)

Age Group	*Cancer Patients*	*Control Patients*	*Significance*
Under 40	40% (2/5)	44% (11/25)	N.S.
40–49	82% (23/28)	43% (20/46)	p <0.001
50+	72% (33/46)	30% (6/20)	p <0.002

case of release of other feelings, there were only minimal differences between cancer patients and controls aged under 40; but in patients over 40, the cancer patients were, as before, significantly more likely than controls to show abnormal release of feelings other than anger (Table 5).

CONCLUSIONS

"Anger is one of the sinews of the soul;
He that lacks it hath a maimed mind."

Thomas Fuller 1608–61.

We were unable to confirm earlier reports, based upon uncontrolled or inadequately controlled studies, of associations between cancer and such variables as previous stress – particularly loss of a loved person – habitual use of denial in the face of stress, and depression. Nor were we able to confirm previous findings of a correlation between breast cancer and extraversion, possibly for the reasons tutlined earlier.

The discovery that approximately one-third of women in both the experimental and control groups had suffered from depressive illnesses within 5 years preceding the appearance of the breast lump is, perhaps, surprising. But no interpretation of this result can be made in the absence of any accurate data concerning the incidence of depressive illnesses among women of similar age distribution in the general population. In this connection, it is interesting to note that Kerr *et al.* (1969) reported a significant relationship between a form of depressive illness and subsequent death from cancer in males. However, this statistical association was not confirmed in a later study which showed that the observed number of deaths from malignant disease in both sexes after depressive illness did not exceed the expected rate for the general population (Evans *et al.*, 1974).

The main positive finding of this investigation is a statistically significant association between the diagnosis of breast cancer and abnormal release of emotions. This abnormality, in the majority of cases, was extreme suppression of anger and of other feelings, but extreme expression of these emotions – though less common – also occurred in a higher proportion of cancer patients than controls. The results applied to patients in all age groups except for cancer patients and controls under 40 years who differed significantly only in terms of release of anger but were similar with respect to release of feelings other than anger. The present findings held good when the assessments of type of emotional release by each of the three interviewers were analysed separately, suggesting a reasonable degree of reliability of these assessments in this study.

We cannot prove conclusively that this behaviour pattern in the patients is an antecedent, rather than a concomitant, of breast cancer.

Nevertheless, we were able to establish by careful questioning of patients and their close relatives that the pattern had persisted at least throughout adult life, and often since childhood. Consequently, it seems probable that these patterns antedated the onset of cancer.

It must be admitted that women with benign breast disease do not provide an ideal control group in every respect, since they differ in age and also because a small proportion of benign breast conditions may be precancerous. Pathologists are agreed, however, that the vast majority of benign breast tumours do not proceed to malignancy (Sandison, 1974).

In designing this controlled study, we were then faced with the choice of either age-matching or conducting our psychological investigations preoperatively without prior knowledge of the diagnosis. It was considered more important to ensure that we remained "blind" with regard to diagnosis when making psychological assessments of patients. In the present study, we have therefore obviated major sources of bias in the following respects: (i) neither the patient nor the investigators knew the diagnosis at the time of examination and interview; (ii) all patients were examined under identical conditions in hospital on the day before operation when they were facing the stress of uncertainty about their diagnosis and possible mastectomy; (iii) the date obtained from structured clinical interviews with patients were corroborated by interviews with husbands or close relatives.

This study is based on the hypothesis that impairment of homeostatic regulation of cell growth and function plays a part in the development and course of breast cancer, and that psycho-social variables may be among the factors which contribute, possibly via neuro-endocrine and immunological mechanisms, to such disorganization of homeostatic controls. In order to examine the roles and interaction of psycho-social, hormonal and immunological variables in women with breast cancer, a multidisciplinary study has been set up (Greer, 1971) to carry out concurrent measurements of these variables before operation and postoperatively. The results of the pre-operative psychological enquiry have been reviewed here. Correlations with the physiological measures will be reported as they become available.

SUMMARY

Psychological investigation of a consecutive series of 160 women admitted to hospital for breast tumour biopsy was carried out by means of detailed structured interviews and standard tests. Interviews and testing were conducted on the day before operation, without knowledge of the provisional diagnosis. Information obtained from patients was verified in almost all cases by separate interviews with husbands or close relatives. Present results are based on statistical comparisons between 69 patients found at operation to have breast cancer and a control group comprising the remaining 91 patients with benign breast disease.

The principal finding was a significant association between the diagnosis of breast cancer and a behaviour pattern, persisting throughout adult life, of abnormal release of emotion. This abnormality was, in most cases, extreme suppression of anger and, in patients over 40, extreme suppression of other feelings. Extreme expression of emotions, though much less common, also occurred in a higher proportion of cancer patients than controls. Previous reports of correlations between breast cancer on the one hand, and extraversion, previous emotional stress and depressive states on the other, were not confirmed.

Acknowledgements

The work reviewed here is part of an interdisciplinary study being conducted in the Faith Courtauld Unit for Human Studies in Cancer at King's College Hospital Medical School, London. I am grateful to the patients for their willing cooperation, to all my colleagues on the Unit for their help, and especially to Tina Morris who collaborated with me in this study. My thanks are due to the editor of the *Journal of Psychosomatic Research* and to its publishers, Pergamon Press, for permission to reproduce parts of the data and text previously published in that Journal.

REFERENCES

Caine, T. M. and Foulds, G. A. (1967): Personality Questionnaire (H.D.H.Q.). University of London Press, London.

Coppen, A. and Metcalfe, M., (1963): Cancer and extraversion. *Br. Med. J.*, **2**, 18.

Evans, N. J. R., Baldwin, J. A. and Gath, D. (1974): The incidence of cancer among in-patients with affective disorders. *Brit. J. Psychiat.*, **124**, 518–25.

Eysenck, H. J. and Eysenck, S. B. G., (1964): Manual of the Eysenck Personality Inventory. University of London Press, London.

Greer, H. S. (1971): Women with breast cancer: a psychosomatic approach. In Cancer Priorities, edited by G. Bennette. The British Cancer Council, London.

Greer, H. S. (1974): Delay in the treatment of breast cancer. *Proc. R. Soc. Med.*, **67**, 470.

Greer, H. S. and Morris, T. (1975): Psychological attributes of women who develop breast cancer: A controlled study. *J. Psychosom. Res.*, **19**, 147.

Guy, R. (1759): An essay on scirrhus tumours and cancers. Churchill, London. Cited in Goldfarb, C., Driesen, J. and Cole, D. (1967). Psychophysiologic aspects of malignancy. *Am. J. Psychiat.*, **123**, 1545.

Hamilton, M. (1967): Development of rating scale for primary depressive illness. *Br. J. Soc. Clin. Psychol.*, **6**, 278.

Kerr, T. A., Schapira, K. and Roth, M. (1969): The relationship between premature death and affective disorders. *Brit. J. Psychiat.*, **115**, 1277–82.

Kissen, D. M., (1963): Personality characteristics in males conducive to lung cancer. *Br. J. Med. Psychol.*, **36**, 27.

Kissen, D. M. (1964): The influence of some environmental factors on personality inventory scores in psychosomatic research. *J. Psychosom. Res.*, **8**, 145.

Kissen, D. M., Brown, R. I. F. and Kissen, M. A. (1969): A further report on personality and psychosocial factors in lung cancer. *Ann. N.Y. Acad. Sci.*, **164**, 535.

Le Shan, L. L. and Worthington, R. E. (1956): Personality as a factor in the pathogenesis of cancer: a review of the literature. *Br. J. Med. Psychol.*, **29**, 49.

Le Shan, L. L. (1959): Psychological states as factors in the development of malignant disease: a critical review. *J. Natn. Cancer Inst.*, **22**, 1.

Muslin, H. L., Gyarfas, K. and Pieper, W. J. (1966): Separation experience and cancer of the breast. *Ann. N.Y. Acad. Sci.*, **125**, 802.

Paget, J. (1870). Surgical Pathology. 2nd edition, p. 800. Longmans Green, London.

Raven, J. C. (1958): The Mill Hill Vocabulary Scale. H. K. Lewis, London.

Sandison, A. T. (1974): Limited surgical treatment of carcinoma of the breast: Pathological aspects. *Proc. Roy. Soc. Med.*, **67**, 469–70.

Snow, H. L. (1893): Cancer and the cancer process. (1893). p. 33. Churchill, London. Cited in Goldfarb, C., Driesen, J. and Cole, D. (1967). Psychophysiologic aspects of malignancy. *Am. J. Psychiat.*, **123**, 1545.

Section 2
PROGNOSTIC FACTORS

6

Prognostic Significance of Histopathology

Edwin R. Fisher, Remigio Gregorio and Bernard Fisher

During the past 3 years we have been concerned with the systematic study of 32 histopathologic features in 1000 cases of invasive breast cancer. We have examined their interrelationships, and also their relationship to certain clinical parameters, including stage (clinical status of the axilla), race and age of patient, duration of symptoms, and breast and quadrant involved by the primary tumor. The material utilized was derived from patients with invasive mammary cancer entered in the National Surgical Adjuvant Breast Project, protocol 4 of the National Cancer Institute, Bethesda. Maryland, U.S.A.

These women were prospectively randomized so that those with clinically negative axillae were treated by either radical mastectomy, total (simple) mastectomy and irradiation, or total mastectomy only. Those with clinically positive axillae were also randomized and subjected to either radical mastectomy, or total mastectomy and irradiation. The relatively short duration of this prospective study has allowed us to correlate these histopathologic and clinical discriminants only with early tumor recurrence (6, 12, 18 and 24 months). The significance of these interrelationships was computed by means of contingency table analysis using the Statistical Package of the Social Sciences computer programs. Associations with a p value of 0.05 or less were regarded as significant.

In this presentation we shall be principally concerned with the possible prognostic significance of histopathologic discriminants such as histologic tumor type, histologic and nuclear grade. Also with those responses which may in some manner reflect host resistance or immunologic responsiveness to tumor growth, such as cell reaction, regional lymph nodal sinus histiocytosis and nodal involvement by metastasis. In addition, the significance of tumor size will also be evaluated since it has been found in our study to be consistently related to early tumor recurrence.

This presentation will include a brief description of the various pathologic features, a historical review of prior pertinent studies, and the results obtained in our continuing study, which are limited so far to early tumor recurrence. The detailed results of the comprehensive study of all of the pathologic material in the National Surgical Adjuvant Breast Project study will appear in another communication (Fisher, Gregorio and Fisher, 1975).

HISTOLOGIC TYPES

The prognostic significance of morphologic or histologic typing of breast cancer has been suggested by a number of investigators. A variety of classifications has resulted from attempts to classify breast cancer on the basis of its histopathologic features. Most use either descriptive terminology for the various patterns of tumor growth, or a numerical grade representing an index of malignancy. In some instances the classifications appear to reflect both characteristics. We have found that a simple listing of histopathologic types based principally on growth pattern and/or special histopathologic features is both practical, inclusive and reproducible.

No special significance has been given to oxyphilic or apocrine change or squamous metaplasia in our system except to note their presence. Indeed, such changes may occur in tumors exhibiting a variety of different growth patterns. Those recognizing an "apocrine" form of mammary cancer note its clinical behavior to be comparable to that encountered with mammary carcinoma in general (Lee, Pack and Scharnagel, 1933; Higginson and McDonald, 1949; McDivitt, Stewart and Berg, 1968). A similar judgement may be made regarding squamous metaplasia, a change which may occur in a wide variety of malignant neoplasms. On the other hand, squamous cell carcinoma would be regarded as a distinct entity in our scheme, although its occurrence in a pure form in the breast may be regarded with some skepticism.

The incidence of the various histopathologic types of carcinomas encountered in our study are presented in Table 1. It is imperative to recognize that the various designations are based upon the invasive component of the neoplasm.

Infiltrating duct carcinoma, not otherwise specified (NOS)

This is the most common histologic type of mammary carcinoma and appears as solid cords or groups of tumor cells varying in size and stromal content. These tumors are devoid of the special features characteristic of the other types encountered. Because of this, the designation NOS (not otherwise specified) is utilized.

The combination of NOS with other tumor types was not infrequent. It is interesting to compare the correlations of the pure NOS type with those of the combination forms. Notable differences between them are the more frequent occurrence of lymphatic invasion, clinically positive axilla, more malignant histologic grade and occurrence of non-invasive multi-centric

Table 1 Incidence of Histologic Types of Breast Cancer (1000 cases)

		%
Pure Tumor Groups		
Infiltrating duct NOS (not otherwise specified)	526	52.6
Medullary	62	6.2
Lobular invasive	49	4.9
Mucinous	24	2.4
Tubular	12	1.2
Adenocystic	4	0.4
Papillary	3	0.3
Carcinosarcoma	1	0.1
Paget's Disease	23	2.3
With intraductal carcinoma	2	0.2
Infiltrating duct NOS	16	1.6
Infiltrating duct NOS + tubular	4	0.4
Infiltrating duct NOS + mucinous	1	0.1
Combinations with infiltrating Duct NOS	280	28.0
Infiltrating duct NOS		
+ Tubular	165	16.5
+ Lobular invasive	33	3.3
+ Mucinous	16	1.6
+ Lobular invasive + tubular	16	1.6
+ Papillary	12	1.2
+ Adenocystic	10	1.0
+ Tubular + adenocystic	8	0.8
+ Tubular + papillary	8	0.8
+ Mucinous + papillary	4	0.4
+ Adenocystic + mucinous	2	0.2
+ Lobular invasive + adenocystic	1	0.1
+ Lobular invasive + mucinous	1	0.1
+ Lobular invasive + papillary	1	0.1
+ Tabular + mucinous	1	0.1
+ Adenocystic + papillary	1	0.1
+ Lobular invasive + tubular + adenocystic + mucinous	1	0.1
Other Combinations of Tumor Types Exclusive of NOS	16	1.6
Tubular + papillary	5	0.5
Lobular invasive + tubular	4	0.4
Tubular + mucinous	2	0.2
Lobular invasive + mucinous	1	0.1
Tubular + adenocystic	1	0.1
Adenocystic + mucinous	1	0.1
Mucinous + papillary	1	0.1
Lobular invasive + tubular + adenocystic + papillary	1	0.1
	1,000	100.0

cancer in the case of the pure type. On the other hand, NOS combination tumors exhibited a greater correlation with factors other than those which are usually related to the degree of malignancy.

This information raises the question as to whether it is appropriate to judge breast tumors with varied histologic structure according to their most malignant appearing elements. However, in support of such a practice was the similarity of the early tumor recurrence rates for the two groups. The results of longer follow-up studies should help to resolve this problem.

Medullary carcinoma

The significance of this tumor type was first clearly indicated by Moore and Foote in 1949 although earlier reference to this form of mammary cancer was made by Geschickter (1945). Such tumors are often large but generally circumscribed. Histologically, they appear to comprise anastamosing cords and masses of large cells with vesicular, often pleomorphic nuclei containing prominent nucleoli. Mitotic forms are frequent. Their fibrous stoma is scanty but a lymphoid infiltrate is striking. Despite the ominous cytological features of such tumors, their prognosis is said to be better than that observed with tumours of the more usual NOS appearance, at least after radical mastectomy (Moore and Foote, 1949; Richardson, 1956; Bloom, Richardson and Field, 1970; Hutter, 1971).

In our study, in accordance with conventional criteria, only those highly cellular non-papillary tumors that were histologically circumscribed, contained a moderate or marked lymphoid stroma with a scant fibrous component and whose nuclei were regarded as either grade 1 or 2, were regarded as medullary carcinomas. During the review it became apparent that some highly cellular tumors exhibited the general appearance of medullary carcinoma, but were either devoid of lymphoid stroma or exhibited a stellate or infiltrating border; in essence they were lacking one or the other of two important diagnostic features of the classical medullary cancer. This provoked the dilemma, whether to designate such aberrant forms as medullary carcinomas or infiltrating duct carcinomas, NOS type.

By strict definition they qualified as belonging to the latter group. However, it was observed that the atypical medullary tumors possess certain clinical and pathologic correlations, sufficiently different from those encountered in the more classical form, to warrant their distinction. Atypical medullary carcinoma had a significantly greater likelihood of clinically positive nodes, 4 or more nodes being pathologically positive for metastases, and lymphatic invasion being present.

A comparison of atypical medullary tumors with NOS duct carcinoma revealed the former to have a greater likelihood of clinically positive nodes, a severe cell reaction, gross and microscopic circumscription, and nuclear and histologic grades of I and III respectively. There was no difference between atypical medullary cancer and its classical form or NOS tumors in regard to early tumor recurrence up to a period of 24 months.

The data collected thus far suggests that the atypical medullary tumors may be pathologically distinct from the classical form. Whether they are more appropriately regarded as a form of NOS tumor or a separate entity is not certain at this time. However, our observations suggest that careful histological analysis of the medullary group of tumors is essential to any consideration of its prognosis.

Lobular invasive carcinoma

In 1941, Foote and Stewart, as well as Muir (1941) called attention to an in situ form of carcinoma of the breast apparently arising within the end parts of the lobule, which they designated as lobular carcinoma in situ. Subsequent to their reports and those of others, it became recognized that in situ carcinoma may develop into, or at least be associated with, an infiltrating form – so-called lobular infiltrating or lobular invasive carcinoma. The frequency of such a development from in situ carcinoma is unknown (Godwin, 1952; Miller and Kay, 1956; Benfield, Jacobson and Warner, 1965; Newman, 1966; McDivitt *et al.*, 1967).

Despite its apparent derivation and the association of lobular invasive cancer with its in situ analogue, retrospective studies have disclosed that this type of carcinoma is associated with a relatively poor prognosis (Ashikari *et al.*, 1973). There are several excellent accounts of the histopathologic features of lobular invasive carcinoma (Godwin, 1952; Miller and Kay, 1956; Newman, 1966; McDivitt *et al.*, 1967; Ackerman, 1968), and its appearance is usually sufficiently distinctive to allow for its recognition. We suspect that most, if not all, scirrhous carcinomas of the older terminology represent examples of this type of invasive carcinoma. As noted in Table 1, examples of the lobular invasive type of cancer are relatively frequently combined with other types of invasive carcinoma.

It is of interest that despite the purported bad prognosis of this tumor type, evidence of lymphatic invasion was notably absent in our study. However, the combination of lobular invasive cancer with the tubular type was associated with lymphatic invasion within the tumor, a feature not present in either type in their pure forms.

Mucinous carcinoma

Mucinous carcinoma, also designated as mucoid, gelatinous or colloid carcinoma, represents a distinct histopathological type of mammary cancer. It may occur in pure form or in association with other types, a feature noted by other investigators as well as in our study (Norris and Taylor,

1965; Silverberg *et al.*, 1971). Pure mucinous carcinomas have been observed to occur in older women with a relatively long duration of symptoms (Silverberg *et al.*, 1971), and they are also associated with a lesser tendency to axillary metastases and a pushing rather than an infiltrating border. The survival rate has been noted to be appreciably greater in patients with the pure type than in those with the mixed type or other infiltrating duct carcinomas of the breast (Geschickter, 1938; Melamed, Robbins and Foote, 1961; Norris and Taylor, 1965; Silverberg *et al.*, 1971).

Many of these features as well as the differences between pure and mixed varieties were confirmed in our study. In addition, we have noted that there is a greater likelihood that such tumors are devoid of a cell reaction. Necrosis and lymphatic invasion within the tumor are also usually absent. The mucinous tumors comprise aggregates of cells, usually with well differentiated features and high nuclear grade, lying in pools of mucin.

Tubular carcinoma

Tubular carcinoma of the breast, also known as well differentiated (Taylor and Norris, 1970) or orderly carcinoma (McDivitt, Stewart and Berg, 1968), has only recently received attention. Prognosis in this form of carcinoma is regarded as excellent, as emphasized by the studies of Taylor and Norris (1970) and Carstens and associates (1972), even though axillary metastases may be present.

Histologically, this form of cancer may superficially mimic benign sclerosing or blunt duct adenosis. It is comprised of tubular structures which are typically lined by a single layer of well differentiated epithelium. The surrounding stroma is abundant and may exhibit the green fluorescence of amyloid after Congo red staining (Carstens *et al.*, 1972). Illustrations in all reports also include tubular elements arranged in multiglandular, cribriform or adenocystic configurations. We have chosen to regard the presence of these latter foci as evidence of an adenocystic component and have reserved the designation tubular for those tumors exhibiting only the more simple structure.

That tubular elements may be found in association with other histopathologic types of cancer is apparent from Table 1. Indeed, the association of tubular and NOS carcinoma represented the second most frequent form of mammary carcinomas in our series. Carstens and associates (1972) noted such combinations in 80% of the 35 cases of tubular carcinoma they studied. According to them, the other element apparently had no effect on the favorable prognosis of tubular carcinoma.

It is of interest that we found this type of carcinoma more likely to be associated with perineural extension although this is usually found in association with features which suggest the likelihood of poor prognosis.

The low degree of pathologic malignancy as reflected by histopathologic grade, and the presence of mucin and calcifications within these tumors, have been observed previously by others (Taylor and Norris, 1970).

Adenocystic carcinoma

This is a rare form of mammary carcinoma, and less than 100 cases have been recorded. Most accounts emphasize its favorable prognosis, which may be related to the rarity of axillary node involvement associated with it (Groshong, 1966; Galloway, Woolner and Clagett, 1966; Hayes and Brooks, 1967; Ackerman, 1968; Schulenberg and Pepler, 1969; Friedman and Oberman, 1970; Camoun, Contesso and Rouesse, 1972; Carstens *et al.*, 1972). Although distant metastases are likewise said to be rare, Elsner (1970) indicates that the reported follow-up observations on patients with this form of cancer have been for the most part relatively short. He and others have recorded instances in which metastases have developed after long periods of time (Nayer, 1957; O'Kell, 1968; Wilson and Spell, 1967). Axillary metastases were observed in the case recorded by Verani and van der Bel-Kahn (1973).

Some investigators have emphasized the necessity of differentiating the adenocystic form of mammary carcinoma from the less differentiated types of infiltrating carcinoma with a cribriform pattern (Galloway, Woolner and Clagett, 1966; Cavanzo and Taylor, 1969; Friedman and Oberman, 1970). We have concluded from our observations that there is insufficient evidence to warrant such a distinction. Such proponents of histologic grading as Bloom (1956) and Tough *et al.* (1969) depict adenocystic formation as an example of one type of tubule formation in mammary cancers indicating advanced differentiation. The adenocystic pattern is more common than appreciated, and the intraductal component of tumours of the NOS variety may often be truly adenocystic. This association has been commented upon even by some of the investigators who believe the distinction between adenocystic and cribriform infiltrating ductal carcinomas is valid (Cavanzo and Taylor, 1969).

Papillary carcinoma

Although intraductal papillary growth is not an uncommon component of various histologic types of invasive mammary carcinoma, the truly papillary, invasive carcinoma is a rare neoplasm. Some authors refer to its possible derivation and distinction from benign intraductal papilloma (Hart, 1927; Hueper, 1932; Kraus and Neubecker, 1962; Dockerty, 1964). We are unaware of any large scale study of this type of mammary carcinoma and there have been too few examples of its pure form in our series to permit comments on its correlates. Although some have indicated a relatively favorable prognosis (Haagensen, 1956; Dockerty, 1964; McDivitt, Stewart and Berg, 1968; Tomcic, Vukcevic and Vidovic, 1972), the follow-up observations of Kraus and Neubecker (1962) on 21 patients with papillary cancer indicate a disease free survival rate comparable to that of mammary cancer in general.

Paget's disease

There were 23 mammary cancers, accompanied by neoplastic involvement of the epidermis of the nipple, warranting their designation as Paget's disease of the breast. This represents an incidence of 2.4% of the 967 cases in which the nipple was available for examination. Although there has been controversy concerning the derivation of these cells, most investigators subscribe to the view that they represent extensions of neoplastic elements from subjacent ducts in the nipple (Inglis, 1946) and/or metastases from an underlying carcinoma (Simard, 1930; Cheatle and Cutler, 1931; Muir, 1939; Haagensen, 1956). All of the examples of Paget's disease in our study were associated with a clinically evident dominant mass in the underlying breast. The view is often expressed that this is usually of the intraductal type. However, in our study, 16 of the cancers were NOS, 4 were NOS and tubular, and 1 NOS and mucinous, and only 2 were regarded as exclusively intraductal.

It has long been recognized since the original description by Paget (1874) that there is a tendency for the duration of symptoms to be prolonged in patients with Paget's disease. There is also a greater frequency of multicentric cancer. As might be expected, most of the tumours are in the subareolar area of the breast and exhibit other evidence of skin and nipple movement. Although lymphatic invasion is frequent in the mammary tumor, axillary nodal involvement clinically or pathologically does not appear to be especially associated with this type of mammary lesion.

It should be noted that despite the prognostic significance which has been suggested in the literature for various histologic patterns of tumor growth, our study showed no significant statistical association between histologic tumor type and the likelihood of early tumor recurrence.

HISTOLOGIC GRADING

Von Hansemann in 1893 is usually credited with calling attention to a possible relationship between the behavior of malignant neoplasms and their degree of "anaplasia" (Haagensen, 1933) although Tough and associates (1969) note that a similar correlation was suggested even earlier by Dennis in 1891. MacCarty and Sistrunk (1922) and White (1927) considered that it was not only the degree of differentiation of the neoplastic elements which was important in grading mammary carcinomas but also the associated lymphoid infiltration and stromal fibrosis.

Greenough (1925) upon whose method most recent investigators have based their technique of grading mammary carcinomas, divided tumors into three grades of malignancy depending upon the degree of tubule formation, size of cells and nuclei, hyperchromatism and mitoses. That survival might be related to the histologic grade of the tumor was confirmed by Scarff and Patey (1928). However, a subsequent study by Scarff and Handley (1938) led to the conclusion that staging was perhaps a more important factor in prognosis and that the best indicator of survival might be found with the use of both staging and histological grading. Greenough's method of grading was revived by Bloom (1950a and b) who then showed a close correlation between survival rate and tumor grade (Bloom, 1956).

The method employed by most investigators is based upon consideration or scoring of the degree of tubule formation and regularity of nuclei and mitoses. Wolff (1966), Dabska (1968), Tough and associates (1969) and Champion and associates (1972) subsequently confirmed the feasibility as well as prognostic significance of grading as employed by Bloom. However, Wolff (1966) has emphasized that grading combined with pathological staging was more significant than the former alone.

Tough and associates (1969) proposed the addition of tumor size to stage and grade as offering a more comprehensive guide to prognosis, but add that consideration of the tumor characteristics alone is inadequate, and fails to recognize possible host factors. This point may be illustrated by the fact that the medullary form of mammary carcinoma qualifies by most schemes of grading as a highly malignant (Grade III) lesion, yet its favorable prognosis has been repeatedly emphasized. Conversely, the lobular infiltrating form of mammary cancer often exhibits a low histologic grade yet is regarded as having a relatively poor prognosis.

Eichner and associates (1970) compared the results of histological grading as utilized by Bloom, and the assessment of nuclear grade as described by Black and associates (1955, 1956 and 1957), and found the results comparable in relation to survival rates at 5 years. This would not be totally unexpected, for as noted above, much of the Greenough–Bloom criteria of grading is based upon nuclear features.

The method of histological grading of the neoplasms in our study represented a modification of that employed by Bloom and others. Degrees of nuclear differentiation are adequately scored by the relatively simple technique of nuclear grading as employed by Black and associates. Although the latter utilized 4 grades, we have found it practical to combine their grades 0 and 1 into one grade, grade 1. Unfortunately, nuclear grading is numbered in the opposite direction to histological grading and nuclear grade 1 represents the most anaplastic nuclear appearance. Grade 2 nuclei are intermediate in appearance and those designated as grade 3 are the best differentiated forms. A scheme was devised to combine the nuclear grade with the presence or absence of tubule formation in deriving the histological grade (Table 2). As indicated in the Table, the so-called adenocystic pattern is also included as a form of tubule formation.

Table 2 Criteria for Simplified Histological Grading of Mammary Cancer

Tubular Formation	*Nuclear Grade (1–3)*	*Histologic Grade (I–III)*
Pure, or in part tubular	3	I
Pure, or in part adenocystic	3	I
Pure, or in part tubular	1,2	II
Pure, or in part adenocystic	1,2	II
Absent	3	II
Absent	1,2	III

Approximately two thirds of the mammary cancers studied were designated as histologic grade III according to the scheme utilized. Only a relatively small number (2.3%) were regarded as being well differentiated or grade I. Grade I tumors were found to be correlated with older women, absence of nodal involvement, and histologic types said to exhibit a good prognosis. The opposite applied to tumors histologically graded as III (except for the good prognosis with the medullary type), and in addition, it was noted that grade III tumors exhibited a greater frequency of lymphatic invasion.

Noteworthy was the lack of correlation between histologic grade and the likelihood of early tumor recurrence. Perhaps this inconsistency may be related to the fact that the vast majority of mammary cancers are of high or unfavorable histologic grade.

NUCLEAR GRADE

Black and associates (1955, 1956, 1957 and 1959) in several reports have emphasized a clear relationship between nuclear grade of the tumor, sinus histiocytosis of axillary lymph nodes and patient survival. Sommers (1969) found more well differentiated nuclei in intraductal carcinomas as compared to invasive cancers, and related this difference to the invasive ability of the less differentiated mammary carcinoma cells. Tomcic and associates (1972) considered nuclear grade to be useful, but not a certain guide to prognosis. They preferred histological typing, as well as evaluation of other factors including size of tumor, site, infiltrative properties, nodal metastases and other features. Kister and associates (1969) were unable to find any statistically significant relationships between nuclear grade and survival in a clinically favorable (Columbia classification) group of cases.

We have utilized a minor modification of the system of Black and associates for nuclear grading, as noted previously. Slightly less than 10% of all of the tumors in our study exhibited well differentiated nuclei (grade 3). About one-third were considered as poorly differentiated and one-half as intermediate. Most of the features found in association with grade 1 (including positive lymph nodes, blood vessel and lymphatic invasion, large tumor size and young age of the patients) have been reported previously by others as unfavorable prognostic features in mammary cancer. In this study early tumor recurrence was found in association with nuclear grade 1 only at the 24 month interval of follow-up observation.

TUMOR SIZE (MAXIMUM DIAMETER)

Tumor size might be regarded as an obvious discriminant of importance in the prognosis of mammary cancer. The efforts devoted to the "early" detection of mammary lesions certainly impart the impression of an inverse relationship between survival and tumor size. Support for such a view arises from reports indicating the almost three-quarters of patients with tumors larger than 5 cm already have nodal metastases when first examined (Johnstone, 1972). Earlier studies such as that by Eggers and associates (1941) reported a 75% 5 year survival for patients whose tumors were less than 2 cm, 24% for those with lesions measuring 3 to 6 cm, and only 16% when they measured 7 cm or more. These relationships between size of tumor, nodal metastases and prognosis have been for the most part confirmed by more recent studies (Fisher, Slack and Bross, 1969; Brightmore, Greening and Hamlin, 1970; Alderson, Hamlin and Staunton, 1971).

Yet, it is noteworthy that others (Kunath, 1940; Hoopes and McGraw, 1942) have failed to find such a correlation between tumor size and survival. Although in some instances there are apparent reasons for this (e.g. different types of treatment, different stages of disease), in others an explanation is less apparent, suggesting that other factors may affect survival, in addition to or regardless of tumor size. Appreciation of the variety of histologic types and grades of mammary cancers suggest that the doubling times or rates of growth of all mammary cancers are not similar.

Indeed, Bloom (1950) could find no correlation between prognosis and size of tumor in the groups with the lowest or highest grades of malignancy. On the other hand, there was a poorer prognosis in the case of tumors larger than 2 cm when they were of intermediate histologic grade. Hamlin (1968) failed to find a correlation between tumor size and mortality rates in her material although the majority of patients regarded as clinical stage I had small tumors.

Fisher, Slack and Bross (1969) observed poorer survival rates with large tumors when more than 3 axillary nodes exhibited metastases, compared to those with no nodes or only 1 to 3 nodes involved. However, no striking difference in survival rates was observed between patients with small or large tumors when no nodes or 1 to 3 nodes contained metastases. Their data also suggested a greater tendency to axillary metastases with large tumors.

Gold *et al.* (1972) have noted more axillary metastases in patients with large tumors (>6 cm) with an infiltrative border as delineated by mammography, than with tumors measuring less than 4.5 cm with a similar type of border. Complementary to these findings are the observations of Lane and associates (1961) who found a better prognosis in patients with larger, well delimited tumors than those of similar size but an irregular border. They also noted in patients exhibiting a long survival period that tumors with well delimited borders were one-third larger than those that were irregular.

A median size of 3.0 cm for the tumors in our study coincides with that recorded for the period 1948–68 by Cady (1972). This suggests that there has been little or no improvement in the detection of smaller tumors during the past 25 years. Important findings in our study were that tumors greater than 4.0 cm in maximum diameter were found more commonly in younger women (20–44 years), and were consistently associated with multicentric foci of cancer, blood vessel and lymphatic invasion, the presence of 4 or more axillary lymph nodes containing metastases, and a greater likelihood of tumor recurrencce at all time intervals analysed. Tumors larger than 4.0 cm were also associated with a greater likelihood of nipple and skin involvement.

As noted previously by one of us (Fisher and Slack, 1970), there was no correlation between tumor size and involvement of no nodes or 1 to 3 axillary lymph nodes. However, patients with clinically positive axillary nodes showed a greater likelihood of pathological confirmation of metastases when their primary tumors were larger than 4.0 cm. Tumors measuring between 2.1 and 4 cm more frequently exhibited a nuclear grade of 1, whereas those less than 2.1 cm in size were frequently found to be associated with a nuclear grade of 3, and absent cell reaction and a clinically and pathhologically negative axilla.

Surprisingly, no correlation was found between size and any particular tumor type although the impression has been conveyed that medullary and mucinous types are frequently of large size.

CELL REACTION

It has long been recognized that mammary as well as other cancers may have a lymphoid infiltrate at their periphery or among their cellular elements. Sistrunk and MacCarty in 1922 considered the lymphocyte content of tumors as a criterion for their system of grading. Moore and Foote (1949) described the favorable prognosis associated with medullary cancers which contain a marked lymphoid infiltrate. They suggested that this cellular reaction might represent a host response to the tumor, an interpretation offered by many early investigators for the presence of inflammatory cells in other neoplasms.

Subsequently Black and associates (1953, 1956, 1958, 1959, 1960), indicated that the lethality of breast cancer may be determined by the interaction of two groups of factors: those relating to the growth potential of the tumor as reflected by nuclear grade, and those relating to host inhibitory or resistance factors such as lymphoid infiltrate in the tumor and sinus histiocytosis in regional nodes. This conclusion was based upon the study of cases followed either to death or for a minimum of 5 years after operation. It is of interest, however, that tumors from only 11 of the patients in one study (Black, Opler and Speer, 1955) were regarded as having a lymphoid infiltrate greater than 2 plus.

Hamlin (1968), a strong proponent of the theory relating lymphoid infiltrate to host resistance, performed an exhaustive study of the cellular infiltration in 272 tumors, assessing the general pattern, quality and density of infiltrate. There was a close correlation found between this index of "host resistance" and the prognosis, and similarly between cell reaction and the tumor grade. Berg (1959, 1962, 1971) reported that a peripheral plasmacellular infiltrate in poorly differentiated (high grade) carcinomas was associated with an improved survival rate, and that this was directly proportional to the degree of such reaction.

On the other hand, Champion and associates (1972), utilizing a less sophisticated analysis of the lymphoid infiltrate than Hamlin (1962), found this reaction to be more common in tumors of high grade malignancy which exhibited a poorer prognosis. However, the cellular reaction had no influence on prognosis when considered within each grade of malignancy. This view that lymphoid infiltration does not in all instances reflect a good prognosis is similar to that expressed previously by Scarff and Torloni (1968). Sommers (1969) failed to find any difference in cell reaction between incipient intraductal carcinoma and the invasive form, in cases which were regarded as clinical stage I.

Fisher, Saffer and Fisher (1973) have recently attempted to correlate the lymphocyte transformation of regional node cells with various histologic parameters of mammary cancer. Surprisingly they noted a significant statistical relationship between lymphocyte transformation and a mild lymphoid infiltrate, and this would tend to minimize the significance of lymphoid infiltration as a measure of host resistance to tumor growth. This impression receives some support from the study of Richters and Sherwin (1971) who observed a greater degree of lymphocyte activity (including cytotoxicity on tumour cells), in explants of mammary carcinomas containing lymphoid infiltrates, when regional node cells were added.

Three-fourths of the mammary cancers in our study exhibited either slight to moderate or a severe cell reaction, the former in slightly more than half of the cases. An absent or slight to moderate cell reaction was associated in our study with an increased tendency to early tumor recurrence albeit only at the 6 month period of observation. A severe cell reaction tended to be associated with blood vessel invasion, and poor differentiation or high histologic grade (grade III). As suggested previously by us, cell reaction appears more closely related to the histologic degree of malignancy of the breast cancer rather than to an immunologic response by the host. No association with sinus histiocytosis was found.

SINUS HISTIOCYTOSIS

There is accumulating evidence in experimental systems as well as in humans which indicates that the regional lymph nodes are essential for the initiation as well as for the maintenance of tumor immunity (Fisher and Fisher, 1971; Deodhar, Crile and Esselstyn, 1972; Fisher and Fisher, 1972; Fisher, Saffer and Fisher, 1974). Lymph nodes draining experimental tumors in syngeneic systems reveal a marked response of pyroninophilic cells (immunoblasts) as early as 3 days following tumor implantation, with a maximal reaction at 7 to 14 days, at which time tumor immunity may be demonstrated (Fisher, Reidbord and Fisher, 1973). Although lymph follicle formation and sinus histiocytosis are not a conpicuous part of the morphologic expression of such immunity in the regional nodes, they are encountered to some degree in those of non-regional sites.

A variety of nodal changes may be encountered in the axillary lymph nodes of women harboring breast cancer. Lymph follicle formation has been observed in association with tumors of low nuclear grade and mild lymphoid infiltrates, and its absence noted in tumors of high nuclear grade with a marked cell reaction (Fisher, Saffer and Fisher, 1973). Regional nodes draining mammary cancers exhibit transformation of their lymphoid elements with or without stimulation by phytohemagglutinin (Fisher, Saffer and Fisher, 1972).

It is of interest that the uptake of tritiated thymidine by nodal cells is significantly greater in the lower levels of the axilla than in higher or apical regions (Fisher, Saffer and Fisher, 1974). It has been suggested that the high nodes are more closely related functionally to distant or non-regional nodes, and that those low in the axilla more dynamically reflect a response to tumor antigen. Yet, there does not appear to be any significant difference in the presence of lymph follicle formation or sinus histiocytosis between the nodes at the two levels. The observations of Berg and associates (1973) are of interest in this regard. They found the prognosis to be better when there was sinus histiocytosis and/or prominent germinal centers in the apical nodes. This was considered important in accounting for the better survival rates when apical nodes were enlarged but not replaced by cancer (in the presence of other axillary metastases) than if they were small or undetectable.

Due to the efforts of Black and associates (1953, 1955, 1956, 1958, 1959, 1960) considerable attention has been directed to the occurrence and significance of sinus histiocytosis in axillary nodes draining mammary cancers. These investigators as well as others (Wartman, 1959; Masse, Masse and Chassiagne, 1960; Anastassiades and Pryce, 1966; Hamlin, 1968) have observed a correlation between the intensity of this nodal response and survival rates. All have considered this reaction to represent a manifestation of the host immunologic reaction to tumor growth. On the other hand, several investigators (Berg, 1956; Kister *et al.*, 1969) have failed to find any correlation between sinus histiocytosis and survival rates in breast cancer.

Silverberg and associates (1970) concluded that sinus histiocytosis is a valuable prognostic indicator only when other predictive factors are inconclusive. Thus they found assessment of sinus histiocytosis to be of little prognostic value in the case of well differentiated tumors, or when nodal metastases were absent or when there were many nodes involved. On the other hand, the presence of sinus histiocytosis suggested an improved survival for those individuals whose tumors exhibited moderate or poor differentiation or in whom nodal metastases were only moderate in number. Dire and Lane (1963) found its assessment to be of value only in tumors with irregular borders. It is of interest that the cells prominent in sinus histiocytosis ultrastructurally resemble banal macrophages rather than so-called immunoblastic elements (Fisher, Reidbord and Fisher, 1973). Further, from a functional standpoint no relationship between this phenomenon and lymphocyte transformation of nodal cells has been recognized (Fisher, Saffer and Fisher, 1973).

In our study the criteria for grading sinus histiocytosis were based upon those described by Black and associates (1953, 1955, 1956, 1958) with only minor modification. Seventy-five per cent of the cases were found to exhibit either absent or slight to moderate reactions, the latter predominating. The presence of marked sinus histiocytosis was consistently associated with pathologically, but not clinically, negative axillary nodes. When sinus histiocytosis was absent there was a greater likelihood that 4 or more nodes contained metastases. There is no consistent relationship between sinus histiocytosis and necrosis and this would tend to minimize this as a causal factor in its pathogenesis. A correlation between the absence of sinus histiocytosis and early tumor recurrence was also noted, but only at the 12 month interval of follow-up observation.

Most recently Tsakraklides and associates (1974) retrospectively correlated 10 year survival in a group of 227 women with breast cancer with nodal changes other than sinus histiocytosis. They noted that lymphocyte predominance was associated with a high survival rate, whereas an appearance of lymphocyte depletion was common in cases with poor survival. Predominance of germinal centers or an unstimulated pattern was found in those with intermediate prognosis. They speculated that the favorable prognosis in the presence of lymphocyte predominance might be related to augmented T cell activity in these nodes, because they exhibited an abundance of lymphoid elements in thymus dependent areas. On the other hand, a poor prognosis, as was encountered, might be expected when such elements were depleted.

The cells involved in germinal center predominance might represent B cells which are associated with blocking antibody, and these might either augment or inhibit tumor growth, according to whether there was production of cytotoxic or lymphocyte dependent antibody respectively. This scheme of nodal evaluation appears more directly related to recognized immunologic function than does the degree of sinus histiocytosis. Its true value in this regard awaits confirmation.

NODAL STATUS

Although relatively little is known concerning the route of vascular dissemination of mammary cancer, it is widely accepted that the main route of lymphatic spread is by way of the axilla. The significance of the latter as a prognostic discriminant has been repeatedly emphasized, and the presence or absence of palpable lymph nodes within the ipsilateral axilla represents one of the most important criteria for clinical staging. Bloom (1950) as well as Wolff (1966) have indicated that although histologic grading of mammary cancer and clinical staging are comparable from the prognostic standpoint, a more accurate prediction in this regard may be obtained when both are considered. The former also indicated that recognition of the histologic grade might help account for the unexpectedly long survival period exhibited by some patients. This could be associated with an unfavorable clinical stage but a well differentiated tumor.

There are others who have failed to find any correlation between axillary nodal status and the histologic features of the neoplasm (Champion, Wallace and Prescott, 1972). Cutler and associates (1967, 1970) have emphasized the importance of tumor size and skin fixation in the clinical assessment of prognostic factors, features which appear to be adequately noted in the staging systems now employed. Cutler and Myers (1967) also noted a better prognosis for individuals whose nodes were clinically regarded as positive but proven to be negative after pathologic examination, particularly if the contralateral axillary nodes were also palpable. Uninvolved but large nodes were regarded as a host response to the tumor.

On the other hand, Champion and associates (1972) found that a bad prognosis was present in all patients with pathologically proven nodal metastases regardless of their previous clinical assessment. They regarded the relatively poor prognosis of the whole group of patients with clinically palpable nodes as due to the high incidence of metastases in such enlarged nodes. In this regard Cutler and Myers (1967) noted pathologically negative nodes in 35% of the instances in which the axillae were regarded clinically to be positive. False negative evaluation of the axilla was found in 38% of cases. More disagreement between the pathological and clinical evaluation was observed with large primary tumors and clinically negative axillae, than when the nodal status was clinically regarded as positive and the tumours were small.

In our study the incidence of false positive and negative evaluations of the axilla were 24% and 39% respectively and the overall error in clinical staging was 32%. In spite of such findings, reports in the literature show little differences in 5 year survival rate between patients with pathologically negative nodes and those in whom clinical estimation of such involvement was also negative. This same relationship also obtains between patients with positive clinical and pathological assessment of the nodal status. This information confirms the prognostic value of clinical staging in breast cancer.

In our study the presence of clinically positive axillary nodes was associated with a greater likelihood that the tumor was of the NOS histologic type, measured 2.1–4.0 cm in greatest diameter, exhibited lymphatic invasion and had a nuclear grade of 1. There was a likelihood that the axillary lymph nodes exhibited either marked or absent sinus histiocytosis and were pathologically positive for metastases. Further, this parameter was associated with a likelihood of early tumor recurrence at all intervals studied (6, 12, 18 and 24 months).

On the other hand, in those instances where the axillary nodes were considered to be clinically negative there was a greater frequency of NOS + tubular, pure tubular and lobular invasive types of cancer with better differentiated nuclei (grades 2 and 3). The tumors were likely to be smaller, measuring up to 2.0 cm, and lymphatic invasion absent. The nodes were likely to exhibit slight or moderate degrees of sinus histiocytosis and to be free of metastases.

The pathologic status of the lymph nodes was classified according to whether no nodes were positive, 1 to 3 were positive or 4 or more contained metastases. The correlations noted in the presence of 4 or more pathologically positive nodes are similar to those noted with a clinically positive axilla. In addition such nodal involvement was likely to be associated with blood vessel invasion and perineural extension. The tumors were likely to be larger than those found with the clinically positive nodes, measuring 4.1 cm or more and exhibiting a histologic grade of III. Sinus histiocytosis was likely to be absent, unlike the biphasic pattern noted in clinically positive axillary nodes.

The direct relationship between pathologic nodal status and histologic grade of the primary tumor is similar to that noted by Haagensen (1956) and indicates that nodal status may be predicted, at least to some extent, from the histologic grade of the tumor. On the other hand, the histologic type of the tumor could not be related to the presence or absence of nodal metastases.

LYMPHATIC INVASION

Although it has long been recognized that mammary cancer has a predilection for lymph nodal metastases, little attention has been directed to the phenomenon of lymphatic invasion within the tumor. This oversight might be related to the uncertainty in the identification of emboli in such structures. In our study, lymphatic invasion was more likely to be associated with non-circumscribed, large tumors (4.1 cm or more) of high histologic grade and of the NOS type, with blood vessel and perineural space invasion, and nipple involvement. This strongly implicates lymphatic invasion as an unfavorable pathologic finding in mammary cancer, a conclusion which is confirmed by noting its association with early tumor recurrence at 6 and 18 months.

BLOOD VESSEL INVASION

There have been relatively few reports concerning the incidence and possible significance of blood vessel invasion in mammary carcinoma, but a few investigations report the incidence to vary from 21 to 46% (Friedell, Betts and Sommers, 1965; Kister *et al.*, 1966; Bell, Friedell and Goldenberg, 1969; Ruiz *et al.*, 1973). Such vascular involvement has been claimed to affect survival rates adversely. In at least one of the studies, blood vessel invasion was prognostically significant only in the presence of nodal metastases, whereas in others significance was encountered only in the absence of such metastases.

It is our impression that the incidence of blood vessel invasion cited above is inordinately high. This is in large part due to the difficulty of distinguishing intravascular extension from intraductal involvement by neoplasm in the breast. Elastic tissue stains for the assessment of blood vessel invasion are advisable in the case of tumors in other organs but may be misleading in mammary cancer since the larger ductal structures of this organ also contain a relatively marked mantle of elastic fibers.

Forty-seven tumors revealed evidence of blood vessel invasion in our study representing an incidence of 4.7%. Blood vessel invasion was more likely to be associated with a severe cell reaction in the tumour, lymphatic invasion, metastases in 4 or more axillary nodes, tumors with marked necrosis, nuclear grades of 1, but surprisingly, not with evidence of early tumor recurrence.

PERINEURAL SPACE INVASION

Although extension of mammary carcinoma into perineural spaces is well recognized, little information is available concerning its significance or association with other pathologic features. In some organs such as salivary glands, demonstration of perineural extension is often useful in establishing the malignancy of such well differentiated carcinomas as the cylindromatous or adenocystic type. In other sites such as the prostate, this feature may have some diagnostic value, although its significance in this regard, as well as its relationship to prognosis, is not as meaningful as was once considered (Byar and Mostofi, 1972).

In our study, perineural space involvement was present in 104 of 378 cases in which such structures were recognized, representing an incidence of 27.8%. Tumours with perineural space invasion were more likely to be associated with lymphatic invasion, nipple involvement, and the presence of metastases in axillary lymph nodes. Early tumor recurrence was also noted more frequently at the 18 month period of observation in its presence.

CONCLUSION

An attempt has been made to evaluate the possible prognostic significance of certain histopathologic features of mammary carcinoma. These include histologic type, histologic and nuclear grade, cell reaction to tumor, lymph nodal sinus histiocytosis and metastases, tumor size, blood and lymphatic vessel and perineural extension. The investigation has been made on the basis of a review of the pertinent literature as well as on data derived from the prospective study of 1,000 cases of invasive mammary cancer. In the latter, the interrelationship of these parameters, as well as their relationship to early tumor recurrence, were ascertained by contingency table analysis. The following conclusions appear warranted.

1. Retrospective investigations indicate that such histopathologic types of mammary carcinoma as the tubular, mucinous, medullary and adenocystic types may be associated with a better prognosis than the more common forms without special histopathological features. However, there was no significant relationship between histologic tumor type and early tumor recurrence in our own prospective series of cases.

2. Although there is evidence to indicate that prognosis may, at least to some degree, be related to the histological grade of mammary carcinoma, this was not found in our own material in the short term follow-up period of 24 months. On the other hand, tumors of high histologic grade (those

appearing to be most malignant), are more likely to be associated with nodal metastases than those of lower grades. The medullary carcinoma with its reputation of a good prognosis and the lobular infiltrating type, with its ominous prognosis, appear as paradoxes in widely utilized grading schemes, since the former reveals high grade features and the latter usually those of low grade.

3. The nuclear grade of tumors has similar interrelationships to those of histologic grade. This is not unexpected since nuclear grade represents an important feature of histologic grading schemes.

4. The presence of blood vessel, lymphatic and perineural space invasion was more likely to be associated with the presence of positive axillary nodal metastases but not with early tumor recurrence.

5. A severe cell reaction to breast cancer appears to be more closely related to the histologic degree of malignancy of the tumor, rather than to an immunologic response by the host.

6. Some degree of sinus histiocytosis, another purported feature of host immunologic responsiveness, was encountered in three-quarters of the cases in our series. Although no evidence was obtained from our studies to confirm or deny the immunologic nature of this reaction, its absence was more likely to be associated with the presence of 4 or more nodes involved by metastases. A new method for evaluating prognosis based on other histopathologic features of the regional nodes has been recently proposed. The patterns utilized appear to have a greater immunologic relevance than does the degree of sinus histiocytosis. Its value in this regard awaits confirmation.

7. The number of axillary nodes involved by metastases may be a better indicator of prognosis than the proportion of positive nodes among the total number removed. The presence of 4 or more involved nodes or a clinically positive axilla was consistently related to early tumor recurrence. This finding agrees with other studies and indicates the prognostic importance of clinical staging and pathological evidence of nodal metastases in mammary cancer.

8. In our study the presence of a clinically positive axilla, 4 or more nodal metastases, or a tumor 4.1 cm or larger, all favoured early tumor recurrence at all periods of observation. Lack of circumscription, lymphatic invasion of the quadrant as well as in the tumor, age 20–54 or proliferative fibrocystic disease in the quadrants remote from the primary cancer all favored early tumor recurrence at several but not all intervals. Nipple or skin involvement, the absence of sinus histiocytosis, perineural extension, marked tumor necrosis, presence of glycogen, nuclear grade 1 or black race were found to favor early tumor recurrence at only one time interval of observation.

9. Whether any of the less recognized histologic features will be significant prognostic factors for mammary cancer remains to be demonstrated

after longer periods of follow-up. Nevertheless, it would appear that some previously unemphasized histopathologic features may be of equal or even greater significance as prognostic discriminants of breast cancer, than are those which are conventionally recognized.

10. It also becomes evident, that there is not necessarily a direct relationship between some of the so-called histopathologic discriminants and survival rates. For instance, in our study histologic grade was related to nodal metastases but although the latter was related to early tumor recurrence, the former was not. The inquiry into this inconsistency should provide significant information concerning the relationship between the pathologic characteristics of mammary cancer and factors relating to survival.

11. Lastly, and perhaps most important is a possible explanation for the divergence between some of our findings and those recorded in the literature. Retrospective analyses of data including those of a pathologic nature frequently suffer from inadequate information concerning treatment and staging and as a result, the uniformity of such analyses may be questioned. The advantage of prospective studies is that they yield not only more meaningful therapeutic data but also the possibility of accurate pathologic discriminants of prognostic value.

Acknowledgement

Supported by USPHS Grant CA-12027; Contract NOI-CB23876 (Breast Cancer Task Force).

REFERENCES

Ackerman, L. V. (1968): Surgical Pathology. 4th ed. St. Louis, C. V. Mosby Co.

Alderson, M. R., Hamlin, I. and Staunton, M. D. (1971): The relative significance of prognostic factors in breast carcinoma. *Br. J. Cancer,* **25,** 646.

Anastassiades, O. T. and Pryce, D. M. (1966): Immunological significance of the morphological changes in lymph nodes draining breast cancer. *Br. J. Cancer,* **20,** 239.

Ashikari, R., Huvos, A. G., Urban, J. A. and Robbins, G. F. (1973): Infiltrating lobular carcinoma of the breast. *Cancer,* **31,** 110.

Bell, J. R., Friedell, G. H. and Goldenberg, I. S. (1969): Prognostic significance of pathologic findings in human breast carcinoma. *Surg. Gynecol. Obstet.,* **129,** 258.

Benfield, J. R., Jacobson, M. and Warner, N. E. (1965): *In situ* lobular carcinoma of the breast. *Arch. Surg.,* **91,** 130.

Berg, J. W. (1956): Sinus histiocytosis: a fallacious measure of host resistance to cancer. *Cancer,* **9,** 935.

Berg, J. W. (1959): Inflammation and prognosis in breast cancer. A search for host resistance. *Cancer,* **12,** 714.

Berg, J. W. (1962): Active host resistance to breast cancer. *Acta. Un. Int. Cancr.,* **18,** 854.

Berg, J. W. (1971): Morphological evidence for immune response to cancer. An historical review. *Cancer,* **28,** 1453.

Berg, J. W., Huvos, A. G., Axtell, L. M. and Robbins, G. F. (1973): A new sign of favorable prognosis in mammary cancer: hyperplastic reactive lymph nodes in the apex of the axilla. *Ann. Surg.,* **177,** 8.

Black, M. M., Kerpe, S. and Speer, F. D. (1953): Lymph node structure in patients with cancer of breast. *Am. J. Pathol.,* **29,** 505.

Black, M. M., Opler, S. R. and Speer, F. D. (1955): Survival in breast cancer cases in relation to the structure of the primary tumor and regional lymph nodes. *Surg. Gynecol. Obstet.,* **100,** 543.

Black, M. M. and Speer, F. D. (1957): Nuclear structure in cancer tissues. *Surg. Gynecol. Obstet.,* **105,** 97.

Black, M. M. and Speer, F. D. (1958): Sinus histiocytosis of lymph nodes in cancer. *Surg. Gynecol. Obstet.,* **106,** 163.

Black, M. M. and Speer, F. D. (1959): Immunology of cancer. *Int. Abstr. Surg.,* **109,** 105.

Black, M. M. and Speer, F. D. (1960): Lymph node reactivity in cancer patients. *Surg. Gynecol. Obstet.,* **110,** 477.

Black, M. M., Speer, F. D. and Opler, S. R. (1956): Structural representations of tumour–host relationships in mammary carcinoma: biologic and prognostic significance. *Am. J. Clin. Path.,* **26,** 250.

Bloom, H. J. G. (1950): Prognosis in carcinoma of the breast. *Br. J. Cancer,* **4,** 259.

Bloom, H. J. G. (1950): Further studies on prognosis of breast carcinoma. *Br. J. Cancer,* **4,** 347.

Bloom, H. J. G. (1956): The role of histology in the treatment of breast cancer. *Brit. J. Radiol.,* **29,** 488.

Bloom, H. J. G., Richardson, W. W. and Field, J. R. (1970): Host resistance and survival in carcinoma of breast: study of 104 cases of medullary carcinoma in a series of 1411 cases of breast cancer followed for 20 years. *Br. Med. J.,* **3,** 181.

Brightmore, T. G., Greening, W. P. and Hamlin, I. (1970): An analysis of clinical and histopathological features in 101 cases of carcinoma of breast in women under 35 years of age. *Br. J. Cancer,* **24,** 644.

Byar, D. P. and Mostofi, F. K. (1972): Carcinoma of the prostate: prognostic evaluation of certain pathologic features in 208 radical prostatectomies. *Cancer,* **30,** 5.

Cady, B. (1972): Changing patterns of breast cancer. A point of view. *Arch. Surg.,* **104**, 266.

Cammoun, H., Contesso, G. and Rouesse, J. (1972): Les adenocarcinomes cylindromateaux du sein. *Ann. Anato. Pathol.* (Paris), **17**, 143.

Carstens, P. H. B., Huvos, A. G., Foote, F. W., Jr. and Ashikari, R. (1972): Tubular carcinoma of the breast: a clinicopathologic study of 35 cases. *Am. J. Clin. Pathol.,* **58**, 231.

Cavanzo, F. J. and Taylor, H. B. (1969): Adenoid cystic carcinoma of the breast. An analysis of 21 cases. *Cancer,* **24**, 740.

Champion, H. R., Wallace, I. W. and Prescott, R. J. (1972): Histology in breast cancer prognosis. *Br. J. Cancer,* **26**, 129.

Cheatle, G. L. and Cutler, M. (1931): Paget's disease of the nipple. *Arch. Path.,* **12**, 435.

Cutler, S. J., Axtell, L. M., Schottenfeld, D. and Farrow, J. H. (1970): Clinical assessment of lymph nodes in carcinoma of the breast. *Surg. Gynec. Obstet.,* **131**, 41.

Cutler, S. J. and Myers, M. H. (1967): Clinical classification of extent of disease in cancer of the breast. *J. Nat. Cancer Inst.,* **39**, 193.

Dabska, M. (1968): Prognosis in breast cancer on the basis of histological evaluation of malignancy according to the criteria of Bloom. *Pol. Med. J.,* **7**, 908.

Deodhar, S. D., Crile, G., Jr. and Esselstyn, C. G., Jr. (1972): Study of the tumor cell–lymphocyte interaction in patients with breast cancer. *Cancer,* **29**, 1321.

DiRe, J. J. and Lane, N. (1963): The relation of sinus histiocytosis in axillary lymph nodes to surgical curability of carcinoma of the breast. *Am. J. Clin. Pathol.,* **40**, 508.

Dockerty, M. B. (1964): The grading and typing of carcinoma of the breast. *J. Iowa Med. Soc.,* **54**, 289.

Eggers, C., deCholnoky, T. and Jessup, D. S. (1941): Cancer of the breast. *Ann. Surg.,* **113**, 321.

Eichner, W. J., Lemon, H. M. and Friedell, G. (1970): Tumor grade in the prognosis of breast cancer. *Nebr. Med. J.,* **55**, 405.

Elsner, B. (1970): Adenoid cystic carcinoma of the breast. Review of the literature and clinico-pathologic study of seven patients. *Pathol. Eur.,* **5**, 357.

Fisher, B. and Fisher, E. R. (1971): Studies concerning the regional lymph node in cancer. I. Initiation of immunity. *Cancer,* **27**, 1001.

Fisher, B. and Fisher, E. R. (1972): Studies concerning the regional lymph node in cancer. II. Maintenance of immunity. *Cancer,* **29**, 1496.

Fisher, B., Saffer, E. A. and Fisher, E. R. (1972): Studies concerning the regional lymph node in cancer. III. Response of regional lymph node cells from breast and colon cancer patients to PHA stimulation. *Cancer,* **30**, 1202.

Fisher, B., Saffer, E. A. and Fisher, E. R. (1974): Studies concerning the regional lymph node in cancer. VII. Thymidine uptake by cells from nodes of breast cancer patients relative to axillary location and histopathologic discriminants. *Cancer,* **33,** 271.

Fisher, B., Saffer, E. A. and Fisher, E. R. (1974): Studies concerning the regional lymph node in cancer. IV. Tumor inhibition by regional lymph node cells. *Cancer,* **33,** 631.

Fisher, B. and Slack, N. H. (1970): Number of lymph nodes examined and the prognosis of breast carcinoma. *Surg. Gynecol. Obstet.,* **131,** 79.

Fisher, B., Slack, N. H., Bross, I. D. J. *et al.* (1969): Cancer of the breast: size of neoplasm and prognosis. *Cancer,* **24,** 1071.

Fisher, E. R., Gregorio, R. M. and Fisher, B. (1975): The Pathology of Invasive Breast Cancer. A Syllabus Derived from Findings of the National Surgical Adjuvant Breast Project (Protocol #4). *Cancer Supplement* in Press.

Fisher, E. R., Reidbord, H. and Fisher, B. (1973): Studies concerning the regional lymph node in cancer. V. Histologic and ultrastructural findings in regional and nonregional nodes. *Lab. Invest.,* **28,** 126.

Fisher, E. R., Saffer, E. and Fisher, B. (1973): Studies concerning the regional lymph node in cancer. VI. Correlation of lymphocyte transformation of regional node cells and some histopathologic discriminants. *Cancer,* **32,** 104.

Foote, F. W., Jr. and Stewart, F. W. (1941): Lobular carcinoma in situ. A rare form of mammary cancer. *Am. J. Path,* **17,** 491.

Friedell, G. H., Betts, A. and Sommers, S. C. (1965): The prognostic value of blood vessel invasion and lymphocyte infiltrates in breast carcinoma. *Cancer,* **18,** 164.

Friedman, B. and Oberman, H. A. (1970): Adenoid cystic carcinoma of the breast. *Am. J. Clin. Pathol.,* **54,** 1.

Galloway, J. R., Woolner, L. B. and Clagett, O. T. (1966): Adenoid cystic carcinoma of the breast. *Surg. Gynecol. Obstet.,* **122,** 1289.

Geschickter, C. F. (1938): Gelatinous mammary cancer. *Ann. Surg.,* **108,** 321.

Geschickter, C. F. (1945): Diseases of the Breast; Diagnosis, Pathology, Treatment, 2nd ed. Philadelphia, J. B. Lippincott Co.

Godwin, J. T. (1952): Chronology of lobular carcinoma of the breast. Report of a case. *Cancer,* **5,** 259.

Gold, R. H., Main, G., Zippin, C. and Annes, G. P. (1972): Infiltration of mammary carcinoma as an indicator of axillary node metastasis. A preliminary report. *Cancer,* **29,** 35.

Greenough, R. B. (1925): Varying degrees of malignancy in cancer of the breast. *J. Cancer Res.,* **9,** 453.

Groshong, L. E. (1968): Adenocystic carcinoma of the breast. *Arch. Surg.,* **92,** 424.

Haagensen, C. D. (1933): The bases for the histologic grading of carcinoma of the breast. *Am. J. Cancer,* **19,** 285.

Haagensen, C. D. (1956): Diseases of the Breast. Philadelphia, W. B. Saunders Co.

Hamlin, I. M. E. (1968): Possible host resistance in carcinoma of the breast, a histological study. *Br. J. Cancer,* **22,** 383.

Hart, D. (1927): Intracystic papillomatous tumors of the breast, benign and malignant. *Arch. Surg.,* **14,** 793.

Hayes, J. A. and Brooks, V. (1967): Adenoid cystic carcinoma of the breast. *Arch. Surg.,* **94,** 134.

Higginson, J. F. and McDonald, J. R. (1949): Apocrine tissue, chronic cystic mastitis and sweat gland carcinoma of the breast. *Surg. Gynecol. Obstet.,* **88,** 1.

Hoopes, B. F., and McGraw, A. B. (1942): The Halsted radical mastectomy. Five-year results in 246 consecutive operations at the same clinic. *Surgery,* **12,** 892.

Hueper, W. C. (1932): The clinical significance and application of histologic grading of cancers. *Ann. Surg.,* **95,** 321.

Hutter, R. V. P. (1971): The pathologist's role in minimal breast cancer. *Cancer,* **28,** 1527.

Inglis, K. (1946): Paget's disease of the nipple with special reference to the changes in the ducts. *Am. J. Pathol.,* **22,** 1.

Johnstone, F. R. (1972): Carcinoma of breast. Influence of size of primary lesion and lymph node involvement based on selective biopsy. *Am. J. Surg.,* **124,** 158.

Kister, S. J., Sommers, S. C., Haagensen, C. D. and Cooley, E. (1966): Reevaluation of blood vessel invasion as a prognostic factor in carcinoma of the breast. *Cancer,* **19,** 1213.

Kister, S. J., Sommers, S. C., Haagensen, C. D., Friedell, G. H., Cooley, E. and Varma, A. (1969): Nuclear grade and sinus histiocytosis in cancer of the breast. *Cancer,* **23,** 570.

Kraus, F. T. and Neubecker, R. D. (1962): The differential diagnosis of papillary tumors of the breast. *Cancer,* **15,** 444.

Kunath, C. A. (1940): Problem of cancer of the breast; radical mastectomy in 90 cases. *Arch. Surg.,* **41,** 66.

Lane, N., Goskel, H., Salerno, R. A. and Haagensen, C. D. (1961): Clinico-pathologic analysis of the surgical curability of breast cancers: a minimum ten-year study of a personal series. *Ann. Surg.,* **153,** 483.

Lee, B. J., Pack, G. T. and Scharnagel, I. (1933): Sweat gland cancer of the breast. *Surg. Gynecol. Obstet.,* **56,** 975.

MacCarty, W. C. and Sistrunk, W. E. (1922): Life expectancy following radical amputation for carcinoma of the breast; a clinical and pathological study of 218 cases. *Ann. Surg.,* **75,** 61.

Masse, L., Masse, C. and Chassiagne, J. P. (1960): Le prognostic de cancers du sein en function de la surcharge en histiocytes des sinus des ganglions axillaires. *Mem. Acad. Chir.*, **86**, 940.

McDivitt, R. W., Hutter, R. V., Foote, F. W., Jr. and Stewart, F. W. (1967): *In situ* lobular carcinoma. A prospective follow-up study indicating cumulative patient risks. *JAMA*, **201**, 82.

McDivitt, R. W., Stewart, F. W. and Berg, J. W. (1968): Tumors of the Breast. Washington, D.C., *Armed Forces Inst. of Path.*

Melamed, M. R., Robbins, G. F. and Foote, F. W., Jr. (1961): Prognostic significance of gelatinous mammary carcinoma. *Cancer*, **14**, 699.

Miller, H. W., Jr. and Kay, S. (1956): Infiltrating lobular carcinoma of the female mammary gland. *Surg. Gynecol. Obstet.*, **102**, 661.

Moore, O. S. and Foote, F. W., Jr. (1949): The relatively favorable prognosis of medullary carcinoma of the breast. *Cancer*, **2**, 635.

Muir, R. (1939): Further observations on Paget's disease of the nipple. *J. Pathol. Bacteriol.*, **49**, 299.

Muir, R. (1941): The evolution of carcinoma of the mamma. *J. Pathol. Bacteriol.*, **52**, 155.

Nayer, H. R. (1957): Cylindroma of the breast with pulmonary metastases. *Dis. Chest*, **31**, 324.

Newman, W. (1966): Lobular carcinoma of the female breast. *Ann. Surg.*, **164**, 305.

Norris, H. J. and Taylor, H. B. (1965): Prognosis of mucinous (gelatinous) carcinoma of the breast. *Cancer*, **18**, 879.

O'Kell, R. T. (1964): Adenoid cystic carcinoma of the breast. *Mo. Med.*, **61**, 855.

Paget, J. (1874): On disease of the mammary areola preceding cancer of the mammary gland. *St. Barth. Hosp. Statistical Reports*, **10**, 86.

Richardson, W. W. (1956): Medullary carcinoma of the breast; a distinctive tumour type with a relatively good prognosis following radical mastectomy. *Br. J. Cancer*, **10**, 415.

Richters, A. and Sherwin, R. P. (1971): The significance of autochthonous lymphocyte interactions with human breast cancer cells in primary tissue cultures. *Cancer*, **27**, 274.

Ruiz, U., Babeu, S., Schwartz, M. S., Soto, E., McAuley, R. A. and Friedell, G. H. (1973): Blood vessel invasion and lymph node metastasis: two factors affecting survival in breast cancer. *Surgery*, **73**, 185.

Scarff, R. W. and Handley, R. S. (1938): Prognosis in carcinoma of the breast. *Lancet*, **ii**, 582.

Scarff, R. W. and Patey, D. H. (1928): The position of histology in the prognosis of carcinoma of the breast. *Lancet*, **i**, 801.

Scarff, R. W. and Torloni, H. (1968): Histological typing of breast tumours. Geneva, World Health Organization.

Schulenburg, C. A. and Pepler, W. J. (1969): Adenoid cystic carcinoma of the breast. *Br. J. Surg.*, **56**, 395.

Silverberg, S. G., Chitale, A. R., Hind, A. D., Frazier, A. B. and Levitt, S. H. (1970): Sinus histiocytosis and mammary carcinoma: Study of 366 radical mastectomies and an historical review. *Cancer,* **26**, 1177.

Silverberg, S. G., Kay, S., Chitale, A. R. and Levitt, S. H. (1971): Colloid carcinoma of the breast. *Am. J. Clin. Pathol.*, **55**, 355.

Simard, C. (1930): La maladie de Paget du mamelon; cancer epidermotrope. *Bull de l'Assoc franc p l'etude du cancer,* **19**, 50.

Sistrunk, W. E. and MacCarty, W. C. (1922): Life expectancy following radical amputation for carcinoma of the breast: A clinical and pathologic study of 218 cases. *Ann. Surg.*, **75**, 61.

Sommers, S. C. (1969): Histologic changes in incipient carcinoma of the breast. *Cancer,* **23**, 822.

Taylor, H. B. and Norris, H. J. (1970): Well-differentiated carcinoma of the breast. *Cancer,* 687.

Tomcic, S., Vulkcevic, S. and Vidovic, Z. (1972): Histolski i drugi faktori u prognozi raka dojke i histoloski tip raka dojke i prognoza. *Med. Arh.*, **26**, 3.

Tough, I. C., Carter, D. D., Fraser, J. and Bruce, J. (1969): Histological grading in breast cancer. *Br. J. Cancer,* **23**, 294.

Tsakraklides, V., Olson, P., Kersey, J. H. and Good, R. A. (1974): Prognostic significance of the regional lymph node histology in cancer of the breast. *Cancer,* **34**, 1259.

Verani, R. R. and Van der Bel-Kahn, J. (1973): Mammary adenoid cystic carcinoma with unusual features. *Am. J. Clin. Pathol.*, **59**, 653.

Wartman, W. B. (1959): Sinus cell hyperplasia of lymph nodes regional to adenocarcinoma of the breast and colon. *Br. J. Cancer,* **13**, 389.

White, W. C. (1927): Late results of operations for carcinoma of the breast. *Ann. Surg.*, **86**, 695.

Wilson, W. B. and Spell, J. P. (1967): Adenoid cystic carcinoma of the breast: A case with recurrence and regional metastasis. *Ann. Surg.*, **166**, 861.

Wolff, B. (1966): Histological grading in carcinoma of the breast. *Br. J. Cancer,* **20**, 36.

7

Clinical Prediction of Growth Behaviour

James E. Devitt

When confronted with a patient with breast cancer, we do not know whether, when or where she will develop metastatic disease. Because of the remarkable variability in the course of the disease from patient to patient, MacDonald (1966) has suggested that breast cancer can be regarded as a number of entities masquerading under a single name. In each individual, the biologic balance between tumor and local and systemic host factors, will have determined the course of the patient's disease, long before the clinician can exert any influence on it.

However, the effect of such factors can be estimated. The purpose of this chapter is to review the available clinical observations on the growth behaviour and pattern of spread of breast cancer. By applying this knowledge to the observed behaviour of a tumor, it is possible to predict the likelihood of various clinical courses.

GROWTH RATES OF BREAST CANCER

The growth rates of human breast cancer have been studied in several ways. Collins, Loeffler and Tivey (1956) observed the growth of pulmonary metastases and calculated the time necessary for the tumor to double its volume. They assumed a constant growth rate, and by extrapolating this backwards to the point where the volume equalled that of a single cell, they deduced that most metastases had a lengthy preclinical duration.

Gershon-Cohen, Berger and Klickstein (1963) had the opportunity to study several untreated primary breast cancers by mammography. Assuming a constant growth rate, they calculated the tumor doubling times to vary from 2.3 to 209 days, while Philippe and Le Gal (1968) calculated the average doubling time of recurrent skin and subcutaneous nodules to be 40 days (range of 3 to 211 days).

Slack, Blumenson and Bross (1969) analysed the data of the National Surgical Adjuvant Breast Project Protocol and developed a mathematical model characterizing the course of breast cancer. They concluded that there were two distinct diseases, one with a doubling time of 3 weeks and a less malignant kind with a doubling time of 6 weeks.

Kusama *et al.* (1972) observed 163 primary breast cancers and 57 metastases at various sites. They too assumed that the doubling time was constant, and calculated that except for some stationary tumors, the median doubling time was 3 to 5 months with a range of 0.2 to 18 months. The frequency distribution of all doubling times formed a log normal distribution. There was no correlation between the calculated length of doubling time and the presence of axillary node metastases, though tumors with short doubling time were associated with a poor prognosis.

The short-comings of assuming a constant growth rate have been reviewed by Smithers (1968). Most measurements have been made late in the course of the disease and these may not represent the growth rates in the much longer pre-clinical period, which of course, cannot be measured. He described a young woman with a metastatic tumor that grew so slowly that, had it been growing at a constant rate, it would need to have originated long before she was conceived. Ingleby and Moore (1956) had observed one patient's breast cancer, by mammography, for two years. They reported that the growth during the final 11 months was considerably greater than in the first 11 months, but that there was a decrease in the rate of growth in the last $2\frac{1}{2}$ months of study.

Brennan (1966) describes a growth curve for breast cancer which increases progressively until it passes through a point of inflection at about 37% of the final or limiting tumor size. Then growth declines gradually until it reaches zero. He describes the empirical upper limit in size of 90% of skin and subcutaneous metastases as 3 cm, and by the time they reach a diameter of 2 cm, subcutaneous nodules are usually in a plateau phase of growth. Brennan describes the cell population doubling times for skin, subcutaneous and lymph node metastases of 0.5 to 1.5 cm diameter as varying from 15 to 120 days with a modal value of approximately 80 days.

Brennan claims that the upper limit in the size of 90% of pulmonary metastases is 4 cm. He reports doubling times for pulmonary metastases to be much shorter than for skin metastases, with a median of 20 days. This indicates that growth rates may vary with the site of the metastasis as well as with the size of the cell populations. Brennan also points out that new lesions can appear while earlier ones remain stationary. Skipper (1971) also considers the doubling time of breast tumors to be an ever changing value, in that doubling time increases and growth rates slow with advance of the disease.

Devitt (1971a) has recorded the great variation in the relative time of appearance of metastases in the interval between primary treatment and death. Not only is there a variation in the relative time of appearance of any one type of metastasis, but there are differences in the *patterns* of

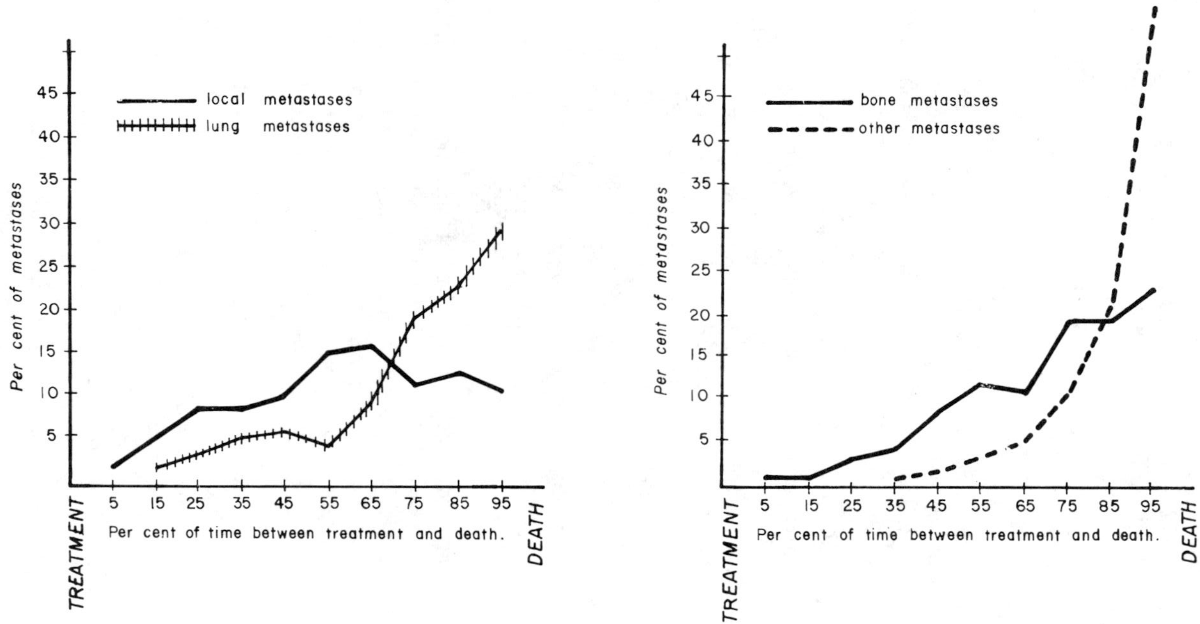

Fig. 1. The relative time of appearance of metastases in the initial treatment-to-death interval in breast cancer.

(Reproduced from Devitt (1971a) by courtesy of the Editor of Cancer)

timing distribution. These differences can be shown between the different metastatic sites (Fig. 1); between metastases appearing within 18 months and those after 36 months (Fig. 2); and between patients whose primary tumors were stage I compared with those in stage III (Fig. 3). If tumor

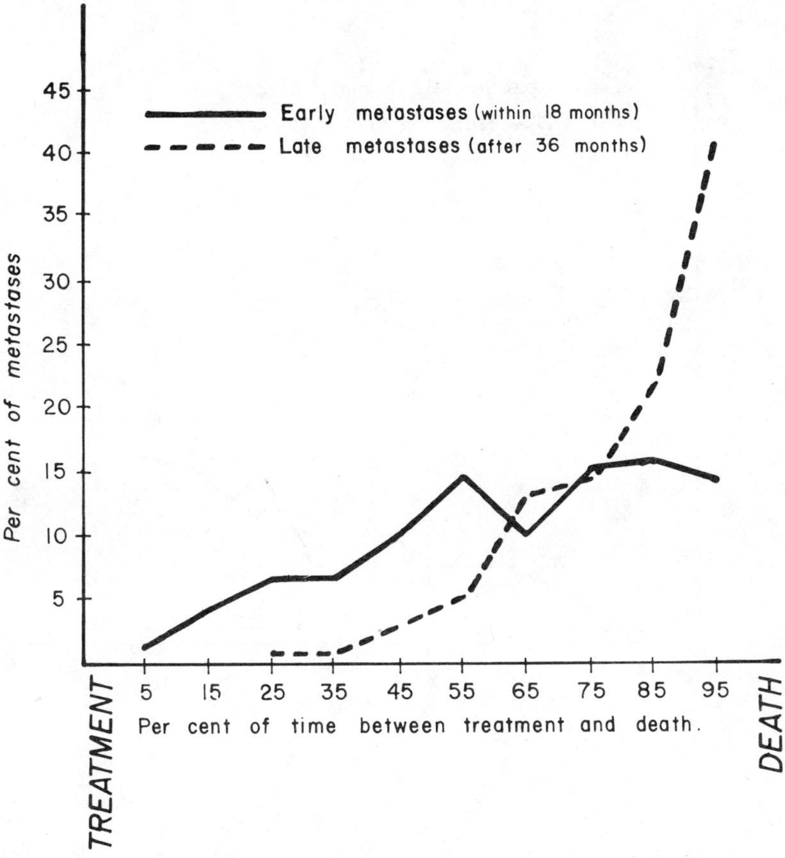

Fig. 2. The relative time of appearance in the initial treatment-to-death interval of early and late metastases in breast cancer.

(Reproduced from Devitt (1971a) by courtesy of the Editor of Cancer)

doubling times and growth rates were constant, metastases should have appeared at the same narrow point in the treatment-to-death interval.

The report of Edwards, Baum and Magarey (1972) that most axillary lymph nodes in Stage II patients either regress or remain stationary after simple mastectomy, and the somewhat similar statement by Bond (1972), is discussed later. It cannot be reconciled with the concept of a constant growth rate. Laird (1965) studying the growth of various laboratory animal tumors, observed growth rates to decrease constantly as growth progressed. She did not regard this as the fortuitous result of the failure of a

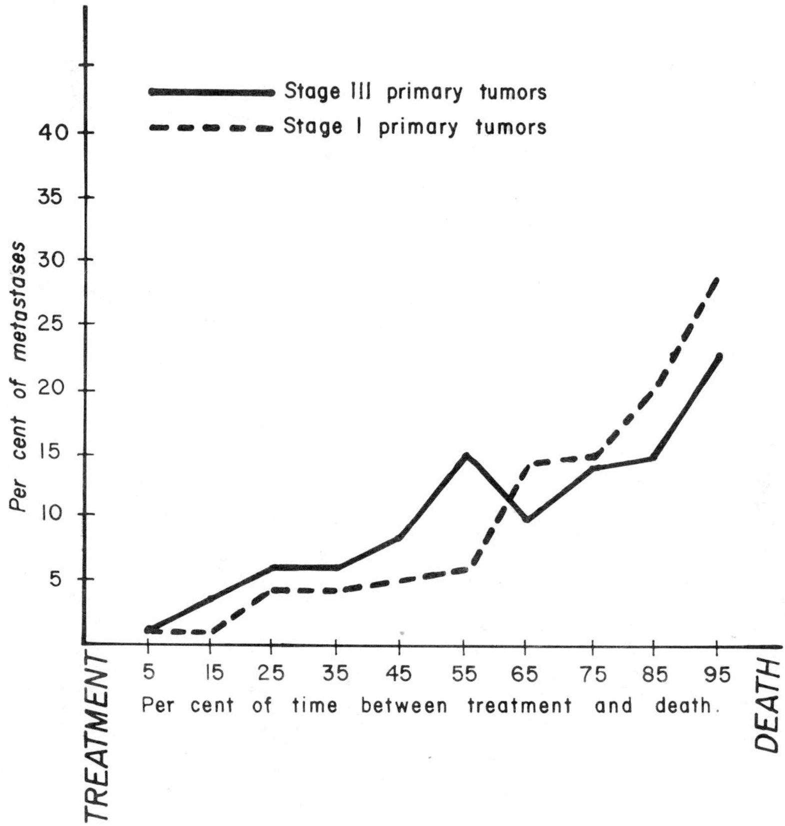

Fig. 3. The relative time of appearance in the initial treatment-to-death interval of metastases from Stage I and Stage III primary breast cancers.

(Reproduced from Devitt (1971a) by courtesy of the Editor of Cancer)

dying host to afford nutritional support, but as a growth characteristic of tumors in the animal host. Each tumor and each species had fairly characteristic growth curves.

All of these observations suggest that growth rates (tumor doubling times) do indeed vary markedly under differing circumstances. Though the concept of constant tumor doubling times has been useful in indicating the likelihood of a long pre-clinical duration of neoplastic change, it is quite wrong to apply it to all tumors at all times or at all sites.

DORMANT BREAST CANCER

All clinicians dealing with breast cancer have observed patients who apparently remain free of disease for many years before reactivation occurs, and Herrmann (1972) collected a group of patients with a free interval of 20 or more years. Schwartz (1961) claimed that apparent dormancy is actually very slow subclinical growth, and that what appears to be a sudden change in clinical growth rates when metastasis appears, is an illusion resulting from the tumor's constant geometric increase. Most, however, would concur with Hadfield (1954) who commented that when the interval between excision and the appearance of secondary tumors reaches four or more years, it becomes increasingly difficult to believe that cellular proliferation in the residual tumor fragments has been continuous and uninhibited.

Devitt (1965) reported that ipsilateral or contralateral axillary lymph node metastases may manifest long after the appearance of distant metastases (Devitt and Michalchuk, 1969), and suggested that they were unlikely to be a tertiary form of spread. Different rates of tumor growth at different metastatic sites could account for the observation but in view of the fact that five to ten years may have elapsed from the initial treatment, it seems more likely that the axillary lymph node metastases have remained in a dormant state until local conditions permit further growth.

Crile (1967) studying patients who developed axillary lymph node recurrences after simple mastectomy, found no discernible tendency for cancer to metastasize from the involved nodes after the primary tumor was removed. In fact, Edwards, Baum and Magarey (1972) have reported regression and apparent dormancy of enlarged axillary lymph nodes after simple mastectomy.

Another observation that may represent a form of dormancy is the discrepancy between the reported incidence of histological carcinoma and clinical carcinoma in the remaining breast after mastectomy. Urban (1969) routinely biopsied the remaining breast in 73% of a series of breast cancer patients. Though only five patients were suspected clinically of having a cancer, 17 infiltrating and 31 non-infiltrating cancers were found—a total incidence of 14%. This is more than twice the incidence of carcinoma of the remaining breast usually reported in 10 year follow-ups (Robbins and Berg, 1964; Devitt, 1971b), but it matches the cumulative 30 year rate reported by Adair *et al.* (1974).

It therefore seems likely that a state of dormancy may exist, both before the recognition of the primary tumor as well as before the appearance of secondary lesions.

GROWTH BEHAVIOUR AND MORTALITY RATES

Survival/mortality rates of breast cancer patients must bear some relationship to growth rates, though they also reflect the tumor's ability to metastasize. Thus a study of survival or mortality rates and of those factors which influence the rates, should provide some insight into the nature of mammary cancer.

Jones (1956) concluded that groups of breast cancer patients maintained the same annual death rate throughout the disease and that it did not increase with longer duration of the disease. He also concluded that the survival tendency in four treated and four untreated series of breast cancer were statistically not significantly different. Devitt (1967) studying the annual mortality rates of patients in the different clinical stages of primary breast cancer, observed that in the first 10 years after treatment, the mortality rates were surprisingly constant and specific for each stage. Patients with (Manchester) Stage I lesions had approximately a 6% annual mortality. For Stage II patients it was 12% and for Stage III it was approximately 21% each year.

Cutler, Asire and Taylor (1969) studying patients with metastatic breast cancer found constant annual mortality rates, which could be correlated with the recurrence-free period. Campos (1972) reported that the number of breast cancer patients who died during equal periods was a fixed proportion of those alive at the beginning of the period. Each category of breast cancer may have its particular slope. While the half-lethality period for patients without axillary lymph node metastases was 27.4 months, that for patients with axillary metastases was 31.8 months.

What do these constant mortality rates mean? Presumably that the factors responsible for the reactivation of breast cancer growth continue to operate with exactly the same force. Alternatively, one might suggest that the factors responsible for the restraint of tumor growth continue to decay at the same rate. The metastases presumably remain in a state of relative dormancy until the restraints reach the critical level of failure.

CLINICAL STAGE, "FREE" INTERVAL AND SURVIVAL AFTER METASTASES

The clinical stage at presentation correlates fairly well with the eventual outcome in breast cancer patients. The "earlier" the presenting stage, the more likely the patient is to be "cured". The "later" the stage of the tumor, the more likely the patient will succumb to her disease. Assuming a step-by-step progression of breast cancer, this has led to hope that earlier treatment would cure more patients and has created an impetus for the screening of non-symptomatic women. There is, however, increasing evidence that initial clinical stage is more an indication of the tumor–host potential than of the length of time that the tumor has been present.

Shimkin *et al.* (1954) observed that the median time before appearance of metastatic or recurrent disease was 30 months for patients who presented with Stage I primary tumors, 21 months for Stage II and 12 months for Stage III patients. They also reported that the median survival of patients after the development of metastases was 19 months for Stage I patients and only 13 months for Stage II and III patients.

Berg and Robbins (1966) observed that the 15 year mortality rate of five year survivors is lower for patients with earlier staged lesions. They suggested that lethal cancers tend to remain lethal, and low grade cancers kill less frequently in later years as well as in earlier years. Tough (1966) observed that the time from treatment to recurrence showed a significant difference in the different clinical stages, being longer in the Stage I patients. However, his analysis of the recurrence-to-death interval by clinical stages showed no difference between the stages.

Table 1 Time of Appearance of Metastases in Months (Devitt, 1971a)

Type	*Stage of primary*	*No. of patients*	*Median*	*Range*
Local	I	86	35.5	3 to 126
	II	69	20	2 to 108
	III	99	9	2 to 71
Bone	I	89	38	2 to 165
	II	81	24	2 to 120
	III	72	18.5	3 to 104
Lung	I	63	47	4 to 165
	II	67	23	4 to 215
	III	66	14	2 to 102
Other	I	54	45	3 to 204
	II	54	25.5	4 to 215
	III	38	11	2 to 81

Devitt (1967, 1971a) reported that not only did patients with early stage primary lesions develop local, bony, lung or other metastases later (Table 1), but they survived the metastases longer than did patients with advanced primary lesions (Table 2). Also, patients who developed early metastases (within 18 months) did not survive their metastases nearly as long as did patients who developed metastases after 36 months (Table 3).

Cutler, Asire and Taylor (1969) noted that the longer the time between primary treatment and the recurrence, the longer the survival after recurrence. Myers, Hankey and Mantel (1973) confirmed this. Haagensen (1971) reported that parasternal and chest wall recurrences appeared later in patients with Stage A primaries, and that such patients survived their metastases longer. Bengmark, Hafstroem and Olsson (1972) found that liver metastases appeared later in patients with tumors presenting at an earlier stage, but that survival after the appearance of metastases was not very different.

Herrmann (1972) reported that delayed reactivation of breast cancer

Table 2 Survival Time after the Development of the Metastases in Months (Devitt, 1971a).

Type	*Primary Stage*	*Median*	*Range*
Local	I	23	1 to 172
	II	10	1 to 203
	III	8	1 to 52
Bone	I	10	1 to 83
	II	9	1 to 72
	III	5.5	1 to 104
Lung	I	8	1 to 72
	II	7	1 to 62
	III	4	1 to 42
Other	I	3.5	1 to 38
	II	2	1 to 57
	III	2	1 to 15

Table 3 Survival Time after Metastases Related to Time of Appearance of Metastasis (Devitt, 1971a).

	Median Survival Time after Appearance Metastases	
	Within 1–18 mos.	*After 36 mos.*
Local	8 mos.	24 mos.
Bone	6 mos.	12 mos.
Lung	3 mos.	10 mos.
Other	1 month	4 mos.

(20 or more years after treatment) usually manifested itself in the lungs, osseous metastases being relatively infrequent. Papaioannou, Tang and Volk (1967) however, in describing 57 patients whose first recurrence appeared more than five years after primary therapy, observed 24 of these to be local, 20 osseous and 13 in various visceral sites.

In a retrospective review Stoll and Ackland (1970) observed that the average rate of growth of scar recurrences, as measured by the mean recurrence free period was not significantly different between patients who had received post-operative radiotherapy and those who had not.

Thus, the overall impression is that the growth behaviour of breast cancer is somewhat predictable in an odds-quoting way. The patient who is fortunate enough to have a good tumor–host relationship will present with an "early" clinical stage. She is less likely to develop local recurrence or distant metastases. If metastases develop, they will occur after a relatively longer "free" interval and she will survive the metastases for a longer period of time. These observations and the constant annual mortality rate strongly hint that it is biologic predeterminism (Macdonald, 1966) that is largely responsible for what happens to patients with breast cancer.

GROWTH BEHAVIOUR AND THE INFLUENCE OF TREATMENT

The few prospective randomized clinical trials of breast cancer therapy that have been reported have all shown that conservatively treated patients invariably have as good survival rates (although possibly not as good local control rates), as aggressively treated patients. This raises the question as to what aggressive treatment will accomplish other than better local control.

Kaae and Johansen (1968) compared simple mastectomy with postoperative irradiation, to extended radical mastectomy. Brinkley and Haybittle (1971) compared simple or modified simple mastectomy with postoperative irradiation, to radical mastectomy. Atkins *et al.* (1972) compared extended tylectomy, thioTEPA and postoperative irradiation, to radical mastectomy, thioTEPA and postoperative irradiation. Except for the Stage II patients in the last study, there were no differences of statistical significance in any of the reports. As the five year survival rate for the Stage II patients treated by radical mastectomy was 72% in the Guy's trial, the possibility of this being a fortuitous group of 80 patients is considerable.

The Manchester radiation trial (Gibb, 1969) compared two different techniques of postoperative prophylactic radiotherapy, to a control group that was not irradiated, all patients having had a radical mastectomy. The National Surgical Adjuvant Breast Project Protocol No. 2 reported by Fisher *et al.* (1970) compared postoperative irradiation after radical mastectomy, to a control group receiving thioTEPA or a placebo. The differences in survival rates between any of the groups was not statistically significant.

The National Surgical Breast Project Protocol No. 1 reported by Fisher *et al.* (1968) compared thioTEPA after radical mastectomy to a placebo. The differences in survival rates between the various groups compared were not statistically significant. It was stated that thioTEPA-treated premenopausal patients with more than 4 metastatic lymph nodes showed a better survival rate, but the 57% five year survival in the 23 reported patients, could probably not be reproduced in a larger series.

The Manchester ovarian irradiation trial compared radiation castration to a control group (Cole, 1968), and the National Surgical Adjuvant Breast Project Protocol No. 3 reported by Ravdin *et al.* (1970) compared surgical castration to a control group. Again no statistically significant differences in survival were noted.

Each of these therapeutic interventions can, sometimes at least, be seen to make malignant tumors disappear. Yet paradoxically, the randomized clinical trials show that eventually death occurs at the same time in spite of the aggressiveness of the therapy offered, and in spite of somewhat better local control. Is this related to the same factors that are responsible for the constant mortality rates?

INFLUENCE OF TREATMENT DELAY

Many studies have failed to show a close relation between survival rates and the length of time the patient admits to being aware of the tumor (Robbins and Bross, 1957; Humphrey and Swerdlow, 1963; Bloom, 1965; Brinkley and Haybittle, 1968; Handley, 1972). Consequently many reviews have concluded that it is the biologic features of the tumor and host which are the major determinants of the clinical course, rather than the time at which therapy is applied (Devitt, 1967; Fisher *et al.*, 1969).

Retrospective reviews of untreated patients have been used to exemplify the natural history of breast cancer. But the material in such studies usually consists of patients who, when they present for the first time, are in the terminal stages of the disease. Thus Bloom's (1962) well documented series had no patients presenting in (Manchester) Stage I, 2.4% were Stage II, 23.2% Stage III and 74.4% Stage IV.

Jones (1956) claimed that a comparison of four untreated and four treated series of breast cancer patients showed no significant differences in their survival tendency. However, he calculated the five year survival rate of breast cancer to be of the order of 25%, which is only one half of what most series report. MacKay and Sellers (1965) observed 145 untreated patients and reported five year survival in 35.2% from the first recorded symptom, compared to 52.3% for all breast cancer patients registered at the Ontario clinics during the period studied. Although recognizing that a group of only 145 patients is small, they observed that except for patients with lymph node metastases, the differences in survival after the first symptom between the treated and untreated patients were not significant.

Strax, Venet and Shapiro (1973) have been conducting a prospective study to determine the value of screening and earlier treatment in reducing mortality from breast cancer. When studies such as this have been completed and confirmed by others, it will become clear whether, and to what extent, the time of treatment influences the mortality patterns of patients with breast cancer. It will also be clearer whether early treatment improves survival rates other than by merely starting the observation period that much earlier.

In the present state of our knowledge, we can only say that the timing of initial treatment appears to have little influence on the growth behaviour of breast cancer, as reflected in survival rates. This is parallel to our previous observation that the type of initial treatment seems to be of unproven importance.

REGIONAL LYMPH NODE METASTASES

The earliest clinical evidence of metastases is usually recognized in the axillary lymph nodes. The larger the primary tumor the more likely that the regional lymph nodes will contain metastases (Fisher *et al.*, 1969; Handley, 1972). The likelihood of regional lymph node metastases varies with the histology of the primary tumor (McDivitt, Stewart and Berg, 1968), but does not necessarily correspond to the length of time the primary tumor has been present (Robbins and Bross, 1957; Bloom, 1965; Handley, 1972).

Edwards, Baum and Magarey (1972) observed 40 clinical Stage II patients treated by simple mastectomy alone. In 28 there was regression of the axillary nodes within three months, in 5 patients there was no change, in 2 the nodes enlarged and required treatment, in 3 there was regression but distant metastases developed, and in 2 the nodes enlarged and distant metastases developed. Bond (1972) has stated that 40% of axillary nodes enlargements will disappear after simple mastectomy without other treatment, and relatively few will enlarge. It has to be assumed that some of these represent axillary metastases which regress after mastectomy.

Irradiating regional lymph node areas after radical mastectomy does not improve survival rates (Gibb, 1969; Fisher *et al.*, 1970). Radical surgical excision of lymph nodes does not improve survival rates (Kaae and Johansen, 1968; Brinkley and Haybittle, 1971; Bruce, 1971). Atkins *et al.* (1972) does report better survival rates for Stage II patients treated by radical mastectomy as opposed to extended tylectomy but as mentioned earlier, their 5 year survival rate of 72% for Stage II patients may have been fortuitous.

These and other observations related to regional lymph node metastases and recurrence have led Copher, Chenard and Butcher (1962) and Devitt (1965) to suggest that regional lymph node metastases are not responsible for the poor prognosis with which they are associated, but rather that they reflect a poor tumor–host relationship. It is this biologic phenomenon that determines the outlook.

Fisher, Saffer and Fisher (1974) studying mouse tumor models, suggested that disseminated tumor cells gaining access to regional lymph nodes may be destroyed in those structures. They postulate that the finding of negative lymph nodes may be the result of just such a circumstance.

SIGNIFICANCE OF REGIONAL RECURRENCE

The likelihood of regional recurrence is increased in the more "advanced" clinical stages (Devitt, 1967; Haagensen, 1971). This is indicated by the presence (Chu *et al.*, 1967; Bruce, Carter and Fraser, 1970) and the number (Donegan, 1967) of metastatic axillary lymph nodes, and to a lesser extent by the size of the primary tumor (Donegan, 1967; Fisher *et al.*, 1969). Most regional recurrences appear within two or three years of therapy (Devitt, 1963, 1971 a; Spratt, 1967). Patients with more advanced primary tumors have earlier regional recurrences than patients with "early" primaries (Shimkin *et al.*, 1954; Tough, 1966; Devitt, 1967).

The development of a regional recurrence is usually an ominous portent. Though the disease may remain localized for a long period (Herrman, 1972), the more common experience is that distant metastases become evident, if not simultaneously, within a few months (Stoll, 1965; Spratt, 1967; Bruce *et al.*, 1970). The 5 year survival rates after regional recurrence are in the range between 4% and 9% (Devitt, 1967; Spratt, 1967).

As a rule then, the development of a regional recurrence indicates that the patient will soon die from her breast cancer although there are exceptions. Thus, Atkins *et al.* (1972) and Crile (1967) report that 5 year survival rates are not apparently affected by the higher incidence of local recurrence after 'extended tylectomy' or simple mastectomy, and that when not part of widespread metastatic disease, the recurrence can be dealt with successfully by local measures.

In a retrospective study Devitt (1963) also observed that the higher incidence of axillary lymph node recurrence after conservative surgery did not apparently influence 5 year survival rates, although all patients with such recurrence ultimately died of breast cancer. The higher regional recurrence rates observed after conservative surgery, and when prophylactic radiotherapy is witheld (Gibb, 1969; Fisher *et al.*, 1970) do not apparently worsen survival rates either.

Thus it would seem that regional recurrences identify patients with a poor tumor–host relationship, but the recurrences are not in themselves responsible for the death that will follow. For this reason, only palliative therapy for regional recurrence is appropriate.

The propensity for local recurrence is not readily explained. Though in experimental animals trauma of a part will increase the number of metastases (Fisher, Fisher and Feduska, 1967), this does not seem to be the case in humans. Thus, the local recurrence rate is not worse after supraradical mastectomy compared to simple mastectomy (Kaae and Johansen, 1968), but is actually somewhat worse after "lumpectomy" than after radical mastectomy (Atkins *et al.*, 1972). Nor is radical skin excision and skin grafting followed by worse (or better) local recurrence rates (Spratt, 1967). Indeed these studies suggest that the extent of surgical excision has no effect on the incidence of local recurrence except in the case of "lumpectomy" where the high local recurrence rate may well be due to the greater possibility of "new" tumor arising in the remaining breast tissue.

On rare occasions irradiation determines the site of recurrence. Cole and Halnan (1971) have described patients in whom the recurrent tumor appeared selectively in areas previously treated by prophylactic irradiation. Yet, prophylactic irradiation has also been shown to reduce the incidence of local recurrence (Gibb, 1969; Fisher *et al.*, 1970).

SELECTIVITY OF METASTATIC SITES

The pattern of metastases of breast cancer in no way corresponds to the distribution of the cardiac output of blood, which is approximately – liver 30% (most of which has traversed the gastrointestinal tract), kidney 20%, muscle 15%, brain 15%, skin and skeleton 10%, heart 5% and bronchi 5%. All blood goes through the lungs (Detweiler, 1973).

The different incidence of breast cancer metastases in the bones, lungs, pleura, liver and brain, presumably indicates the importance of local site factors in determining that a metastasis thrives. That site factors are a major determinant in metastasis is indicated by the observation that the numbers of circulating tumor cells are of little prognostic significance (Webster and Sabbadini, 1967). Moreover, there must be a close to total destruction of circulating tumor cells, since relatively few metastases ultimately do develop.

Approximately one-half of patients with distant metastases already have evidence of regional recurrence. The local manifestation of active disease may precede, occur simultaneously with, or follow the distant metastases (Devitt, 1965; Spratt, 1967; Bruce *et al.*, 1970). There is no regular pattern of distant metastases and it is possible to die with only one or any combination of the common sites of metastases involved with tumor.

In general, patients with skeletal metastases (or with local recurrence) survive longer than patients with other sites of systemic spread (Shimkin *et al.*, 1954; Papaioannou *et al.*, 1967). The longer survival of patients with bone metastases may result from their ease of treatment, the less vital function of the skeleton, or to their being involved by a less aggressive form of the disease.

The "earlier" the stage of the initial tumor, the longer the interval before the appearance of metastases. The later the appearance of the metastases, the longer the median survival afterwards (Shimkin *et al.*, 1954; Cutler, Asire and Taylor, 1969; Devitt, 1971a; Bengmark *et al.*, 1972). Larger numbers of metastatic sites are, not surprisingly, associated with shorter post-metastatic survivals (Donegan, 1967; Myers *et al.*, 1973).

"New" primary cancer in the remaining breast does not behave as might be expected. Robbins and Berg (1964) found that the annual incidence was fairly constant over a 20 year follow-up period, instead of the increasing incidence with age that is observed with first breast cancers. They and Devitt (1971b) found that the survival curves after the second "primary" drop more rapidly in the early years of follow-up. Nearly as many "new primary" breast cancers occur in patients with other evidence of active breast cancer, as in patients without such evidence.

The latter two observations suggest that some "new primary" lesions represent a deterioration in the tumor–host relationship rather than a new and entirely separate development. It is perhaps not surprising that the general factors which permit or encourage metastases to grow, may also do the same for a tumor in the remaining breast.

CONCLUSION

Breast cancer should be regarded as a number of entities, masquerading under a single name. Those factors causing an increased incidence of breast cancer do not affect its behaviour after it is established. As it appears that a large part of the life cycle of a mammary cancer has gone by before the clinical diagnosis, it is obvious that the biologic balance between host and neoplasm has become established long before the clinician can influence it. The biologic balance involves on the one hand, host factors which are both local and systemic, and on the other, tumor factors.

The effect of these factors can be estimated clinically by the presenting clinical stage, the "free" interval between treatment and appearance of metastases, and the number and site of metastases. The biological balance will determine whether metastases occur, and if and when and at what rate subsequent tumor growth takes place. It is likely that the same factors do *not* control each of these events.

It is these host–tumor factors which largely determine the outcome of the disease rather than the type of treatment or when it is provided. Although local or systemic therapy can be associated with dramatic local success, it is not clear to what extent, if at all, it is capable of delaying eventual death. As clinicians we should not allow our urge to treat or the patients' urge to be treated, to cause us to inflict regimens that may do no more than increase the total patient suffering, or needlessly consume society's resources.

REFERENCES

Adair, F., Berg, J., Joubert, L. and Robbins, G. E. (1974): Long-term follow-up of breast cancer patients: the 30-year report. *Cancer,* **33,** 1145.

Atkins, H., Hayward, J. L., Klugman, D. J. and Wayte, A. B. (1972): Treatment of early breast cancer: a report after ten years of a clinical trial. *Brit. Med. J.,* **2,** 423.

Bengmark, S., Hafstroem, L. and Olsson, A. (1972): The natural history of primary and secondary liver tumours. V. The prognosis for conventionally treated patients with liver metastases from breast cancer. *Digestion,* **6,** 321.

Berg, J. W. (1959): Inflammation and prognosis in breast cancer. *Cancer,* **12,** 714.

Berg, J. W. and Robbins, G. F. (1966): Factors influencing short and long term survival of breast cancer patients. *Surg. Gynec. Obstet.,* **122,** 1311.

Bloom, H. J. G. (1962): The natural history of untreated breast cancer. *Brit. Med. J.,* **2,** 213.

Bloom, H. J. G. (1965): The influence of delay on the natural history and prognosis of breast cancer. *Brit. J. Cancer,* **19,** 228.

Bond, W. H. (1972): Treatment of Carcinoma of the breast in: Modern Trends in Radiotherapy, 2, p. 165. Edited by Deeley, T. V., London: Butterworths.

Brennan, M. J. (1966): Indices of Response to Breast Cancer Therapy in: Clinical Evaluation in Breast Cancer, p. 141. Edited by J. L. Hayward and R. D. Bulbrook, Academic Press, London.

Brennan, M. J. (1973): Breast Cancer, p. 1769, in: Cancer Medicine. Edited by Holland, J. F. and Frei, E., Lea and Febiger, Philadelphia.

Brinkley, D. and Haybittle, J. L. (1968): A 15-year follow-up study of patients treated for carcinoma of the breast. *Br. J. Radiol.,* **14,** 215.

Brinkley, D. and Haybittle, J. L. (1971): Treatment of stage II carcinoma of the female breast. *Lancet,* **2,** 1086.

Bruce, J. (1971): Operable cancer of the breast. A controlled clinical trial. *Cancer,* **28,** 1443.

Bruce, J., Carter, D. C. and Fraser, J. (1970): Patterns of recurrent disease in breast cancer. *Lancet,* **1,** 433.

Campos, J. L. (1972): Observations on the mortality from carcinoma of the breast. *Brit. J. Radial.,* **45,** 31.

Chu, F. C. H., Lucas, J. C., Farrow, J. H. and Nickson, J. J. (1967): Does prophylactic radiation therapy given for cancer of the breast predispose to metastases. *Am. J. Roentgenol., Rad. Therapy and Nuclear Med.,* **99,** 987.

Cole, M. P. (1968): Suppression of ovarian function in primary breast cancer; in Prognostic Factors in Breast Cancer. Editors Forrest, A. P. M. and Kunkler, P. B., p. 146, E. and S. Livingstone Ltd., Edinburgh and London.

Cole, H. and Halnan, K. E. (1971): Facilitation of tumour spread in irradiated tissue after prophylactic postoperative x-ray therapy for breast cancer. *Clin. Radial.,* **22,** 133.

Collins, V. P., Loeffler, R. K. and Tivey, H. (1956): Observations on growth rates of human tumors. *Am. J. Roentgen. & Rad. Therapy,* **76,** 988.

Copher, G. H., Chenard, J. and Butcher, H. R., Jr. (1962): Factors influencing mortality from mammary cancer. *Arch. Surg.,* **85,** 73.

Crile, G., Jr. (1967): A biological consideration of treatment of breast cancer, p. 62. Charles C. Thomas, Springfield.

Cutler, S. J., Asire, A. J. and Taylor, S. G. (1969): Classification of patients with disseminated cancer of the breast. *Cancer,* **24,** 861.

Detweiler, D. K. (1973): Circulation in: Best and Taylor's Physiological Basis of Medical Practice, ninth edition. Edited by J. R. Brobeck, P.3–2, The Williams and Wilkins Co., Baltimore.

Devitt, J. E. (1963): The local control of carcinoma of the breast. *Can. J. Surg.,* **6,** 316.

Devitt, J. E. (1965): The significance of regional lymph node metastases in breast carcinoma. *Can. Med. Assn. J.,* **93,** 289.

Devitt, J. E. (1967): The clinical stages of breast cancer – what do they mean? *Can. Med. Assn. J.,* **97,** 1257.

Devitt, J. E. (1971a): The enigmatic behaviour of breast cancer. *Cancer,* **27,** 12.

Devitt, J. E. (1971b): Bilateral Mammary Cancer. *Ann. Surg.,* **174,** 774.

Devitt, J. E. and Michalchuk, A. W. (1969): Significance of contralateral axillary metastases in carcinoma of the breast. *Can. J. Surg.,* **12,** 178.

Donegan, W. L. (1967): Local and regional recurrence in major problems in clinical surgery. p. 190, Vol. 5, Cancer of the Breast, W. B. Saunders Company, Philadelphia and London.

Edwards, M. H., Baum, M. and Magarey, C. J. (1972): Regression of axillary lymph nodes in cancer of the breast. *Brit. J. Surg.,* **59,** 776.

Fisher, B., Fisher, E. R. and Feduska, N. (1967): Trauma and the localization of tumour cells. *Cancer,* **20,** 23.

Fisher, B., Ravdin, R. G., Susman, R. K., Slack, N. H., Moore, G. E. and Noer, R. J. (1968): Surgical adjuvant chemotherapy in cancer of the breast: results of a decade of cooperative investigation. *Ann. Surg.,* **168,** 337.

Fisher, B., Saffer, E. and Fisher, E. R. (1974): Studies concerning the regional lymph node in cancer, *Cancer,* **33,** 631.

Fisher, B., Slack, N. H., Bross, I. D. J. and Cooperating Investigators (1969): Cancer of the breast: size of neoplasm and prognosis. *Cancer,* **24,** 1071.

Fisher, B., Slack, N. G., Cavanagh, P. J., Gardner, B., Ravdin, R. G. (and Cooperating Investigators), (1970): Postoperative radiotherapy in the treatment of breast cancer: results of the N.S.A.B.P. clinical trial. *Ann. Surg.,* **172,** 711.

Gershon-Cohen, J., Berger, S. M. and Klickstein, H. S. (1963): Roentgenography of breast cancer moderating concept of "biologic predeterminism". *Cancer,* **16,** 961.

Gibb, R. (1969): Discussion of "Taking it that removal of the breast is required for the primary tumour, how should one treat the axillary nodes – by surgery, by radiotherapy, or by both?" *Brit. J. Surg.,* **56,** 791.

Haagensen, C. D. (1971). Diseases of the Breast, second edition. W. B. Saunders Company, Philadelphia, London, Toronto.

Hadfield, G. (1954): The dormant cancer cell. *Brit. Med. J.,* **2,** 607.

Handley, R. S. (1972): Observations and thoughts on cancer of the breast. *Proc. R. Soc. Med.,* **65,** 437.

Herrmann, J. B. (1972): Chronicity of mammary carcinoma. *New York State J. Med.,* **72,** 2310.

Humphrey, L. J. and Swerdlow, M. (1963): Factors influencing the survival of patients with carcinoma of the breast. *Am. J. Surg.,* **106,** 440.

Ingleby, H. and Moore, L. (1956): Periodic roentgenographic studies of a growing human mammary cancer. *Cancer,* **9,** 749.

Jones, H. B. (1956): Demographic consideration of the cancer problem. *Trans. N.Y. Acad. Sc.,* **18,** 298.

Kaae, S. and Johansen, H. (1968): Simple versus radical mastectomy in primary breast cancer; Prognostic Factors in Breast Cancer. Editors: Forrest, A. P. M. and Kunkler, P. G., p. 93, E. and S. Livingstone Ltd., Edinburgh and London.

Kusama, S., Spratt, J. S., Donegan, W. L., Watson, F. R. and Cunningham, C. (1972): The gross rates of growth of human mammary carcinoma. *Cancer,* **30,** 594.

Laird, A. K. (1965): Dynamics of tumour growth: comparison of growth rates and extrapolation of growth curve to one cell. *Brit. J. Cancer,* **19,** 278.

Macdonald, I. (1966): The natural history of mammary carcinoma. *Am. J. Surg.,* **111,** 435.

MacKay, E. N. and Sellers, A. H. (1965): Breast Cancer at the Ontario Cancer Clinics 1938–1956: a statistical review. *Can. Med. Assn. J.,* **92,** 647.

McDivitt, R. W., Stewart, F. W. and Berg, J. W. (1968): Tumors of the Breast. Atlas of tumor pathology, second series, fascicle 2, Armed Forces Institute of Pathology, Washington, D.C.

Myers, M. H., Hankey, B. F. and Mantel, N. (1973): A logistic-exponential model for use with response-time data involving regressor variables. *Biometrics,* **29,** 257.

Papaioannou, A. N., Tang, F. J. and Volk, H. (1967): Fate of patients with recurrent carcinoma of the breast. *Cancer,* **20,** 371.

Philippe, F. and Le Gal, Y. (1968): Growth of seventy-eight recurrent mammary cancers. *Cancer,* **21,** 461.

Ravdin, R. G., Lewison, E. F., Slack, N. H., Dao, T. L., Gardner, B., State, D. and Fisher, B. (1970): Results of a clinical trial concerning the worth of prophylactic oophorectomy for breast carcinoma. *Surg. Gynec. Obstet.,* **131,** 1055.

Robbins, G. F. and Berg, J. W. (1964): Bilateral primary breast cancers. *Cancer,* **17,** 1501.

Robbins, G. F. and Bross, I. (1957): The significance of delay in relation to prognosis of patients with primary operable breast cancer. *Cancer,* **10,** 338.

Shimkin, M. B., Lucia, E. L., Low-Beer, B. V. A. and Bell, H. G. (1954): Recurrent cancer of the breast. *Cancer,* **7,** 29.

Skipper, H. E. (1971): Kinetics of mammary tumor cell growth and implications for therapy. *Cancer,* **28,** 1479.

Slack, N. G., Blumenson, L. E. and Bross, I. D. J. (1969): Therapeutic implications from a mathematical model characterizing the course of breast cancer. *Cancer,* **24,** 960.

Smithers, D. W. (1968): Clinical assessment of growth-rate in human tumors. *Clin. Radiol.,* **19,** 113.

Spratt, J. S. (1967): Locally recurrent cancer after radical mastectomy. *Cancer,* **20,** 1051.

Stoll, B. A. (1965): Pleural effusion and breast cancer. *Brit. Med. J.,* **1,** 658.

Stoll, B. A. and Ackland, T. H. (1970): Management of breast cancer in old age, *Brit. Med. J.,* **4,** 201.

Strax, P., Venet, L. and Shapiro, S. (1973): Value of mammography in reduction of mortality from breast cancer in mass screening. *Am. J. Roentgenol. Rad. Therapy & Nuclear Med.,* **117,** 686.

Tough, I. C. K. (1966): The significance of recurrence in breast cancer. *Brit. J. Surg.,* **53,** 897.

Urban, J. A. (1969): Bilateral breast cancer. *Cancer,* **24,** 1310.

Webster, D. R. and Sabbadini, E. (1967): The prognostic significance of circulating tumour cells. *Can. Med. Assn. J.,* **96,** 129.

8

Effect of Age on Growth Pattern

Basil A. Stoll

INTRODUCTION

It is almost universally accepted that the malignancy of breast cancer in women varies according to age group. Most clinicians would state with confidence that in the young woman (under the age of 35), breast cancer behaves in a more malignant manner, while in the elderly patient (over the age of 70) it behaves in a less malignant manner, than in the intermediate age group. These opinions have been supported by many authorities, yet a study of the literature shows that clear differences have not been demonstrated in the parameters of malignancy which have been compared.

Does this mean that there is no factual basis for the impression, apart from the poorer prognosis associated with pregnancy? Alternatively, have we so far failed to define the criteria which give the impression of malignant behaviour in breast cancer?

BIOLOGICAL VARIABILITY OF BREAST CANCER

Both in the young patient and in the older patient, there appears to be an almost infinite range of malignant behaviour in breast cancer. It affects every phase of the disease including, (a) clinical pattern at presentation, (b) length of recurrence-free interval, (c) number of sites of recurrence and metastasis, (d) length of survival subsequent to tumour dissemination and (e) histopathological pattern. Moreover, the manifestation of aggressive or indolent behaviour by a tumour in one phase is not necessarily reflected by similar behaviour in another. It is becoming increasingly recognized that in each individual there is a dynamic and precarious balance between the agressive potential of the tumour on the one hand, and host defence factors on the other (Stoll, 1975). Breast cancer is simply a nosological heading.

In the past, the mean or median values of some of the above parameters have been compared in the young and elderly age groups. They have provided conflicting reports and no evidence of clear differences between the age groups. It is however still possible that there may be differences in the malignant behaviour of breast cancer between the young and old. The following study presents evidence of a marked change in the clinical growth rate of breast cancer at specific times in its life history. Some of the changes observed are related to known endocrine factors, some to presumed immunological factors, while others may be due to variations in tumour cell kinetics. Changes in growth pattern may be more prominent in certain age groups.

Mammary cancer can be regarded as a spectrum of tumours of widely differing biological potential, ranging from the acutely "inflammatory" type at one extreme to the indolent "dormant" type at the other. These different growth characteristics are thought to result from interaction between the proliferative and invasive potential of the tumour cells on the one hand, and changeable host factors on the other. It is now widely accepted that the host factors include both immunological and endocrinological factors. There is, in addition, a likelihood that they involve psychosomatic factors (see Chapters 5 and 12), and the release by injury of unidentified growth factors (Crile, 1975), which can stimulate the tumour to metastasise.

Not only endocrinological activity, but also immunological activity can vary with the age of the patient (Roberts-Thomson *et al.*, 1974), and differences in the behaviour of breast cancer between young and elderly patients might therefore be attributable to either factor. There is another possible explanation. Postmenopausal breast cancer may have a biological activity different from that of premenopausal breast cancer.

In Western women, a distinctive feature of the incidence of breast cancer is the progressive increase in risk with advancing age, even into the eighth and ninth decades of life (Fig. 1). Among the populations of Asia, Africa and Latin America on the other hand, the overall incidence of breast cancer is low and is associated with a risk increasing only until the age of 45, after which it plateaus or may even show a fall (Doll, Payne and Waterhouse, 1966).

There is increasing epidemiological evidence that the development of premenopausal breast cancer is mainly influenced through genetic and ovarian influences, while the tumour appearing after the menopause is more influenced by socio-environmental and adrenal influences (see Chapter 2). This has led to the suggestion that the growth of the universal premenopausal type of breast cancer depends on the relative proportions of the ovarian oestrogen fractions. The postmenopausal type on the other hand (confined mainly to the Western world) is thought to be influenced by steroids originating in the adrenal cortex (Hems, 1967; de Waard, 1969).

There seem to be consequent differences in the hormonal requirements for growth between premenopausal and postmenopausal breast cancers.

Whereas the administration of physiological doses of oestrogen may stimulate tumour growth in the premenopausal woman, high doses of oestrogen can cause regression of tumour growth in a proportion of older patients. Although stressed by Hems (1967), this difference between oestrogen "dependent" and oestrogen "responsive" types of tumour is by no means absolute. Very high dosage of oestrogen has been reported to cause regression of premenopausal breast cancer also (Kennedy, 1962), while oestrogen therapy can stimulate tumour growth occasionally in the older age group also, although it is increasingly less likely with advancing age (Stoll, 1972).

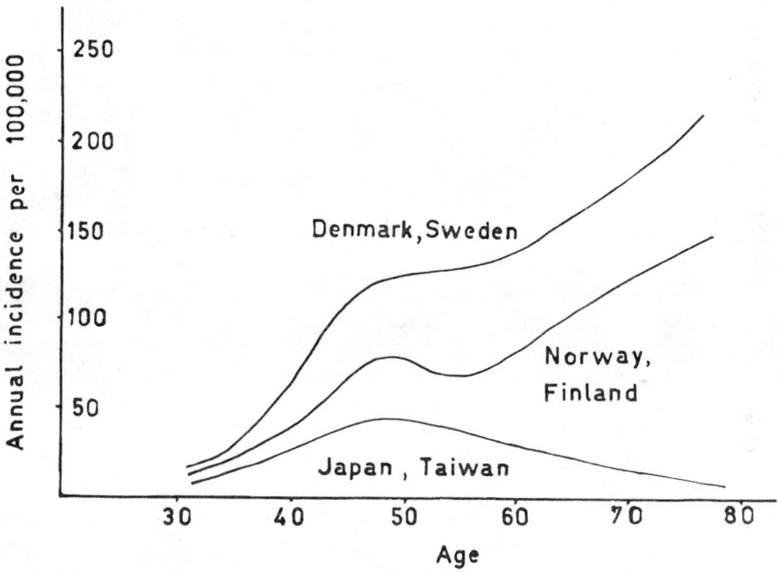

Fig. 1. Diagrammatic representation of age specific incidence of breast cancer in six countries (data from Doll *et al.*, 1966).

In some populations a trough or depression has been observed in the incidence curve of breast cancer, usually occurring in the age group between 50 and 55 (Clemmesen, 1948; de Waard, Baanders van Halewijn and Huizinga, 1964). The trough in the incidence curve is not seen in all of the high incidence populations (Fig. 1). It may be a gap between the incidence of the two aetiological types of tumour. Alternatively, it may be due to slowing up of the tumour growth around the time of the menopause (Clemmesen, 1948). This is the view adopted in this section and the evidence for it is discussed in detail later.

PROGNOSIS IN RELATION TO AGE

Is breast cancer in the young woman more aggressive and associated with a relatively poor prognosis? There is no firm evidence to support such a belief apart from the somewhat poorer prognosis associated with breast cancer complicating pregnancy which is discussed in Chapter 10. Haagensen (1971) mentions "the clinical impression that the prognosis from breast cancer in young women is not as good as in older patients". Support for this view is provided by the survival rates quoted in some of the earlier reported breast cancer series (Taylor and Wallace, 1947; Smithers *et al.*, 1952; Lewison, Trimble and Griffith, 1953; Kleinfeld, Haagensen and Cooley, 1963).

However, the vast majority of recent series report 5 year survival rates in young women which are not significantly different from those of other age groups (MacDonald and Wilcox, 1956; Moore and Lewis, 1964; Lefall, Ewing and White, 1965; Byrd *et al.*, 1966; Watson, 1966; Horsley, Alrich and Wright, 1969; Peters, 1970). The only large reported series of patients under the age of 35 is of 549 cases treated at the New York Memorial Center (Treves and Holleb, 1958). Their 5 year clinical cure rate was 30.7%, which is similar to that of patients of other age groups treated at the Center at the same time.

The stage of the disease at presentation is probably the most important factor which can be correlated with prognosis in breast cancer. If the survival and cure rates are no different, is it possible that the common assumption of a more malignant character to breast cancer in the young woman is based upon a more florid presentation, such as an "inflammatory" appearance or a larger tumour? Many clinicians have the impression that an inflammatory appearance in the primary tumour is seen more commonly in the young patient. However, it has been authoritatively stated that the age distribution of the inflammatory type of breast cancer is no different from that of the other clinical types (Haagensen, 1971). Moreover, in spite of a general belief to the contrary, there is no increase in the proportion of women with inflammatory carcinoma presenting either in pregnancy or in lactation.

Haagensen (1971) notes that at presentation, the average diameter of breast cancer found in the young woman is larger than in other age groups, and deduces that this is a sign of more rapid tumour growth. Fisher finds similarly that larger tumours are more common in the younger patient (Chapter 6). On the other hand, many clinicians report that cancer of the breast at presentation shows a higher proportion of locally more advanced cases in the elderly woman than in other age groups (Kraft and Block, 1962; Philip, 1967; Schottenfeld and Robbins, 1967). This is confirmed in a personal series of 1141 breast cancer patients followed until death which showed the proportion with locally advanced tumours at presentation to be almost twice as high in the oldest age group as in the youngest (Table 1). Nor can one assume that a larger tumour at presentation necessarily reflects a more rapidly growing tumour. Larger tumours (in elderly patients, at least) are often associated with a longer history of tumour growth and may represent a slowly mitosing tumour (Delarue *et al.*, 1965; Bloom, 1965; Fisher, 1969; Bond, 1975).

Table 1 Proportion of locally advanced cases at presentation among 1141 women with breast cancer. Subdivided according to age group.

Age Group	*Locally advanced Percentage*	*Numbers*
Under 40	18%	19/109
40 to 49	14%	30/221
50 to 59	20%	50/248
60 to 69	27%	71/262
Over 70	35%	106/301

So far, therefore, we have found no clear evidence of either a poorer survival or a more advanced presentation of the tumour to account for the more malignant behaviour which is commonly ascribed to breast cancer in the young woman. No more is there clear evidence of the less malignant behaviour which is usually ascribed to breast cancer in the elderly woman. Although locally advanced disease appears to be more common at presentation, the mortality rate from breast cancer in the elderly patient is reported to be no different from that in younger age groups (Bloom, 1950; Ratzkowski and Hochman, 1961; Kraft and Block, 1962).

One factor may give the clinician the *impression* that breast cancer is less malignant in the elderly woman. Deaths from intercurrent disease in the elderly group would eliminate patients who might otherwise have shown evidence of recurrent disease. When however, allowance is made for deaths from intercurrent disease, the breast cancer mortality in the elderly is no different from that in other age groups (Devitt, 1970).

HISTOPATHOLOGY IN RELATION TO AGE

Having so far discovered no firm clinical evidence of a difference between the behaviour of breast cancer in the young woman and that in the elderly, is there any histopathological evidence of such a difference? It is now believed by many that histological examination of the excised tissue at mastectomy may reflect not only the proliferative and invasive potential of the tumour, but also the degree of host resistance in the breast cancer patient (see Chapter 6).

Although histological grading of breast cancer may be a somewhat subjective procedure, it is thought to reflect the aggressive potential of the tumour, and several reports have claimed that it can be correlated with the prognosis (Scarff and Patey, 1928; Bloom, 1950; Champion, Wallace and Prescott, 1972). According to the earlier reports, the proportion of the various histological grades was said to show little variation with age (Lees and Park, 1949; Bloom, 1950). Later reports disagree however, and suggest a somewhat greater proportion of higher grade tumours in women under the age of 30 (Brightmore, Greening and Hamlin, 1970), or a greater proportion of lower grade tumours in elderly women (Berg and Robbins, 1961; Barnett and Eisenberg, 1964). Fisher (1975) confirms in his series a higher proportion of more anaplastic tumours with decreasing age.

Pathologists recognize that in addition to grading, the structural type of breast cancer may give a clue to its clinical behaviour. Thus, some types rarely metastasize widely and of these, the intraductal and medullary types are said to represent a relatively higher proportion of tumours in young woman (Norris and Taylor, 1970). On the other hand, the papillary and colloid types are said to be more common in elderly women (Schottenfeld and Robbins, 1967).

We noted at the beginning of this chapter that the prognosis of breast cancer depends on host factors as well as on the aggressive potential of the tumour. The presence of a lymphoid infiltrate in and around the tumour, and of sinus histiocytosis in the regional nodes, is thought by some to be a manifestation of host defence (Black, Opler and Speer, 1955; Black, 1975). Little information is so far available as to the comparative prominence of such histopathological evidence of host defence in young and elderly women respectively.

Some have claimed that both sinus histiocytosis of the draining nodes and plasma cell infiltrates around breast cancers are better developed in premenopausal women than in older women (Berg and Robbins, 1970). Fisher (1975) has found no relationship between age and the presence of sinus histiocytosis, although he confirms the significantly greater likelihood of lymphoid infiltrates in the younger patient. This latter reaction he believes to be more closely related to the histological degree of malignancy of the tumour than it is to an immunological response by the host (see Chapter 6). This would explain its greater frequency in the younger patients in his series.

It has been suggested by some that a "discriminant" based on the histopathology of the primary tumour at the time of primary surgery may be able to predict the clinical progress of the disease (Hartveit, 1971). Its inherent limitation is that it takes no account of host defence factors either in the blood or lymph nodes at the time of the operation. It also ignores subsequent changes in the endocrinological or immunological milieu of the tumour which can influence the course of the disease. The importance of these factors will now be discussed.

CLINICAL GROWTH RATE IN RELATION TO AGE

It has been suggested that the clinical growth rate of breast cancer can be used to compare the degree of malignancy of tumours. One supposed measure of clinical growth rate is the delay between primary resection of a breast cancer and the first clinical manifestation of recurrence or metastasis. Haagensen's group have suggested that the clinical growth rate of breast cancer is slower in the older patient because they found the average time before the appearance of recurrence or metastasis to be more prolonged in women over the age of 65 (Papadrianos, Cooley and Haagensen, 1965).

However, different site factors may influence the development of scar, lymph node and blood borne metastases respectively, and subclinical metastases at the latter sites may already be present at the time of primary treatment. For this reason, I have restricted the comparison of recurrence-free intervals to scar recurrences only (Stoll and Ackland, 1970), and showed no significant differences between the various age groups. The percentage of women showing the first scar recurrence within 3 years of mastectomy was not significantly different between the age groups (Table 2). This observation suggests that the *average* rate of tumour growth in the scar from microscopic size to minimum measurable lesion, is similiar in young, middle aged and elderly women.

Table 2 Proportion of women developing the first scar recurrence within 3 years of mastectomy, subdivided according to age group. Personal series of 1141 breast cancer patients (from Stoll and Ackland, 1970, with permission).

Age Group	*Scar Recurrence within 3 years* *Percentage*	*Numbers*
Under 50	20%	74
50 to 59	23%	57
60 to 69	22%	50
Over 70	29%	24

It is remarkable however that the *range* of recurrence free intervals found in these cases varied over a hundredfold, from 2 months to over 20 years. Does each breast cancer maintain its individual aggressive potential throughout its subclinical and clinical course? Alternatively, does the growth rate change at specific times in its clinical life history in some individuals? The following evidence suggests that changes in growth rate might result from changes in the endocrinological or immunological status of the host or from other factors, such as variations in tumour cell kinetics.

(a) Retardation of growth

It is well established that in some patients, the recurrence-free interval may show considerable prolongation when the natural menopause intervenes some time after the primary treatment (Clemmesen, 1948; Smithers *et al.*, 1952; Hadfield and Holt, 1956; AMA Committee on Research, 1960). The mechanism is not clear and it is uncertain whether the implantation of metastases is delayed in such cases, or whether their subclinical growth is delayed. The latter seems more likely as the menopause can cause measurable slowing also in the *clinical* growth of metastases (Stoll, 1972). Moreover, the average survival time after the diagnosis of disseminated disease is prolonged in such patients (Cutler, Asire and Taylor, 1969, 1970).

In a series of 8481 breast cancer patients, Peters (1970) has found the highest survival rates (corrected for other causes of death) at 15 to 20 years after primary treatment, to be in women presenting between the ages of 45 and 59. It is important to note that the improved survival rate in this group of patients was not apparent at 5 years after treatment. The best survival rates in all the group were in patients presenting within 5 years after an artificial menopause. Mustakallio (1972) also has observed that the corrected survival rate at 15 to 20 years after excision of breast cancer combined with radiation, was greater in women who were under 65 years of age at the time of treatment than in those over 65 years of age.

Herrmann (1972) in a review of 34 patients manifesting their first metastasis or recurrence more than 20 years after mastectomy, notes that the average age of these patients was 43.1 at the time of the first treatment. This is about 10 years younger than the median age at presentation in most reported series of breast cancer. In my personal series there were 21 who showed the first evidence of clinical recurrence 10 years or longer after the primary treatment. Of the 21 cases, 19 were aged between 40 and 59 at the time of presentation.

These reports point to the age group between 40 and 59 as that when a proportion of women with breast cancer show considerable slowing in the clinical growth rate of their tumours. However, it seems that the change in growth rate will not normally be reflected in the 5 year survival rate, but is best demonstrated either by considerable delay in the appearance of metastasis or recurrence, or by an improvement in the corrected survival rate after the lapse of 10 to 15 years. There is little to confirm the

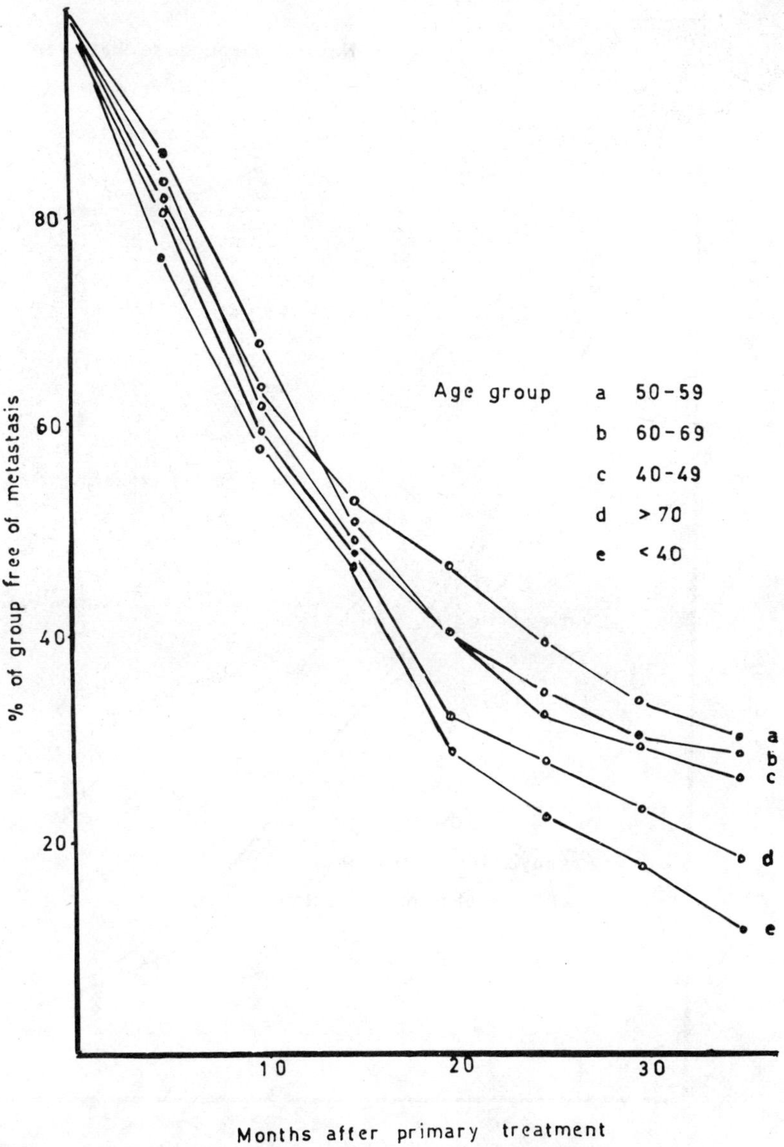

Fig 2. Duration of freedom from metastases after primary treatment in breast cancer, according to age group (in 786 patients who died of the disease).

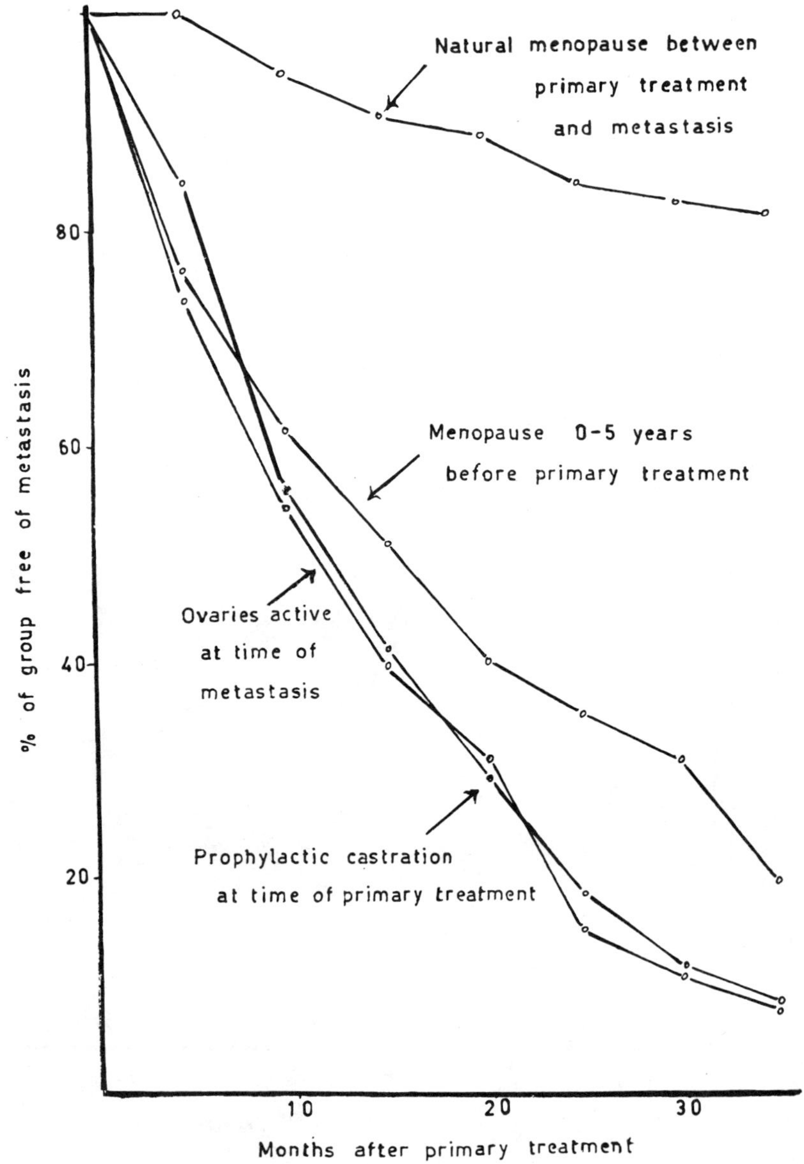

Fig. 3 Duration of freedom from metastases after primary treatment in breast cancer, according to ovarian status (in 409 patients who died of the disease).

suggestion of Peters (1970) that this flattening of the survival curve after 15 years in women between 40 and 59 may represent evidence of clinical *cure*. Many of these patients ultimately die of their disease (Herrman, 1972).

The above observations suggest that it should be possible to identify a slowing up of tumour growth in a selected group of breast cancer patients at the approach to the menopause. It is not surprising from what has been said above that some writers have found no improvement in the overall 5 year survival rate of women presenting in the premenopausal age group (MacMahon, List and Eisenberg, 1968; Singer *et al.*, 1972). Only a small proportion of such a group are affected by endocrinological control of tumour growth. It should be possible however, to show evidence of delayed recurrence after primary treatment if women approaching the menopause are subdivided according to their ovarian status *at the time of tumour dissemination.*

This was done in a personal series of 1141 breast cancer patients followed until death. First of all, the proportion of women remaining recurrence free month by month was plotted separately for each decade of age. It is seen in Fig. 2 that the recurrence-free curves for women under 40 and for those aged over 70 are slightly lower than those for the other age groups, but the difference is small. However, when recurrence-free curves were plotted for women under the age of 59, subdivided according to their ovarian status, marked differences became apparent bettween the various categories (Fig. 3).

Of the women in whom the natural menopause occurred subsequent to the primary treatment but before the appearance of metastases, 80% were still recurrence-free at 3 years after the primary treatment. This is in marked contrast to those women whose ovaries remained active, of whom only 8% were recurrence-free after 3 years. At five years after primary treatment, 46% of the former group were still recurrence free. It should be noted that the two groups mentioned were in no way distinguishable at primary treatment except that the mean age was higher in the former group. These figures are intended to show delayed recurrence in certain groups, but do not represent the overall salvage rate. The analysis is only of women who died of the disease.

When the crude survival curves for the period after the appearance of metastases were plotted for the women under the age of 59, differences were again apparent according to their ovarian status (Fig. 4). The longest survival was in women in whom the natural menopause occurred between the time of primary treatment and the appearance of metastases. Of the groups whose ovaries were still active at the time of the first metastasis, the ones who were healther were selected for therapeutic castration and are obviously a selected group compared to those who were not castrated.

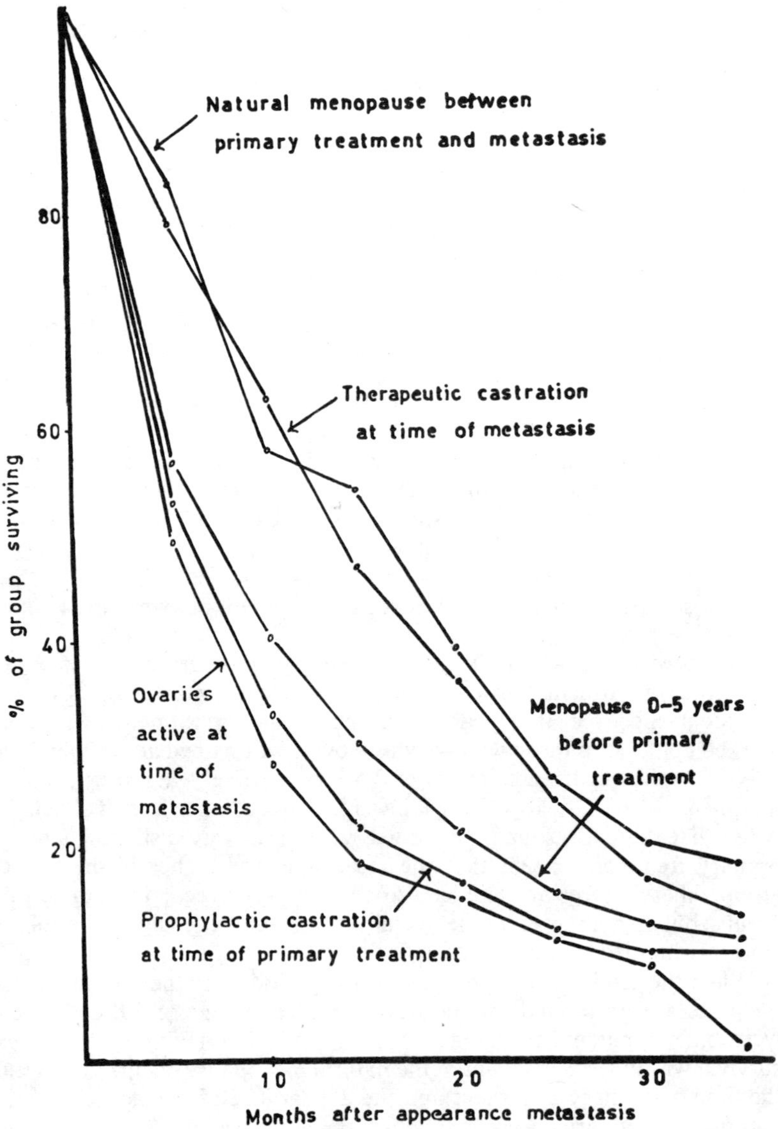

Fig 4. Duration of survival after appearance of metastases in breast cancer, according to ovarian status (in 409 patients who died of the disease).

(b) The "shower of metastases"

Most clinicians have a clear impression that breast cancer may suddenly throw off growth restraint at a particular point in its clinical life history. It is common to see a sudden shower of metastases and early death, even in patients who have been free from recurrence for a very long time after primary treatment. Expressed more scientifically, the ratio between the recurrence-free interval and the interval from metastasis to death varies widely from patient to patient. Yet, if the growth curve of breast cancer were of an exponential type, one would expect the ratio to be fairly constant (Devitt, 1971).

Devitt has made a similar observation based on mortality rates in breast cancer (see Chapter 7). He notes the constant annual mortality rate for each stage which has been reported by many observers, and suggests that the factors responsible for the restraint of tumour growth appear to decay at a constant rate. When the restraints reach a critical level of failure, the existing metastatic foci show sudden activation of growth.

Table 3 Proportion of women surviving more than 2 years after the first metastasis in relation to the recurrence-free interval (Numbers of patients in brackets). From a personal series of 1141 breast cancer patients.

	Recurrence-free interval	
	Under 12 months	*Over 5 years*
Surviving over 2 years after mets.	13% (41/318)	26% (20/76)
Total surviving	16% (61/394)	

This change in growth rate is demonstrated in Table 3 in figures derived from a personal series of breast cancer patients followed up until death. Whether the first metastasis appears within 12 months after primary treatment or is delayed for 5 years or more, does not make a great difference to the length of the subsequent survival in the majority of cases. Similar observations have been made by others (Pawlias, Dockerty and Ellis, 1958; Papaioannou, Tang and Volk, 1967).

My personal experience had given me the impression that sudden activation of growth was a more prominent feature of breast cancer in the younger woman. This would give the clinician the impression of a more malignant behaviour of the disease, but how could it be defined and measured?

Every clinician is familiar with the breast cancer patient who shows in rapid succession the involvement of two or more of the three major localizations of metastases (regional, osseous and visceral), and dies within 18 months of the first metastasis. Applying this criterion to the 21 patients in my series who had survived without recurrence for 10 years or longer following primary treatment, I found that 14 of the 21 had behaved in this fashion. I named this pattern "a shower of metastases" and looked for it in the 764 patients in my series treated primarily for Stage 1 or 2 breast cancer.

Table 4 Proportion of women developing a "shower of metastases" within 18 months preceding death. Subdivided according to age group. (Numbers of patients in brackets.) From a personal series of 1141 breast cancer patients.

	"Shower of metastases"	
Age group	*Total*	*Within 3 years of primary treatment*
Under 40	62% (50/81)	46% (37/81)
40 to 49	52% (91/175)	34% (60/175)
50 to 59	48% (88/181)	28% (52/181)
60 to 69	38% (60/159)	25% (40/159)
Over 70	14% (23/168)	9% (15/168)

The results are shown in Table 4 where the patients are subdivided according to age group. A shower of metastases occurs within 18 months of death in 62% of women under the age of 40 at the time of treatment. The proportion decreases steadily with each decade so that in women over 70, the proportion is only 14%. The difference between the age groups is statistically significant at the $p<0.01$ level. It is not less marked in cases with short recurrence-free intervals because I have also recorded the proportion for each decade showing a shower of metastases within 36 months of primary treatment, and we find the differences between the age groups to be equally marked.

This sudden failure of host defence is not confined to the perimenopausal group and it probably reflects immunological rather than endocrinological factors. It is generally accepted that immunological responses are normally stronger in the younger patients (Robert–Thomson *et al.*, 1974). They may possibly also be more easily damaged in the younger patient. Stjernswaard (1974) points out that the addition of radiotherapy after mastectomy for breast cancer decreased the survival rates in five controlled studies and comments that when the patients were subdivided according to age, it was found that the effect was confined to younger premenopausal patients. This aspect of breast cancer management is deserving of considerably more investigation.

The localization of metastases in breast cancer is probably determined by site factors. Some of these also may have an immunological basis, and thus can be influenced by the patient's age group. Peters (1970) has noted that initial skeletal metastases after radical treatment in Stage 1 were more than twice as common in younger patients as in those aged over 60. The more frequent diagnosis of liver metastases in younger patients is stressed by Bengmark, Hafstroem and Olsson (1972) who noted that only 20% of patients with clinical evidence of liver metastases were aged over 60.

Other observations also suggest a relatively greater failure of immunological defences in younger patients dying of breast cancer. Patients under the age of 50 have been found at autopsy to have a larger number of sites involved by metastases than did patients over 50 (Viadana *et al.*, 1973). This was most evident for metastases in bone, liver and endocrine glands. It may be relevant that autopsy findings in breast cancer patients treated with corticosteroids show an unusual distribution of metastases also (Iversen and Hjort, 1958: Sherlock and Hartmann, 1962).

More observations are needed to investigate age-related differences in the spread of metastases and the suggestion of a possible relationship to immunological factors. In particular, we should establish whether a sudden shower of metastases is due to sudden breakdown of host resistance and confirm that this is the reason for the more malignant reputation of breast cancer in the younger patient.

(c) Changes in tumour doubling time

In the case of experimental tumours it has been established that as the tumour increases in size, so there is a tendency for tumour growth to slow up (Laird, 1965). This almost certainly applies to human cancer also (Hall and Laing, 1968; Skipper, 1971), and measurements confirming this have been shown in superficial and pulmonary tumours in breast cancer (Brennan, 1966). Slowing up of tumour growth can occur either as a result of changes in tumour kinetics or host factors. The mechanism may be a prolongation of the intermitotic interval or a reduction in the proportion of the cells dividing at any one time (Hall and Laing, 1968).

Yet surprisingly, there is a widespread assumption among clinicians that the growth of breast cancer proceeds at a constant rate. On this basis, several investigators (detailed in Chapter 7) have stressed the importance of calculating tumour doubling times, using serial measurements of the volume of the primary growth or of its metastases. It should be stressed that the tumour volume does *not* reflect the rate of tumour cell proliferation as over 90% of the cell proliferation may be lost.

A recent investigation of this type calculated the doubling time for primary breast cancer and its metastases to be less than three months in half the cases examined, and less than eight months in three quarters of all cases

(Kusama *et al.*, 1972). Tumour doubling time was said to be shorter in patients under the age of 30 and longer in patients over the age of 60, and the report concluded that the tumour doubling time could be related to the duration of survival after treatment.

Can such observations have any prognostic significance if there is a tendency for tumour growth to slow up with advancing disease or at the time of the menopause, and accelerate at the time of metastasis? These questions are even more relevant when it is even possible that the primary tumour and the various metastases may represent different clones, and that tumour doubling time may differ between the primary tumour and its metastases (Kusama *et al.*, 1972), or even between different metastases in the same organ (Macdonald, 1966).

Just as it cannot be assumed that all the clones of the patient's tumour have a similar doubling time, so it cannot be assumed that they all have a similar capacity to establish or maintain metastases (Carter, 1975). Nor that they all have similar hormone dependence or are all similarly capable of stimulating cell mediated or humoral defence factors. These may be some of the reasons why the clinical behaviour of breast cancer presents such a varied pattern, and why age related trends are so difficult to demonstrate.

CONCLUSION

No factual basis has been shown in the past for the common belief that breast cancer in the younger woman behaves in a more malignant manner than the average, or that in the elderly patient it behaves in a less malignant manner. There are almost infinite variations in the biological behaviour of breast cancer and no clear differences have been shown between the various age groups either in survival rate, clinical presentation, recurrence-free interval or histopathological picture.

Nevertheless, it is clear that changes in the tumour-host relationship at specific times can lead to changes in the rate of tumour growth – either retardation or acceleration. Such changes in tumour growth rate are reviewed critically in this section and are related as far as is possible, to known endocrinological factors or to presumed immunological factors. A sudden "shower of metastases" is shown to be more prominent in younger age groups.

If it is established that changes in host defence can lead to changes in the pattern of tumour growth, then a tumour doubling time derived from the primary tumour, or a "histopathological discriminant" derived at the time of primary treatment, can be of only limited usefulness in providing a pointer to the prognosis in the individual patient.

REFERENCES

A.M.A. Committee on Research (1960): Androgen and estrogen in the treatment of disseminated mammary carcinoma. *J. Amer. Med. Assoc.* **172,** 1271.

Barnett, R. N. and Eisenberg, H. (1964): Histopathological grading in breast cancer. *Conn. Med.* **28,** 123.

Bengmark, S., Hafstroem, L. and Olsson, A. (1972): The natural history of primary and secondary liver tumours. *Digestion,* **6,** 321.

Berg, J. W. and Robbins, G. F. (1961): Modified mastectomy for older poor risk patients. *Surg. Gynec. Obst.,* **113,** 631.

Berg, J. W. and Robbins, G. F. (1970); In *Breast Cancer, Early and Late.* Year book Medical Publishers, Chicago, p. 19.

Black, M. M. (1975): In *Host Defence in Breast Cancer.* Ed. B. A. Stoll, Heinemann medical, London, p. 48.

Black, M. M., Opler, S. R. and Speer, F. D. (1955): Survival in breast cancer cases in relation to structure of the primary tumour and regional lymph nodes. *Surg., Gynec. Obst.,* **100,** 543.

Bloom, H. J. G. (1950): Further studies on prognosis of breast cancer. *Brit. J. Cancer,* **4,** 347.

Bloom, H. J. G. (1965): The influence of delay on the natural history and prognosis of breast cancer. *Brit. J. Cancer,* **19,** 228.

Bond, W. H. (1975): In *Host Defence in Breast Cancer.* Ed. B. A. Stoll, Heinemann Medical, London, p. 95.

Brennan, M. J. (1966): In *Clinical Evaluation in Breast Cancer.* Eds. J. E. Hayward and R. D. Bulbrook, Academic Press, London, p. 141.

Brightmore, T. G. J., Greening, W. P. and Hamlin, I. (1970): An analysis of clinical and histopathological features in 101 cases of carcinoma of the breast in women under 35 years of age. *Brit. J. Cancer,* **24,** 644.

Byrd, B. F., Stephenson, S. E., Burch, J. C. *et al.* (1966): Type of mastectomy in cancer of the breast. *Ann. Surg.,* **163,** 746.

Carter, R. L. (1975): In *Host Defence in Breast Cancer.* Ed. B. A. Stoll, Heinemann Medical, London, p. 6.

Champion, H. R., Wallace, I. W. and Prescott, R. J. (1972); Histology in breast cancer prognosis. *Brit. J. Cancer,* **26,** 129.

Clemmesen, J. (1948): Carcinoma of the breast. Results from statistical research. *Brit. J. Radiol.,* **21,** 583.

Crile, G. Jr. (1975): In *Host Defence in Breast Cancer.* Ed. B. A. Stoll, Heinemann Medical, London, p. 121.

Cutler, S. J., Asire, A. J. and Taylor, S. G. (1969): Classification of patients with disseminated cancer of the breast. *Cancer (Phil.)* **24,** 861.

Cutler, S. J., Asire, A. J. and Taylor, S. G. (1970): An evaluation of ovarian status as a prognostic factor in disseminated cancer of the breast. *Cancer (Phil.),* **26,** 938.

Delarue, W. C., Ash C. L., Peters, V. and Fielden, R. (1965): Preoperative irradiation in management of locally advanced breast cancer. *Arch. Surg.,* **91,** 136.

Devitt, J. E. (1970): The influence of age on the behaviour of carcinoma of the breast. *Canad. Med. Assoc. J.,* **103,** 923.

Devitt, J. E. (1971): The enigmatic behaviour of breast cancer. *Cancer (Phil.)* **27,** 12.

De Waard, F. (1969): The epidemiology of breast cancer: Review and prospects. *Int. J. Cancer.* **4,** 577.

De Waard, F., Baanders-van Halewijn, E. A. and Huizinga, J. (1964): The bimodal age distribution of patients with mammary carcinoma. *Cancer (Phil.),* **17,** 141.

Doll, R., Payne, P. and Waterhouse, J. (1966): *Cancer incidence in 5 continents.* Springer Verlag, Berlin.

Fisher, B. (1969): Prospects for the control of metastases. *Cancer (Phil.),* **24,** 1263.

Fisher, B. (1975): Personal communication.

Haagensen, C. D. (1971): Diseases of the Breast, 2nd Edition, W. B. Saunders Co. Philadelphia, London.

Hadfield, G. J., and Holt, J. A. G. (1956): The physiological castration syndrome in breast cancer. *Brit. Med. J.,* **2,** 972.

Hall, E. J. and Laing, A. H. (1968): In *Prognostic Factors in Breast Cancer.* Eds. A. P. M. Forrest and P. B. Kunkler, E. and S. Livingstone, Edinburgh, p. 275.

Hartveit, F. (1971): Prognostic typing in breast cancer. *Brit. Med. J.* **4,** 253.

Hems, G. (1967): Two types of breast cancer. *Brit. Med. J.,* **3,** 496.

Herrmann, J. B. (1972): Chronicity of mammary carcinoma. *New York State, J. Med.,* **72,** 2310.

Horsley, J. S., Alrich, E. M. and Wright, C. B. (1969): Carcinoma of the breast in women 35 years of age or younger. *Ann. Surg.,* **169,** 839.

Iversen, H. G. and Hjort, G. H. (1958): The influence of corticosteroids on the frequency of spleen metastases in patients with breast cancer. *Acta Path. Microbiol. Scand.,* **44,** 205.

Kennedy, B. J. (1962): Massive estrogen administration in premenopausal women with metastatic breast cancer. *Cancer (Phil.),* **15,** 641.

Kleinfeld, G., Haagensen, C. D. and Cooley, E. (1963): Age and menstrual status as prognostic factors in carcinoma of the breast. *Ann. Surg.,* **156,** 600.

Kraft, R. O. and Block, G. E. (1962): Mammary carcinoma in the aged patient. *Ann. Surg.,* **156,** 981.

Kusama, S., Spratt, J. S., Donegan, W. L. *et al.* (1972): The gross rates of growth of human mammary carcinoma. *Cancer (Phil.),* **30,** 594.

Laird, A. K. (1965): Dynamics of tumour growth and comparison of growth rates. *Brit. J. Cancer,* **19,** 278.

Lees, J. C. and Park, W. M. (1949): The malignancy of cancer at different ages. A histological study. *Brit. J. Cancer,* **3,** 186.

Lefall, L. D., Ewing, J. B. and White, J. L. (1965): Cancer of the breast in young Negro patients. *Amer. J. Surg.,* **109,** 404.

Lewison, E. F., Trimble, F. J. and Griffith, P. C. (1953): Results of surgical treatment of breast cancer at Johns Hopkins Hospital. *J. Amer. Med. Assoc.,* **153,** 905.

MacDonald, J. S. (1966): In *Clinical Evaluation of Breast Cancer.* Eds. J. L. Hayward and R. D. Bulbrook, New York Academic Press, p. 11.

Macdonald, I. and Wilcox, R. E. (1956): Prognosis of mammary carcinoma in young women. *Cancer (Phil.),* **9,** 281.

MacMahon, B., List, N. D. and Eisenberg, H. (1968): In *Prognosttic Factors in Breast Cancer.* Eds. A. P. M. Forrest and P. B. Kunkler, E. and S. Livingstone, Edinburgh, p. 56.

Moore, S. W. and Lewis, R. J. (1964): Carcinoma of the breast in women 30 years and under. *Surg. Gynec. Obstet.,* **119,** 1253.

Mustakallio, S. (1972): Conservative treatment of breast carcinoma. Review of 25 years follow up. *Clin. Radiol.,* **23,** 110.

Norris, M. J. and Taylor, H. B. (1970): Carcinoma of the breast in women less than 30 years old. *Cancer (Phil.),* **26,** 953.

Papadrianos, E., Cooley, E. and Haagensen, C. D. (1965): Mammary carcinoma in old age. *Ann. Surg.,* **161,** 189.

Papaioannou, A. N., Tang, F. J. and Volk, H. (1967): Fate of patients with recurrent carcinoma of the breast. *Cancer (Phil.),* **20,** 371.

Pawlias, K. T., Dockerty, M. B. and Ellis, F. H. (1958): Late local recurrent carcinoma of the breast. *Ann. Surg.,* **148,** 192.

Peters, M. V. (1970): in *Breast Cancer, Early and Late.* Year Book Medical Publishers, Chicago, p. 171.

Philip, J. F. (1967): Results of treatment of breast cancer at Aberdeen Royal Infirmary, *Brit. Med. J.,* **1,** 323.

Ratzkowski, E. and Hochman, A. (1961): Survival of patients with recurrent or inoperable cancer of the breast. *Cancer (Phil.),* **14,** 300.

Roberts-Thomson, I. C., Whittingham, S., Youngchaiyud, V. and Mackay, I. R. (1974). Ageing, immune response and mortality, *Lancet,* **2,** 368.

Scarff, R. W. and Patey, D. H. (1928): The position of histology in the prognosis of carcinoma of the breast. *Lancet,* **1,** 801.

Schottenfeld, D. and Robbins, G. F. (1967): Breast cancer in elderly women. *Geriatrics,* **27** (March) p. 121.

Sherlock, P. and Hartmann, W. H. (1962): Adrenal steroids and the pattern of metastases from breast cancer. *J. Amer. Med. Assoc.,* **181,** 313.

Singer, A. M., Bennett, R. C., Frydenberg, H. *et al.* (1972) Carcinoma of the breast in women aged between 35 and 45 years. *Med. J. Australia,* **1,** 1200.

Skipper, H. E. (1971): Kinetics of mammary tumour cell growth and implications for therapy. *Cancer (Phil.),* **28,** 1479.
Smithers, D. W., Rigby-Jones, P., Galton, D. N. G. and Payne, P. M. (1952): Cancer of the breast – a review. *Brit. J. Radiol.,* Suppl. 1.
Stjernswaard, J. (1974): Decreased survival related to irradiation postoperatively in early operable breast cancer. *Brit. Med. J.,* **4,** 1285.
Stoll, B. A. (1972): In *Endocrine Therapy in Malignant Disease,* Ed. B. A. Stoll, W. B. Saunders, London, Philadelphia, p. 155.
Stoll, B. A. (1975): *Host Defence in Breast Cancer.* Ed. B. A. Stoll, Heinemann Medical, London.
Taylor, G. W. and Wallace, W. R. H. (1947): Carcinoma of the breast. *Surg. Clins., N. America,* **27,** 1151.
Treves, N. and Holleb, A. I. (1958): A report of 549 cases of breast cancer in women 35 years or younger. *Surg. Gynec. Obstet.,* **107,** 271.
Viadana, E., Cotter, R., Pickren, J. W. and Bross, I. D. J. (1973): An autopsy study of metastatic sites of breast cancer. *Cancer Res.,* **33,** 179.
Watson, T. A. (1966): Cancer of the breast, The Janeway Lecture. *Amer. J. Roent.,* **96,** 547.

9

Endogenous Hormones and Prognosis

H. Miller

That oestrogens initiate mammary carcinogenesis in the mouse is beyond doubt (Lacassagne, 1933); that oophorectomy influences the course of established human breast cancer is equally beyond doubt (Lewison, 1965); that the result of hormone ablative surgery for the treatment of advanced human breast cancer – adrenalectomy or hypophysectomy – can be predicted with some degree of accuracy is also beyond doubt (Bulbrook, 1965; Miller and Durant, 1968). It follows that the possibility of oestrogens, and perhaps of other hormones, acting as initiating or modifying factors in the aetiology of human breast cancer has deserved, and has received, serious attention.

From before puberty until up to two years after the menopause – a period of some 40 years – the female breast is subject to a regularly cycling fluctuation of its hormone controllers. In most subjects this pattern is disturbed for up to 15 months at a time, during and after each pregnancy, by even greater hormonal changes.

The commonest malignant growth in the male – of the bronchus – has been shown to be related to a chemical carcinogen. The commonest cancer in the female – of the breast – may equally well be the result of a chemical carcinogen, and our present knowledge, as summarized above, has suggested that it may be of an endogenous hormonal nature.

HORMONAL CONTROL OF BREAST DEVELOPMENT AND FUNCTION

Normal breast development and function is dependent upon a variety of hormones acting in combination or individually. Lyons, Li and Johnson (1958) found that oestrogens were responsible for mammary duct growth in rats and progesterone for the lobular pattern and acinar formation. Corticosteroids and growth hormone were required as synergists and their absence led to a loss of sensitivity of breast tissue to these two principal female sex hormones. Growth hormone caused the secretion of milk in the acini and thence to the duct lumina, provided that the breasts were primed with oestrogens and progesterone. In the human the place of growth hormone is probably taken by its close chemical relative, prolactin. Ejection of milk through the nipple required oxytocin.

Breast function can be modified by thyroid disease (*BMJ Annotation*, 1974). There is an increased incidence of breast cancer in women with reduced thyroid function and a reduced incidence of the disease in thyrotoxic women (Humphrey and Swerdlow, 1964). The effect of thyroid disease may be produced by alteration in prolactin secretion. Thyroid releasing hormone, a simple tripeptide which is secreted in the hypothalamus in response to low circulating thyroid hormone and promotes thyrotrophin secretion, also causes prolactin release. Prolactin, at least in rodents, may be the pituitary factor required for mammary carcinogenesis (Muhlbock and Burt, 1959; Kim and Furth, 1960).

It is apparent therefore that the breast is the target for a variety of hormones from a variety of endocrine tissues (Table 1).

Table 1

Hormones Influencing Mammary Tissue

Hypothalamus	Thyrotrophin releasing hormone Prolactin inhibiting hormone Gonadotrophin releasing hormone Corticotrophin releasing hormone
Pituitary	Follicle stimulating hormone Luteinising hormone Prolactin Growth hormone Corticotrophin Oxytocin
Ovary	Oestrogens, androgens Progesterone
Placenta	Progesterone Chorionic gonadotrophin Placental lactogen
Adrenals	Cortisol Androgens Oestrogens
Thyroid	Thyroid hormone

HORMONES AND THE DEVELOPMENT OF HUMAN BREAST CANCER

Since breast epithelium is so dependent upon the hormone "climate", the discoveries that oestrogens could initiate carcinogenesis in rodents, and that the established human disease could be partially controlled by hormone treatment should have come as no surprise. However it has been a disappointment that it has not proved possible to eradicate the human disease in individual cases except by surgical means in its early stages. Indeed, the ultimate prognosis once the disease is established is still no better than it was at the turn of the century. The main benefit of current hormonal therapy has been amelioration of symptoms rather than useful prolongation of life.

In 1896, Beatson first demonstrated the association between the ovaries and the progression of advanced human breast cancer. This effect was confirmed by Boyd (1900). At this time it was just becoming apparent that certain organs were capable of secreting substances – named 'hormones' by Bayliss and Starling – which were able to influence the activity of other organs. It was soon recognized that the ovaries were hormone secretors and it was a short step to the concept that cancer of the breast might be associated with the ovarian hormones.

In 1919, Loeb demonstrated that it was possible to decrease the incidence of breast cancer in a high risk strain of mice, by oophorectomy, if it was carried out within three months of birth. Subsequently Murray (1928) produced mammary cancer in castrated male mice by grafting ovarian tissue subcutaneously. Lacassagne (1933) finally demonstrated the effect of injected extract of ovarian follicles in producing mammary cancer in male mice. It was clear that the ovarian follicular hormones – oestrogens – were carcinogenic substances in the mouse. It was subsequently shown that the production of experimental mouse mammary cancer by oestrogen implantation was dose related (Shimkin and Wyman, 1946).

The place of hormones in the aetiology of human breast cancer is much more difficult to assess because similar observations are obviously not possible in the human. The evidence therefore for a hormonal cause of human breast cancer is circumstantial and inconclusive.

OESTROGENS AND HUMAN BREAST CANCER

Most studies have been concerned with determining urinary oestrogen patterns in women with breast cancer. Stern *et al.* (1964) found that women with breast cancer excreted significantly greater amounts of oestriol and lesser amounts of oestrone and oestradiol. The changes were most marked in their pre-menopausal patients. However similar results to their post-menopausal patients were found in elderly men with prostatic cancer. Marmorston *et al.* (1965) confirmed these findings in breast cancer patients but found similar patterns in women with benign breast disease.

The position became more confused when Lemon *et al.* (1966) obtained dissimilar results. They found that their breast cancer patients excreted a lesser proportion of total oestrogens as oestriol than healthy women. Further, they suggested that oestriol, which is a metabolite with weak anti-oestrogenic properties, had protective effects against the possibly carcinogenic action of the most active of the classical oestrogens, oestradiol.

Cole and MacMahon (1969) when reviewing the carcinogenic properties of oestrogenic hormones in early reproductive life, were of the opinion that it was more important to study urinary oestrogen excretion patterns in women before they developed breast cancer. This idea certainly seems sensible when the long latent period between the administration of oestrogens and the development of breast cancer in the experimental animal is taken into account. MacMahon *et al.* (1971) followed this up by studying groups of normal women in the early and late stages of reproductive life. They compared Asian with N. American women since the former have a much lower incidence of the disease than the latter group. They found that oestriol excretion was higher, and that oestrone and oestradiol excretion were lower in the Asian women than in the N. American women, and these changes were most marked in the younger age group.

Lipsett (1971) soon challenged these findings. He argued that oestriol was a weak oestrogen as judged by its effects on vaginal epithelial cornification and its capacity to cause withdrawal bleeding, rather than an anti-oestrogen. Further he pointed out that urinary excretion of the three oestrogens have little resemblance to their relative levels in plasma. He conceded, however, that different groups of women might have different metabolic pathways for these natural oestrogens. But Hellman *et al.* (1967) had already shown that both normal women and women with breast cancer metabolized administered oestradiol in similar fashion.

The question whether oestrogens are carcinogenic in women remains unanswered. As will be seen, the progress of human breast cancer is also associated with altered patterns of other hormones of pituitary and adrenocortical origin.

CONCEPT OF HORMONE DEPENDENCY

Beatson's original observations have been amply confirmed by Lewison (1965). In an extensive literature review he found that about one third of women with the advanced disease benefited from surgical or radiotherapeutic castration. Despite the later introduction of the radical endocrine ablative procedures of adrenalectomy and hypophysectomy (Huggins and Bergenstal, 1952; Luft and Olivecrona, 1953), the overall ratio of improvement of one third has not been excelled, although they have helped some women who failed to respond to, or who relapsed after, ovarian ablation.

With the exception of the value of oophorectomy in the premenopausal woman, the greatest benefit of the surgical ablation procedures or of the administration of hormones has been obtained in post-menopausal women (Pearson, 1973). Quite apart from the effects of endogenous hormone interference, beneficial results have been obtained in many cases by hormone administration, although in some cases there appears to have been an acceleration of the disease progress.

The partially satisfactory response to the use of the endocrine ablation procedures, and of administered hormones, has led to the concept that some human mammary cancers are hormone dependent and others are not. The latter are considered to be "autonomous" tumours, i.e. not influenced by circulating hormones. Since even hormone dependent tumours eventually resume their aggressive nature, despite the initial benefit obtained from hormone interference, and become autonomous, it has been considered that even autonomous tumours might have been hormone dependent at some stage during their development.

Even if it is assumed that all tumours are hormone dependent at some stage in their growth, it does not necessarily follow that they were initiated by hormone action. Hormone dependency may be a factor in the tumour development only after its initiation by a non-hormone carcinogen. It is not possible with our present knowledge to confirm or deny that hormones act as mammary carcinogens in the human subject.

HORMONE BINDING SITES

King (1958) had noted the presence of oestrogen receptors in the Dimethylbenzanthrancene (DMBA) induced rat mammary cancers. This tumour is particularly sensitive to the presence of oestrogens. Jensen *et al.* (1972) correlated the concentration of oestrogen receptors in human tumours with the hormonal sensitivity of these tumours. It is curious that both ovariectomy and the administration of oestrogens are effective in producing remissions in tumours with oestrogen affinity (*Lancet Annotation*, 1974).

Braunsberg *et al.* (1974) measured oestradiol uptake by human breast tumour tissue using in-vivo and in-vitro techniques. By the in-vivo techniques, they found that age and menopausal status were not important variables. However, in-vitro techniques did show correlation of oestrogen affinity with the patients' menopausal status. In general, pre-menopausal patients and patients who had achieved the menopause some 20 or more years before, showed greater oestrogen affinity than in the two decades (50–70years) following the menopause. It is of interest that it is in these two decades, that the largest proportion of new cases arise.

THE PLACE OF PROLACTIN IN BREAST CANCER

Despite many dramatic improvements in individual cases, the earlier promise of endocrine surgery and therapy has not been fulfilled. The prognosis of this disease which kills some 10,000 women annually in England and Wales (approximately 5% of all deaths in women) has not changed significantly since the introduction of radical local surgery before the turn of the century. Hope has however been rekindled with the recognition of the pituitary mammotrophic hormone – prolactin. Is this hormone, with its specific mammary function, the actual activator through which other hormones act?

Current knowledge of the physiological function and regulation of secretion of prolactin has been briefly reviewed by Schwartz (1973). The place of prolactin in breast development and function has been described earlier. In physiological doses, oestrogens stimulate prolactin both by direct effect on the anterior pituitary cells and by reduction of hypothalamic "prolactin inhibiting factor" secretion. It is of interest, when one remembers the increased incidence of breast cancer in hypothyroid women, that thyrotrophin releasing hormone stimulates prolactin secretion. In pharmacological doses, oestrogens seem to block the effect of prolactin.

Pearson *et al.* (1954) temporarily reactivated human mammary tumours, after suppression had been obtained by oophorectomy, by the administration of oestrogens. This did not happen however if the patients had been treated successfully by hypophysectomy (Pearson and Ray, 1959). It seemed that oestrogens acted by the stimulation of a pituitary factor. Llerena, Molina and Pearson (1969) later showed the oestrogens caused a surge of prolactin secretion.

Just as some tumours respond unfavourably to administered oestrogens in some cases and favourably in others, so there appear to be some tumours which improve when prolactin secretion is induced; Turkington, Underwood and Van Wyck (1971) showed that in nine subjects treated by pituitary stalk section, five responded with increased prolactin secretion, yet three of these showed clinical improvement. Wilson *et al.* (1974) not only found no significant difference in plasma prolactin levels of healthy women and women with breast cancer, but found increases in prolactin concentration after the use of stilboestrol had produced clinical improvement.

Pearson *et al.* (1969) used the DMBA induced rat mammary adenocarcinoma as a model for their studies of hormone dependency. Oestrogens reactivated the tumour after adrenalectomy and oophorectomy, but not after hypophysectomy. Prolactin however reactivated the tumour after either of the two ablation procedures. In this tumour at any rate, prolactin appears to be the major endocrine controller.

It is perhaps of related interest that Atkins *et al.* (1960) found that hypophysectomy gave marginally better results than combined oophorectomy with adrenalectomy in their series of women with stage IV cancer.

Mioduszewska, Koszarowski and Gorski (1968) grew cell and organ cultures of human mammary cancer tissue, in order to study their behaviour, *in vitro,* in differing hormonal environments. Generally, growth was promoted by a number of hormones. In descending order of activity these were – prolactin, oestrogen, cortisol, testosterone, growth hormone and progesterone. Tumours sensitive to cortisol but not to prolactin were found to have a poor prognosis. Tumours sensitive to prolactin however had a good prognosis. Selwood and Castro (1974) were unable to confirm these findings, but they experienced difficulties in maintaining the organ cultures. Using similar methods, Salih, *et al.*, (1972) found that 16 out of 24 tumours grown by their technique were stimulated – as judged by enzyme activity – by the presence of prolactin.

Jensen *et al.* (1972) have reported that oestrogen sensitive human tumours contained specific oestrogen binding sites within the malignant ephithelial cells. It may well be that those hormones that do influence tumour growth require the presence of binding sites within the tumour cells. What place such sites may have in the initiation of such tumours is not known, but all hormone target cells must have a mechanism for recognizing the hormone for its effects to be exerted, whether through the cyclic AMP mechanism or otherwise.

HORMONES AND PROGNOSIS OF BREAST CANCER

Nathanson (1944) was unable to find any evidence that breast cancer was associated with abnormalities of hormone excretion and concluded that carcinoma of the human breast was independent of hormonal influences once it was established. This view may have been a reflection of the imprecise methods then available for assessing hormonal function by analytical means.

Bulbrook *et al.* (1958 a,b) measured urinary oestrogens pre-operatively in women later to be subjected to adrenalectomy or hypophysectomy for advanced breast cancer and found no correlation with response to adrenalectomy, but some diminution from normal in those responding favourably to hypophysectomy. In 1957, Allen, Hayward and Merrivale had attempted to distinguish pre-operatively between women with the advanced disease who would or would not be found to respond to adrenalectomy or hypophysectomy subsequently. It was clearly desirable to prevent the infliction of additional disability in patients who were not going to respond to this drastic form of therapy. In a small series of patients they found that the ratio of 11-deoxy-17-oxosteroids (11-DKS) – the androgen metabolites – to 11-oxy-17-oxosteroids (11-OKS) – the corticosteroid metabolites, was greater than 1.0 in the responders and in healthy women, but less than 1.0 in the non-responders. Plantin *et al.* (1958) were unable to substantiate these results when they used more specific methods.

This approach was nevertheless pursued by the Bulbrook group and Guy's Hospital, London. Bulbrook, Greenwood and Hayward (1960) elaborated on the Allen *et al.* (1957) work. They widened the study by using more precise methods to measure a greater variety of hormones – oestrogens, fractionated 11-DKS and 11-OKS, corticosteroids (17-OHCS), pregnanediol and total gonadotrophins. Urine samples were obtained from women with advanced breast cancer selected on clinical grounds for adrenalectomy or hypophysectomy. Following operation the women were divided into three groups according to the response to surgery – a "remission" group, an "intermediate" or short-lived remission group, and a group showing no remission. Only three of the parameters were of use in discriminating between the three clinical response groups. These were the 17-OHCS and two of the 11-deoxy-17-oxosteroids – aetiocholanolone and androsterone, the androsterone being slightly less useful than aetiocholanolone. In general, 17-OHCS excretion was raised and aetiocholanolone excretion was reduced in the non-responders.

Table 2 Correlation of Response to Endocrine Ablation and Discriminant Function (Bulbrook *et al.*, 1960)

	No. of Patients	
Response	*Positive Discriminant*	*Negative Discriminant*
Remission	13	1
Intermediate	6	12
Failure	6	21

With the help of Spicer the group devised a mathematical formula 8-80 (17-OHCS(mg/day)) + aetiocholanolone (ug/day), which they called a "discriminant function". A positive number ("positive discriminant") was found in 75% of responders and a negative number ("negative discriminant") in 61% of non-responders (Table 2). Further studies (Hayward and Bulbrook, 1968) with larger series were less promising but showed that whereas 60% of those with positive discriminants gave some improvement only 40% of those with negative discriminants did so. In an attempt to improve the power of the discriminant function, Bulbrook (1965) had already shown that other factors such as the "free-interval" between the initial local treatment and the subsequent recurrence of the disease, and the "menopausal status" of the patient, could be used in conjunction with the discriminant for better selection of cases for surgery. Similar observations were made by other groups (Juret, Hayem and Fleisler, 1964; Kumaoko *et al.*, 1966; Wilson *et al.*, 1966).

Further work from the Guy's Hospital group (Hayward and Bulbrook, 1968) found that nearly one third of all their patients had only a 5% chance of response. These all had negative discriminants and had free intervals of less than two years or were within six years of achieving the menopause. It is also of interest that they had earlier noted (Bulbrook *et al.*, 1962) that it was rare to find a negative discriminant in normal women below the age of 60 and yet half of their early (localized) cancer cases below that age had negative discriminants. Furthermore, Bulbrook, Hayward and Thomas (1965) found that 90% of the stage 2 cancers in women with negative discriminants below 65 years of age, lead to death within three years of the discovery of the disease. It seemed that a negative discriminant was a generally poor prognostic sign.

THE "ALTERNATIVE DISCRIMINANT"

In order to simplify the means of determining the discriminant function, and to widen its application, a group led by Miller in Portsmouth (Miller *et al.* 1967) calculated a new "alternative discriminant" expressed as the ratio 11-DKS: 17-OHCS. They found that a ratio of greater than 0.16 was identical to a positive discriminant, and a figure below 0.13 to a negative discriminant. The two discriminants were found to correlate almost exactly with the response to endocrine ablation (Thomas, Bulbrook and Hayward, 1967).

Table 3 Proportion of Negative Discriminants in Breast Cancer Patients in Portsmouth (Miller and Durant, 1968)

	% with Negative Discriminants
Premenopausal Women	
Normal	0
Local Disease	14
Advanced Disease	36
Menopausal Women	
Normal	44
Local Disease	38
Advanced Disease	56

Using this ratio the Portsmouth group (Miller and Durant, 1968) studied a series of women upon whom the discriminant was calculated when they first presented with the disease and prior to any form of treatment being given. The results are shown in Table 3. In the post-menopausal women, the presence of a negative discriminant was as common in those with breast cancer as it was in the healthy group. In the pre-menopausal women, the incidence of negative discriminants increased with the clinical severity of the disease and none were found in the healthy controls.

They were further able to show that the most important measurement was that of the androgenic metabolites, the 11-DKS (Table 4). It became apparent that although some high 17-OHCS values were present in the advanced disease this was not a significant finding. What was clear, was that all the women with negative discriminants whether healthy and elderly, or young and cancerous, had subnormal excretion of androgenic metabolites. The Portsmouth group's unpublished work shows that 11-DKS excretion drops from a mean of 5.5 mg/day in pre-menopausal women to 2.0 mg/day within two years after the menopause in healthy women, and this then gradually falls to 1.0 mg/day by the age of 70.

Table 4 Mean Urinary Steroid Parameters in Relationship to the Discriminant Ratio in the Portsmouth Series of Breast Cancer Patients (Miller and Durant, 1968)

	17–OHCS (mg./d)		*11–DKS (mg./d)*	
	"Positive" Ratio	*"Negative" Ratio*	*"Positive" Ratio*	*"Negative" Ratio*
Premenopausal				
Normal	15.9 ± 3.1	Nil	5.3 ± 2.2	Nil
Cancer	14.4 ± 5.3	17.9 ± 6.5	4.1 ± 1.8	1.9 ± 0.7
Menopausal				
Normal	13.4 ± 3.2	15.0 ± 4.4	2.6 ± 1.0	1.8 ± 0.7
Cancer	14.2 ± 5.3	17.3 ± 7.9	3.2 ± 1.3	1.6 ± 0.8

(Mean ± 1.S.D.)

They were soon to suggest (Miller and Durant, 1969) that the presence of a negative discriminant in breast cancer was a reflection of the non-specific systemic disturbance produced by the disease which caused a reduction in 11-DKS excretion.

This suggestion was followed up by a study of the various non-specific factors due to the general illness that night be expected to be found in women suffering with advanced breast cancer (Durant and Miller, 1973). Several groups of women were studied and they were all below the age of 50. The groups were – (a) women suffering from chronic debilitating illness due to non-progressive long-standing disease, (b) healthy women who were attempting to lose weight, (c) women with acute infective hepatitis who were followed through to recovery, (d) women with early and advanced non-mammary cancer. In general it was found that there was indeed a reduction in 11-DKS excretion from the normal (Table 5). In the cases of hepatic disease and non-mammary cancer, the changes were most significant in those most severely ill. Indeed 57% of the "ill" hepatitis patients and 50% of the advanced non-mammary cancer cases had negative discriminants. Their figures showed a higher proportion of negative ratios than their earlier series of advanced breast cancer in the pre-menopausal group, (Miller and Durant, 1968).

Table 5 Mean Daily Urinary Excretion of Steroid in Some conditions other than Breast Cancer (Durant and Miller, 1973)

Group	*17–OHCS (mg./day)*	*11–DKS (mg./day)*
Normal	11.2 ± 2.9	5.0 ± 2.7
Chronic Debility	8.3 ± 2.8	2.7 ± 2.0
Hepatic Disease		
Mildly ill	14.4 ± 7.0	3.1 ± 2.3
Severely ill	13.5 ± 7.6	1.2 ± 0.8
Non-Mammary Cancer		
Localized	12.1 ± 5.2	3.7 ± 2.5
Advanced	10.4 ± 4.2	1.4 ± 1.5

(Mean ± 1.S.D.)

Evidence for the non-specifity of these changes originally seen in breast cancer, is strengthened by Rao (1970) in his studies of lung cancer in the male. He found that a correlation existed between poor response to pneumonectomy and pre-operative subnormal androgen and raised corticosteroid excretion. Further, his inoperable cases survived longer if their urinary steroid excretion was normal.

Durant and Miller (1973) concluded that the urinary steroid changes seen in advanced breast cancer were a measure of the general metabolic consequences, or degree of "illness", of the disease. Nevertheless they recognized that the determination of the discriminant in cases of advanced breast cancer was still of some value in selecting women for endocrine surgery.

The Portsmouth group's present opinion is as follows. Women below the age of 50, with negative discriminants and with a "free interval" of less than 2 years should not be selected. Post-menopausal women with positive discriminants are good candidates for endocrine organ ablation; their chances of response improves the older they are. Post-menopausal women with negative discriminants, free-intervals of less than 2 years or who are within six years of having achieved the menopause should not be selected.

What appeared to be a very promising approach to an intractable disease does not seem to have been fully substantiated.

CONCLUSION

There is abundant evidence that breast cancer in the experimental animal depends upon the presence of oestogens and prolactin for the development of the disease. Oestrogens may well be the principal aetiological agents in some species.

In humans, the evidence does not suggest that hormones have prime aetiological place in the genesis of this disease. However, about one third of women with the advanced disease will benefit to some extent either from hormone administration or endocrine organ ablation – oophorectomy, hypophysectomy or adrenalectomy. The response to these forms of treatment may be predicted with a limited degree of accuracy in some groups of women by urinary hormone excretion studies.

Using urinary steroid excretion "discriminant functions" it has been shown that only 5% of patients who have a negative discriminant and a "free period" of less than 2 years or are within 6 years of achieving the menopause, will benefit from hormone therapy. It is considered that pre-menopausal patients with negative discriminants are unlikely to benefit from adrenalectomy or hypophysectomy, and that post-menopausal patients with positive discriminants are worthy of consideration for these operations.

The steroid excretion changes found in breast cancer are believed to be a reflection of the general systemic non-specific metabolic manifestation of the disease.

REFERENCES

Allen, B. J., Hayward J. L. and Merrivale, W. H. H. (1957): The excretion of 17-ketosteroids in the urine of patients with generalised carcinomatosis secondary to carcinoma of the breast. *Lancet,* **1,** 496.

Atkins, H. J. B., Falconer, M. A., Hayward, J. L., Maclean, K. S., Schurr, P. J. and Armitage, P. (1960): Adrenalectomy and hypophysectomy for advanced cancer of the breast. *Lancet,* **1,** 1148.

Beatson, G. T. (1896): On the treatment of inoperable cases of carcinoma of the mamma. *Lancet,* **2,** 104.

Boyd, S. (1900): On oophorectomy in cancer of the breast. *Brit. Med. J.,* **2,** 1161.

Braunsberg, H., James, V. H. T., Jamieson, C. W., Desai S., Carter, A. E. and Hulbert, M. (1974): Effect of age and menopausal status on estimates of oestrogen binding by malignant breast tumours. *Brit. Med. J.,* **4,** 745.

Brit. Med. J. Annotation. (1974): The Thyroid and Breast Cancer. **1,** 472.

Bulbrook, R. D. (1965): Hormone assays in human breast cancer. *Vitamins and Hormones,* **23,** 429.

Bulbrook, R. D., Greenwood, F. C., Hadfield, G. J. and Scowen, E. F. (1958a): Adrenalectomy in breast cancer. An attempt to correlate clinical results with oestrogen production. *Brit. Med. J.,* **1,** 12.

Bulbrook, R. D., Greenwood, F. C., Hadfield, G. J. and Scowen, E. F. (1958b): Hypophysectomy in breast cancer. An attempt to correlate clinical results with oestrogen production. *Brit. Med. J.,* **1,** 15.

Bulbrook, R. D., Greenwood, F. C. and Hayward, J. L. (1960): Selection of breast cancer patients for adrenalectomy or hypophysectomy by determination of urinary 17-hydroxycorticosteroids and aetiocholanolone. *Lancet,* **1,** 1154.

Bulbrook, R. D., Hayward, J. L., Spicer, C. C. and Thomas, B. S. (1962): Abnormal excretion of urinary steroids by women with early breast cancer. *Lancet,* **2,** 1238.

Cole, P. and MacMahon, B. (1969): Oestrogen fractions during early reproductive life in the aetiology of breast cancer. *Lancet,* **1,** 604.

Durant, J. A. and Miller, H. (1973): Non specific factors that may influence significance of urinary steroid excretion in breast cancer. *Brit. Med. J.,* **4,** 767.

Hayward, J. L. and Bulbrook, R. D. (1968): In *Prognostic Factors in Breast Cancer,* p. 383; Forrest, A. P. M. and Kunkler, P. B. (Eds.). E. & S. Livingstone Ltd., Edinburgh and London.

Hellman, L., Fishman, J., Zumoff, B., Cassouto, J. and Gallagher, T. F. (1967): Studies of oestradiol transformation in women with breast cancer. *J. Clin. Endocr.,* **27,** 1087.

Huggins, C. and Bergenstal, D. M. (1952): Inhibition of human mammary and prostatic cancers by adrenalectomy. *Cancer Res.,* **12,** 134.

Humphrey, L. J. and Swerdlow, M. (1964): Relationship of thyroid disease to breast disease. *Cancer,* **17,** 1170.

Jensen, E. V., Block, G. E., Smith, S., Kyser, K. and DeSombre, E. R. (1972): In *Estrogen Target Tissues and Neoplasia,* p. 23. Dao, T. L. (Ed.) University of Chicago Press, U.S.A.

Juret, P., Hayem, M. and Fleisler, A. (1964): A propos de 150 implantations d'yttrium radio-actif intra-hypophysaires dans la traitement du cancer du sein a une étade avancée. *J. Chir* (*Paris*). **87,** 409.

King, R. J. B. (1968): In *Prognostic Factors in Breast Cancer.* p. 354; Forrest, A. P. M. and Kunkler, P. B. (Eds.). E. and S. Livingstone Ltd., Edinburgh and London.

Kim, U. and Furth, J. (1960): Relation of mammary tumours to mammatropes. 1. Induction of mammary tumours in rats. *Proc. Soc. Exp. Biol. and Med.,* **103,** 640.

Kumaoka, S., Sakauchi, N., Abe, O., Kusama, M. and Takatini, O. (1968): Urinary 17-ketosteroid excretion of women with advanced breast cancer. *J. Clin. Endocrin.,* **28,** 667.

Lacassagne, A. (1933): Influence d'un facteur familial dans la production par la folliculine de cancers mammaires chez la souris mâle. *Compt. rend. Soc. de Biol.* **114,** 427.

Lancet Annotation (1974): Oestradiol receptors in human breast cancer. **2,** 631.

Lemon, H. E., Wotiz, H. H., Parsons, L. and Mozden, P. H. (1966): Reduced oestriol excretion in patients with breast cancer prior to endocrine therapy. *J. Amer. Med. Assoc.* **196,** 1128.

Lewison, E. F. (1965): Castration in the treatment of advanced breast cancer. *Cancer,* **18,** 1558.

Lipsett, M. B. (1971): Oestrogen profiles and breast cancer. *Lancet,* **2,** 1378.

Llerena, L., Molina A. and Pearson, O. H. (1969): Radioimmunoassay of rat prolactin. *51st Meeting of the Endocrine Society,* p. 45.

Loeb, L. (1919): Further investigations on the origin of tumours in mice VI: Internal secretions as a factor in the origin of tumours. *J. Med. Res.,* **40,** 477.

Luft, R. and Olivecrona, J. (1953): Experiences with hypophysectomy in man. *J. Neurosurg,* **10,** 301.

Lyons, W. R., Li, C. H. and Johnson, R. E. (1958): Hormone control of mammary growth and lactation. *Red. Prog. Horm. Res.,* **14,** 219.

MacMahon, B., Cole, P., Brown, J. B., Aoki, K., Lin, T. H., Morgan, R. W. and Woo N-C. (1971): Oestrogen profiles of Asian and North American women, *Lancet,* **2,** 900.

Marmorston, J., Crowley, L. G., Myers, S. M., Stern, E. and Hopkins, C. E. (1965): Urinary excretion of oestrone, oestradiol and oestriol by patients with breast cancer and benign breast disease. *Amer. J. Obst. Gynaec.,* **92,** 460.

Miller, H. and Durant, J. A. (1968): The value of urine steroid hormone assays in breast cancer. *Clin. Biochem.,* **1,** 287.

Miller, H. and Durant, J. A. (1969): Discriminants and Breast Cancer. *Lancet,* **1,** 1313.

Miller, H., Durant, J. A., Jacobs, A. G. and Allison, J. F. (1967): Alternative discriminating function for determining hormone dependency of breast cancer. *Brit. Med. J.,* **1,** 147.

Mioduszewska, O., Koszarowski, T. and Gorski, C. (1968): In *Prognostic Factors in Breast Cancer,* p. 347; Forrest, A. P. M. and Kunkler, P. B. (Eds.) E. and S. Livingstone, Edinburgh and London.

Mulhbock, O. and Burt, L. M. (1959): Induction of mammary cancer in mice without the mammary tumour agent by isografts of hypophyses. *Cancer Res.,* **19,** 402.

Murray, W. S. (1928): Ovarian secretion and tumour incidence. *J. Cancer. Res.,* **12,** 18.

Nathanson, I. T. (1944): Relationship of hormones to diseases of the breast. *Surgery,* **16,** 108.

Pearson, O. H. (1973): In *Current Research in Oncology 1972,* p. 125. Anfinsen, C. B., Potter, M. and Schechter, A. N. (Eds.). Academic Press N.Y.

Pearson, O. H., Llerena, O., Llerena, L., Molina, A. and Butler, T. (1969): Prolactin dependent rat mammary cancer: a model for man? *Trans. Assn. Am. Physicians,* **32,** 225.

Pearson, O. H. and Ray, B. S. (1959): Results of hypophysectomy in the treatment of metastatic mammary carcinoma. *Cancer,* **12,** 85.

Pearson, O. H., West, C. D., Hollander, V. P. and Treves, N. (1954): Evaluation of endocrine therapy for advanced breast cancer. *J. Am. Med. Assoc.,* **154,** 234.

Plantin, L. O., Birke, G., Diczfalusy, E., Frankson, C. and Hellstrom, J. (1958): In *Endocrine Aspects of Breast Cancer,* p. 224. A. R. Currie (Ed.). E. and S. Livingstone, Edinburgh.

Rao, L. G. S. (1970): Discriminant function based on steroid abnormalities in patients with lung cancer. *Lancet,* **2,** 441.

Salih, H., Flax, H., Brander, W. and Hobbs, J. R. (1972): Prolactin dependence in human breast cancers. *Lancet,* **2,** 1103.

Schwartz, T. B. (1973): In *The Year Book of Endocrinology 1973,* p. 7. Schwartz, T. B. (Ed.). Year Book Med. Publishers, Chicago.

Sellwood, R. A. and Castro, J. E. (1974): The effect of hormones on organ cultures of human mammary carcinoma. *J. Path.,* **113,** 223.

Shimkin, M. B. and Wyman, R. S. (1945): Effect of adrenalectomy and ovariectomy on mammary carcinogenesis in strain C3H mice. *J. Nat. Cancer. Inst.,* **6,** 187.

Stern, E., Hopkins, C. E., Weiner, J. M. and Marmorston, J. (1964): Hormone excretion patterns in breast and prostatic cancer are abnormal. *Science,* **145,** 716.

Thomas, B. S., Bulbrook, R. D. and Hayward, J. L. (1967): Urinary steroid assays and response to endocrine ablation. *Brit. Med. J.,* **3,** 523.

Turkington, R. W., Underwood, L. E. and Van Wyck, J. J. (1971): Elevated serum prolactin levels after pituitary stalk section in man. *New Eng. J. Med.,* **285,** 707.

Wilson, R. G., Buchan, R., Roberts, M. M., Forrest, A. P. M., Boyns, A. R., Cole, E. N. and Griffiths, K. (1974): Plasma prolactin and breast cancer. *Cancer,* **33,** 1325.

Wilson, R. E., Crocker, D. W., Fairgreave, J., Bartholomew, A. F., Emerson, K. Jr. and Moore, F. D. (1967): Adrenal structure and function in advanced carcinoma of the breast. *J. Am. Med. Assoc.,* **199,** 471.

10

Effect of Pregnancy and Lactation on Prognosis

Basil A. Stoll and Santiago Dexeus

Breast cancer occurring in association with pregnancy is rare. Like male breast cancer it represents a very small proportion of all breast cancers seen by the clinician, and also like male breast cancer, it tends to lead to anecdotal impressions. These led in the past to anecdotal advice, until in 1955, White published his conclusions based upon an analysis of 1375 cases culled from the literature. The only two large personal series reported since then are those of Holleb and Farrow (1962) on 283 patients, and Peters (1968) on 295 patients.

Breast cancer complicates about 3 out of every 10,000 pregnancies, while pregnancy occurs in about 3 out of every 100 cases of breast cancer. The combination presents a special problem either when primary breast cancer manifests during pregnancy or lactation, or when the patient becomes pregnant subsequent to primary treatment of breast cancer. In order to clarify the issues, they will be discussed under the following headings;

(a) Is the prognosis of breast cancer worse in pregnancy?
(b) If so, what is the cause of the poor prognosis?
(c) Is the prognosis affected by the hormonal milieu or by immunosuppression?
(d) Is the prognosis of breast cancer worse in lactation?
(e) Is pregnancy likely to reactivate treated breast cancer?
(f) What is the management of breast cancer in pregnancy and lactation?

IS THE PROGNOSIS OF BREAST CANCER WORSE IN PREGNANCY?

Early reports on the effect of pregnancy on the course of breast cancer stressed that the overall survival rate was poor, and case reports stressed the rapid course of the disease in the individual patient. However, starting with Westberg (1946), more recent reports have shown that if diagnosed early, the individual course of breast cancer treated during pregnancy or lactation is not greatly more malignant than the average (White, 1955; Holleb and Farrow, 1962; Peters, 1963; Devitt *et al.,* 1964).

It is clear that most reported series of breast cancer presenting in pregnancy contain an abnormally high proportion of patients with more advanced disease (White, 1955; Holleb and Farrow, 1964; Peters, 1968). According to Holleb and Farrow (1964), 72% of the operated patients show evidence of axillary node involvement, and in the series reported by Montgomery (1961), 74% of cases showed metastases at the time of operation. The proportion of pregnant patients presenting in Stage 4 is twice as high as in premenopausal patients generally (Peters, 1968).

It is therefore not surprising that the overall 5 year survival for patients with pregnancy complicating breast cancer is only 33% in Peters' series compared to 50% for premenopausal patients generally. The difference in survival is shown to be due partly to the high proportion of advanced cases, because the poorer prognosis among pregnant women is less marked if the group is matched according to stage and age with a group of non pregnant women with breast cancer. However, when this is done the 5 year survival is still only 38% in the pregnant group compared to 45% in the non pregnant group.

WHAT IS THE CAUSE OF THE POOR PROGNOSIS?

There are therefore two questions to answer. Firstly, what is the cause of the higher proportion of more advanced tumours in pregnancy, and secondly, is there another reason for the lower survival rate in patients with breast cancer complicated by pregnancy?

The higher proportion of inoperable tumours is almost certainly associated with delay both in diagnosis and in treatment. The average delay between onset of symptoms and treatment is twice as high in pregnant women as in non pregnant women (Treves and Holleb, 1958). The average delay between onset of symptoms and diagnosis of breast cancer is 11 months in pregnant women compared to 4 months in non pregnant women (Applewhite, *et al.*, 1973). According to Montgomery (1961), the tumour is nearly always first noticed by the patient herself and most of the subsequent delay is created by the attending clinicians.

It has been suggested that breast cancer presenting during pregnancy might have a relatively worse prognosis than those cases where "the tumour was present before the pregnancy had started" (Bloom, 1968; Dao, 1968). The implication is not clear, since it is generally believed that most breast cancers take at least 2 years to develop to the stage when they are clinically palpable and therefore every tumour apparent in pregnancy must have had a prolonged preclinical history before pregnancy started.

Let us turn now to possible causes for the apparently lower intrinsic cure rate in pregnancy complicating the course of breast cancer. White (1955) observed in a series of 1375 patients collected from the literature that patients treated for breast cancer in the second half of pregnancy carried a much worse prognosis than those treated either in the first half of pregnancy or in lactation. He suggested that more advanced disease is likely to be found in the second half of pregnancy because of the greater delay in diagnosis and treatment. It is clear that not only does the larger breast increase the difficulties of diagnosis, but the tendency of the clinician to postpone surgery or radiotherapy until after parturition, often delays treatment (Montgomery, 1961).

On the other hand, Peters (1968) postulates a special "risk" factor in the second half of pregnancy complicated by breast cancer. She confirms in her series the poorer prognosis in Stages 1 and 2 breast cancer treated in the second half of pregnancy. The 5 year survival rate is 14% for this group compared to 57% for similar cases in the first half of pregnancy, and 77% for those operated on in the first 6 months of lactation.

She quotes the following statistics: "Thirteen of the fourteen breast cancer patients in Stages 1 and 2 who were treated during the second half of pregnancy, were treated immediately on discovering, or within 2 months after finding the breast lump, and only two patients survived 5 years (only one free of disease at 5 years). But in Stages 1 and 2, six others who had discovered breast masses during the latter months of pregnancy were treated in the early postpartum period and all have survived 5 to 17 years so far".

It seems more than likely that selection was at work! While the rapidly growing tumours would be operated upon urgently in late pregnancy, the treatment of the more slowly growing tumours (those with an innately lesser biological aggressiveness) would be postponed to the postpartum period. The extraordinarily high survival rate in the latter group confirms this likelihood, and there is no real evidence of a special "risk" factor which affects breast cancer particularly in the second half of pregnancy.

However, there may be other reasons for a lower intrinsic cure rate in patients treated for breast cancer in pregnancy. A possible immunological basis is discussed in the next section. Bloom (1965) has noted an increased proportion of tumours in pregnancy with a higher histopathological grade of malignancy. This has not been confirmed since by any other observer, nor has the degree of host reaction in the tumour or draining nodes in such cases been commented on. It is said that in the higher grade tumours, the degree of host reaction is particularly important (Brightmore, Greening and Hamlin, 1970).

It has been suggested that the greater physiological vascular and lymphatic engorgement of the breast may be a contributory factor to the poorer prognosis of breast cancer treated in the second half of pregnancy (Montgomery, 1961; Miller, 1962). This is unlikely to be a major factor because, as pointed out by Peters (1968), a similar or greater engorgement occurs in the immediate postpartum period, yet the prognosis is relatively good for breast cancer treated in that phase.

IS THE PROGNOSIS AFFECTED BY THE HORMONAL MILIEU OR BY IMMUNOSUPPRESION?

In the human female, a high level of circulating chorionic gonadotrophin is found in the first trimester of pregnancy, but after that it falls rapidly, while the secretion of chorionic somatomammotrophin continues at a high level throughout pregnancy. Radioimmunoassay studies have shown that plasma prolactin levels rise progressively during pregnancy, fall at parturition but rise again during breast feeding. With regard to steroid hormones, placental secretion of oestrogen (particularly oestriol) and progesterone rapidly increases throughout the second and third trimesters.

It is commonly suggested that the very high levels of oestrogen, progesterone or prolactin may be important in stimulating the growth of breast cancer in pregnancy and lactation. This is based mainly on analogy with the hormone sensitive mammary carcinoma induced in Sprague Dawley rats with dimethylbenzanthracene or methyl cholanthrene. Pregnancy and also progesterone administration stimulate the growth of these tumours (Huggins, 1972). Parturition is followed by tumour regression while suckling by the rat will again stimulate the activity of the tumour. These latter observations suggest that prolactin secretion, as well as progesterone, may be important in stimulating the growth of the experimental tumour.

If this applies also to the human tumour, one would expect that the benefit of either castration or termination of pregnancy would be clearly shown in the human. However, the results of prophylactic oophorectomy after the primary treatment of breast cancer in pregnancy are of doubtful value (Peters, 1968), and interruption of pregnancy also is of doubtful value (White, 1955; Miller, 1962; Bunkers and Peters, 1963), although some disagree (Cheek, 1953; Montgomery, 1961; Holleb and Farrow, 1962; Cade, 1964).

Cade (1964) considers that 90% of breast cancers in pregnancy are hormone sensitive. He supports this opinion with the observation that breast cancer has been known to regress after spontaneous abortion or may grow more rapidly when pregnancy supervenes. Such observations are anecdotal. Peters (1962) finds castration to be of little value in the control of *disseminated* breast cancer in pregnancy.

The personal series of one of the writers (B.A.S.) included 15 women treated for breast cancer in pregnancy. Androgen therapy was given in 6 patients and therapeutic castration in 3 patients after termination of pregnancy, but without a single response in the 9 patients. Of the 15 patients, 8 were subjected to prophylactic castration after primary treatment but all died within 3 years. There is little evidence of hormonal sensitivity either in these cases or in the literature. It therefore seems unlikely that the high hormonal levels circulating during pregnancy are directly responsible for stimulating the activity of breast cancer.

It has been suggested by Scholz and Scholz (1971) that following parturition, hormonal therapy with androgens and gestagens is necessary for a prolonged period. The fall in hormonal levels after parturition, following the high levels of pregnancy, is claimed to justify such a procedure. There is no scientific basis for such therapy.

It has recently been shown that certain α2-globulin and macroglobulins occur in the sera of women during pregnancy and may reflect suppression of the normal immune response. Their concentration rises with the course of pregnancy and falls to low levels within a few weeks of parturition. They are not specific to pregnancy and have also been found in women taking oestrogens or oral contraceptives, and in men being treated with oestrogens for prostatic cancer (Stimson, 1974; von Schoultz, 1974).

It has been suggested that the α2-globulins reflect loss of responsiveness to breast cancer. It has been shown that the serum level of α2-globulins is raised in a majority of patients with breast cancer (Minton and Bianco, 1974), and more important, that the level of α2-macroglobulins in breast cancer patients can be correlated with the activity of their disease (Stimson, 1975). Thus the level is found to rise prior to the clinical appearance of metastases and falls when the tumour regresses in size after radiotherapy or cytotoxic chemotherapy. A raised α2-macroglobulin level in the serum may be associated with other types of malignancy also (Stimson, 1975).

It is therefore possible that the increased activity shown by breast cancer during pregnancy might be due to the immunosuppression associated with pregnancy, and not to the raised hormonal levels as such. The latter, especially the raised oestrogen level, may however, be important in causing the suppression of the normal immune response (von Schoultz, 1974). It appears that peripheral blood leucocytes are capable of synthesizing α2-globulin.

IS THE PROGNOSIS OF BREAST CANCER WORSE IN LACTATION?

It is widely believed that breast cancer coexisting with lactation carries a poor prognosis. Peters (1968) has reported the 5 year survival to be 77% in patients treated in the first 6 months of lactation, 14% in those treated between the 6th and 12 months, and 66% in those treated after 12 months. The median delay between the discovery of the lump and treatment in the three groups was 3 months, 6 months and 22 months respectively.

It is obvious from these figures that delay in treatment did not affect the prognosis in these cases, and selection of cases is the only feasible explanation for the widely divergent survival rates. The delay periods suggest that the first and third groups were slowly growing tumours originating in pregnancy, whose treatment was deliberately delayed to a more opportune time. It was therefore the biological characteristics of the tumours and the host defence which determined the prognosis rather than any direct effect of lactation (Peters, 1968).

Inflammatory carcinoma is said to be more common in lactation and is said to reflect a failure of local defence mechanisms. Its prognosis is made even worse by the fact that its diagnosis in lactation is often delayed because of confusion with breast abscess.

IS PREGNANCY LIKELY TO REACTIVATE TREATED BREAST CANCER?

It has been customary for many years to advise women against subsequent pregnancy after treatment for breast cancer (Robinson, 1965) and many would even advise termination of an early pregnancy if it supervenes. There is however, no clear evidence that pregnancy increases the risk of reactivating dormant breast cancer cells. In a review of the literature, White (1954) reported 49% of 5 year survivals among 208 patients who had been permitted to undergo pregnancy after primary treatment for breast cancer. This was similar to the survival rate in a series of women matched for age who did not undergo subsequent pregnancy. Similar findings have been reported by Holleb and Farrow (1962), McWhirter (1968) and Cooper and Butterfield (1970).

Other authors have noted even an improved survival rate in patients who have been permitted to undergo pregnancy subsequent to primary treatment (Westberg, 1946; Richards, 1948; Devitt *et al.,* 1964; Rissanen, 1969). However in such cases it is common practice for clinicians to advise the postponement of pregnancy for several years after the primary treatment of breast cancer while watching for early recurrence. This would tend to eliminate patients with more actively malignant tumours, and it was therefore assumed that the better survival rates which were noted might reflect selection of the naturally slowly growing cancers.

However, Peters (1968) has found the 5 year survival rate in 96 women undergoing pregnancy following primary treatment of breast cancer to be 72% compared to 49.5% in a non pregnant series matched for age and stage. This, in spite of the fact that 47% of the pregnancy group had shown involved axillary nodes at operation. The objection that these might be selected slowly growing tumours could not be levelled, as 50% of the patients had their pregnancies within 1 year and 75% within 2 years of treatment. There is no real evidence therefore that subsequent pregnancy accelerates the growth of metastases from breast cancer.

WHAT IS THE MANAGEMENT OF BREAST CANCER IN PREGNANCY AND LACTATION?

It seems clear from the previous discussion that delayed diagnosis and delayed treatment are a major cause of the poor prognosis associated with breast cancer in pregnancy. It must be stressed therefore that the obstetrician must practise regular palpation of the breasts in every woman who is pregnant. Moreover, surgical treatment should not be delayed in the presence of early breast cancer in pregnancy. Radiation therapy, either primary or supplementary, is, of course, contraindicated unless pregnancy is first terminated, because of the danger of scattered radiation reaching the foetus.

The problems in managing the disease once it is recognized are not inconsiderable. The clinician must take into consideration the psychological attitude of the patient and the religious and moral attitudes of the family, while offering scientifically based advice on the management. The following plan of management is based on that suggested by Peters (1968), but has been modified.

(1) Early cancer of the breast presenting in the first half of pregnancy is treated by radical surgery, without supplementary radiation if the mother is anxious to continue the pregnancy. Alternatively, pregnancy can be terminated and radio-therapy used in conjunction with more limited surgery. Prophylactic castration is not advised although most clinicians would advise delaying pregnancy for about 2 to 3 years. This delay will exclude from pregnancy the patient who is going to show early recurrence and will thus diminish the risk of leaving a motherless infant.

(2) Early cancer of the breast presenting in the second half of pregnancy may be carefully watched if it is of slow growth and delivery of a viable foetus can be expected in the near future. Treatment is then delayed until after delivery.

If tumour growth is rapid however, pregnancy is terminated urgently and treatment of the breast tumour started immediately by surgery in combination with radiation therapy.

Prophylactic castration is not advised but further pregnancy should be delayed as suggested above, whether the tumour was slow or rapid in its growth.

(3) Cancer of the breast presenting during lactation is treated in a routine fashion, after suppressing lactation by antioestrogenic agents rather than by oestrogens.

(4) Late cancer of the breast presenting in pregnancy requires urgent termination of pregnancy, and the use of radiation therapy and cytotoxic chemotherapy. The palliative value of therapeutic castration and additive hormone therapy is doubtful, but further pregnancy will naturally be discouraged.

CONCLUSION

The appearance of breast cancer during pregnancy and lactation is associated with a somewhat poorer prognosis than in the non pregnant patient. This is mainly due to delay both in diagnosis and in treatment but there may be a special risk factor associated with the pregnancy itself. There is little evidence that breast cancer in pregnancy is hormone sensitive or is affected directly by the high hormonal levels associated with pregnancy. It is possible however that the latter may lead to immunosuppression and thus adversely affect the prognosis. There is no evidence that subsequent pregnancy decreases the survival rate or is liable to reactivate the growth of dormant cancer cells after primary treatment of breast cancer.

REFERENCES

Applewhite, R. R., Smith, L. R. and diVincenti, F. (1973): Carcinoma of the breast associated with pregnancy and lactation. *Amer. Surgeon,* **39,** 101.

Bloom, H. J. G. (1965): The influence of delay on the natural history and prognosis of breast cancer. *Brit. J. Cancer,* **19,** 228.

Bloom, H. J. G. (1968): In *Prognostic Factors in Breast Cancer.* Eds. A. P. M. Forrest and P. B. Kunkler, E. & S. Livingstone, Edinburgh, p. 87.

Brightmore, T. G. J., Greening, W. P. and Hamlin, J. (1970): An analysis of clinical and histopathological features in 101 cases of carcinoma of the breast in women under 35 years of age. *Brit. J. Cancer,* **24,** 644.

Bunker, M. L. and Peters, M. V. (1963): Breast cancer associated with pregnancy or lactation. *Amer. J. Obst. Gynec.,* **85,** 312.

Cheek, J. H. (1953): Survey of current opinions concerning carcinoma of the breast occurring during pregnancy. *A.M.A. Arch. Surg.,* **66,** 664.

Cade, S. (1964): Cancer in pregnancy. *J. Obst. Gynae. Brit. Cwlth.* **71,** 341.

Cooper, D. R. and Butterfield, J. (1970): Pregnancy subsequent to mastectomy for cancer of the breast. *Ann. Surg.,* **171,** 429.

Dao, T. L. (1968): In *Prognostic Factors in Breast Cancer.* Eds. A. P. M. Forrest and P. B. Kunkler, E. & S. Livingstone, Edinburgh, p. 88.

Devitt, J. E., Beattie, W. G. and Stoddart, T. G. (1964): Carcinoma of the breast and pregnancy. *Canad. J. Surg.,* **7,** 124.

Holleb, A. J. and Farrow, J. H. (1962): Breast cancer and pregnancy. A report of 283 cases. *Surg. Gynec. Obst.,* **115,** 65.

Holleb, A. J. and Farrow, J. H. (1964): The relation of carcinoma of the breast and pregnancy in 283 cases. *Acta unio Int. Canc.,* **20,** 1480.

Huggins, C. (1972): In *Endocrine Therapy and Malignant Disease.* Ed. B. A. Stoll, W. B. Saunders Co., London, Philadephia, p. 59.

McWhirter, R. (1968): In *Prognostic Factors in Breast Cancer.* Eds. A. P. M. Forrest and P. B. Kunkler, E. & S. Livingstone, Edinburgh, p. 88.

Miller, H. K. (1962): Cancer of the breast during pregnancy and lactation. *Amer. J. Obst. Gynec.,* **83,** 607.

Minton, J. P. and Bianco, M. A. (1974): Serum α2-globulins in breast carcinoma. *Arch. Surg.,* **109,** 238.

Montgomery, T. L. (1961): Detection and disposal of breast cancer in pregnancy. *Amer. J. Obst. Gynec.,* **81,** 926.

Peters, M. V. (1962): Carcinoma of the breast associated with pregnancy. *Radiology,* **78,** 58.

Peters, M. V. (1963): Carcinoma of the breast associated with pregnancy and lactation. *Proc. 10th Clin. Conf. Ontario Res. Foundation,* p. 161.

Peters, M. V. (1968): In *Prognostic Factors in Breast Cancer.* Eds. A. P. M. Forrest and P. B. Kunkler, E. & S. Livingstone, p. 65.

Richards, G. E. (1948): Mammary cancer – the place of surgery and radiotherapy in its management. *Brit. J. Radiol.,* **21,** 109.

Rissanen, P. M. (1969): Pregnancy following treatment of mammary carcinoma. *Acta Radiol. (Ther.),* **8,** 415.

Robinson, D. W. (1965): Breast carcinoma associated with pregnancy. *Amer. J. Obst. Gynec.,* **92,** 658.

Scholz, A. and Scholz, C. (1971): Breast cancer and pregnancy. *Zentralbl. Gynaek.,* **93,** 10.

Stimson, W. H. (1974): Quantitation of a new serum α-macroglobulin in malignant disease, steroid treatment, pregnancy and normal subjects. *J. Endoc.,* **61,** XXX.

Stimson, W. H. (1975): Correlation of the blood level of a pregnancy-associated α-macroglobulin with the clinical course of cancer patients. *Lancet,* **1,** 777.

Treves, N. and Holleb, A. J. (1958): A report of 549 cases of breast cancer in women 35 years or younger. *Surg. Gynec. Obst.,* **107,** 271.

von Schoultz, B. (1974): A quantitative study of the pregnancy zone protein in the sera of pregnant and peuerperal women. *Amer. J. Obst. Gynec.,* **119,** 792.

Westberg, S. V. (1946): Prognosis of breast cancer for pregnant and nursing women. *Acta. Obst. Gyn. Scand. Suppl. No. 4,* 239.

White, T. T. (1955): Carcinoma of the breast in pregnant and nursing women. Review of 1375 cases. *Amer. J. Obst. Gynec.,* **69,** 1277.

11

Factors Provoking Male Breast Cancer

Ole Scheike

The topic will be considered under two headings – the factors which place a male at risk to the development of breast cancer, and the factors which influence prognosis in the male with developed breast cancer.

THE MALE AT RISK TO BREAST CANCER

In the last forty years several theories have been put forward concerning the aetiology of breast cancer in the male. The first section of this chapter assesses these possible aetiological factors on the basis both of our own observations and a review of literature. The Klinefelter syndrome, gynaecomastia, hormonal metabolism and hereditary factors will be considered.

The Klinefelter syndrome

In 1955, Bauer and Erickson submitted the first report on the association between the Klinefelter syndrome and cancer of the breast. Several other case histories followed some years later (Gupta, 1966; Cuenca and Becker, 1968; Robson, Santiago and Huang, 1968; Dodge, Jackson and Muldahl, 1969).

In 1963, Schottenfeld, Lilienfeld and Diamond reported that of 25 male breast cancer patients in whom systematic screening for sex chromatin was carried out, not one showed abnormal sex chromatin. In 1965 however, Jackson *et al.* reported that among 21 male patients with breast carcinoma, 3 were sex chromatin positive and had an abnormal sex chromosome complement. Nadel and Koss (1967) later reported no cases positive for sex chromatin among 16 male patients with breast cancer, but Harnden, Maclean and Langlands (1971) found 5 among 150 patients.

On the basis of these data, a group of 30 male Danish patients with breast cancer was screened for sex chromatin in the buccal smear (Scheike, Visfeldt and Petersen, 1973b), and of these one was found to be sex chromatin positive. In this patient chromosome analysis on peripheral blood showed that the karyotype was 47, xxy, i.e. the chromosome constitution typical of the Klinefelter syndrome.

Table 1 Results of Screening for Sex Chromatin in Males with Mammary Carcinoma (from Scheike, Visfeldt and Petersen, 1973b)

	Number examined	*Number chromatin positive*
Schottenfeld *et al.* (1963)	25	0
Jackson *et al.* (1956)	21	3
Nadel and Koss (1967)	16	0
Harnden *et al.* (1971)	150	5
Present study	30	1
Total	242	9

Thus, by systematic sex chromatic screening, a total of 9 documented cases of the Klinefelter syndrome have been found among 242 males with breast cancer (Table 1). Including the case histories mentioned, 14 documented cases of this association have been reported. In 10 of the cases, the tumour involved the right breast, in 2 the left breast, one was bilateral and in one case the side was not stated. This right-sided predominance, statistically significant at the level of $p < 0.05$, is remarkable. Buccal smears were obtained in 11 cases and chromosome analysis was made in 10 cases. Of these 8 were of the karyotype 47, xxy and 2 were mosaics with 46, xy/47, xxy/48, xxxy and 46, xx/47, xxy respectively.

In order to evaluate its possible aetiological significance, it is essential to estimate the incidence of breast cancer in patients with the Klinefelter syndrome. It was seen (Table 1) that 9 chromatin positive cases were found among 242 men with breast cancer, corresponding to an incidence of 37 per thousand. The incidence of sex chromatin positive individuals in the normal male population is stated to range from 1.9 per thousand (Court Brown, 1969) to 2.2 per thousand (Hambert, 1966).

In Western countries, the incidence of breast cancer in females is about 4,500 per 100,000. The incidence of breast cancer in males is about 1% of that of female and therefore 242 cases of male breast cancer would be expected in a male population of about 500,000. In this size of population one would expect also to find about 1,000 with the Klinefelter syndrome. In the pooled series of 242 cases, 9 cases of breast cancer associated with the Klinefelter syndrome were found, corresponding to an incidence of 0.9% of breast cancer in patients with Klinefelter syndrome (or 9 in 1,000). This is one fifth of the incidence of breast cancer in women and 20 times the incidence of breast cancer in normal men.

The validity of these calculations is based on the following assumptions:

a stationary population (average age being applied); a uniform age distribution for cases of breast cancer in women, men and patients with the Klinefelter syndrome; and a random selection of individuals examined from the cases listed in Table 1 (the mortality in the various age groups exerts an influence in this connection). Therefore, the figures obtained can be considered only approximate. Nevertheless, there is little doubt that patients with the Klinefelter syndrome are at high risk to breast cancer. This may be related to the gynaecomastia and abnormal hormonal metabolism commonly found in these patients.

In the Klinefelter syndrome the gonadotrophin excretion is characteristically increased (Stewart *et al.*, 1959) and measurements showed high excretion levels in 3 out of 6 of the published cases of the Klinefelter syndrome found in association with breast cancer. The excretion of total 17-ketosteroids ranges usually between low and normal in patients with the Klinefelter syndrome. It was measured in 6 of the 14 cases reported, and in 2 cases it was stated to be low. It can hardly be considered relevant in the assessment of testicular function.

The fractionated 17-ketosteroids are of greater interest and in our patient the excretion level was found to be low both for androsterone and etiocholanolone. In addition, a low ratio of 11-desoxy-17-ketosteroids/11-oxy-17-ketosteroids ("11-ratio") was found and this is considered to be a reliable sign of hypogonadism (Johnsen, to be published). The excretion of total oestrogens is usually either normal or decreased in patients with the Klinefelter syndrome (Stewart *et al.*, 1959) but in our patient the value was within normal limits.

In patients with the Klinefelter syndrome, gynaecomastia of long duration is said to occur frequently. In only 4 of the published 14 cases of the Klinefelter syndrome associated with breast cancer was gynaecomastia mentioned. However, in most cases no attempt was made to look for histological evidence of gynaecomastia in the breast tissue removed with the cancer. Such examination requires a reasonable volume of breast tissue.

Gynaecomastia

The possible association between gynaecomastia and breast cancer has been discussed in almost all reports on male breast cancer, and several series mention either a history of, or the co-existence of, clinical and histological signs of gynaecomastia. The reported incidence varies greatly. Gilbert (1933) has reported clinical evidence in 19% of 47 cases while Norris and Taylor (1969) found gynaecomastia in 5% of 108 cases. Out of 40 patients reported by Liechty, Davis and Gleysteen (1967), 17.5% had associated gynaecomastia and of the 7 cases, 5 were clinical and 2 histological diagnoses. On the other hand Huggins and Taylor (1955) reported only one case among 75 patients, and Holleb, Freeman and Farrow (1968a) found clinical evidence of gynaecomastia in only one case and histological evidence in one case among 198 patients.

In order to investigate the possible aetiological relationship between gynaecomastia and breast cancer, a Danish series of 265 cases of male breast cancer (including 8 cases of sarcoma) was reviewed (Scheike and Visfeldt, 1973c). Only one of our patients showed clinical evidence of gynaecomastia coexisting with breast cancer. There were 10 cases with a history of gynaecomastia of which 5 were homolateral and 5 were bilateral. Of the 10 patients 3 gave a history of gynaecomastia during puberty and in 2 of these cases it was irreversible. Seven had gynaecomastia as adults, 5 of them being irreversible. In these 5 patients surgery had been carried out from 5 to 16 years prior to establishment of the cancer diagnosis. In 4 of these cases the histological preparations were available, and the diagnoses were respectively: mastitis, gynaecomastia type I, gynaecomastia type I with mastitis, gynaecomastia type I with pronounced proliferation of epithelium.

A clinical history of gynaecomastia is of doubtful value in the assessment of gynaecomastia as a possible premalignant state, as this condition is fairly frequent not only during puberty but also in adults up to 70 years of age (Nydick *et al.*, 1961; Sirtori and Veronesi, 1957). Histologically verified gynaecomastia, is on the other hand not always associated with enlarged breasts. Williams (1963) found enlargement of the breasts in only 4 out of 178 patients with histologically verified gynaecomastia.

In 79 out of 187 males with operated breast cancer there was sufficient breast tissue in the histological preparations to assess whether a coexisting gynaecomastia was present. This was found in 21 cases, which is 27% of the male breast cancer cases assessed. The histological criteria for gynaecomastia adopted in the examination of the present series were laid down by Williams (1963). Distinction is made between Type I, the florid type, and Type II, the quiescent, fibrous type.

Table 2 Histological Evidence of Gynecomastia co-existing with Male Breast Cancer

Type I (florid type)	6 cases
Type II (quiescent, fibrous type)	15 cases
Total	21 cases

More recent studies indicated that there is a relationship between the histological type of gynaecomastia and the duration of the condition (Nicolis, Modlinger and Gabrilove, 1971). The florid type I is more frequently found in cases of a short duration, and the quiescent, fibrous type II if there is a long history of the condition. Table 2 shows that in the majority of cases the gynaecomastia was of type II. Two of these had shown evidence of type I gynaecomastia, 6 and 16 years respectively prior to the establishment of the diagnosis of breast cancer.

Several authors state that they have observed transition from gynaecomastia to carcinoma by histological examination (Lyall, 1947; Gleichman, 1953; Krückemeyer, 1968). This demonstration is extremely difficult if the criterion is invasive growth of epithelium from the ducts into areas with gynaecomastia. However, the possibility of such a transition is suggested by the demonstration of carcinoma *in situ* in the ductal epithelium. In two of our cases we found ducts with marked atypia of the ductal epithelium in the area with gynaecomastia, coexisting with breast cancer. In spite of examination of serial sections, transition to invasive growth was not demonstrated.

Certain facts appear to support the theory that gynaecomastia may be a premalignant state:

The above-mentioned finding of marked atypia of ductal epithelium in occasional cases with breast cancer and coexisting gynaecomastia.

The average age in 21 patients with breast cancer and coexisting histological gynaecomastia was 55 years. This is significantly lower than the average age for the entire series which is 65 years.

In Egypt and in certain other African areas an incidence of male breast cancer ranging from 6% to 27% is reported (Davies, 1949; El-Gazayerli and Abdel-Aziz, 1963; Bhagwandeen, 1972). In these regions the incidence of gynaecomastia is high and the average age at the appearance of breast cancer is relatively low in these areas.

In patients with the Klinefelter syndrome, the frequency of gynaecomastia is considerably increased, and it is of type II (long duration). The incidence of breast cancer in patients with the Klinefelter syndrome is extremely high compared to the normal male population (Scheike, Visfeldt and Petersen, 1973b).

Hormonal metabolism

The theory that hormonal factors may play an important role in the aetiology of male breast cancer has been discussed for many years. In 1932 Lacassagne proved that breast cancer could be induced in male mice of a certain strain by repeated injections of oestrogen, and since then research has concentrated particularly on the influence of oestrogens. There is very little firm data so far to support the role of oestrogen in the induction of male breast cancer. Some authors maintain that the high incidence of male mammary carcinoma in Egypt and certain tropical regions is due to impairment of the hepatic metabolism of oestrogens because liver damage occurs frequently in these countries (Davies, 1949; Marsden, 1955; El-Gazayerli and Abdel-Aziz, 1963).

In 1968 Symmers reported the remarkable case of two transvestite males. In order to change their appearance to that of women they had themselves castrated, bilateral mammoplasties were performed, and for a long period high doses of oestrogens were administered, orally, by implant and by breast inunction. Each developed a breast carcinoma in their thirties, a very low age for male breast carcinoma.

The popular belief that patients with prostatic cancer receiving oestrogens for a prolonged period might develop breast cancer has however been ruled out by several reports. Campbell *et al.* (1962) proved by histochemical methods that apparently primary breast cancers in these patients were merely metastases from the prostatic cancer, and Berge (1971) found that the primary tumour most often metastasizing to the breast was oestrogen-treated prostatic carcinoma (20 out of 22 cases).

In 1966 Zumoff *et al.* reported abnormal metabolism of labelled oestradiol-17β administered intravenously to patients with male breast cancer. Tritium-labelled oestradiol-17β was administered to 6 men with breast cancer, to 5 healthy men of comparable age and to 9 men with other forms of malignant disease unrelated to the endocrine system. The excretion of oestrone, oestradiol-17β, oestriol, 2-hydroxy-oestrone and 2-methoxyoestrone was measured in 72 hour urine samples. The excretion of oestradiol-17β was found to be identical in the three groups, but the men with breast cancer excreted higher amounts of oestriol and considerably less oestrone, 2-hydroxyoestrone and 2-methoxyoestrone than the other two groups. The authors suggested a relationship between male breast cancer and abnormal oestrogen metabolism.

On the basis of the above data a series of hormone assays was carried out on our male patients with breast cancer (Scheike, Svenstrup and Frandsen, 1973a; Scheike, unpublished results). Firstly, a tracer dose of radioactive oestradiol-17β (2,4,6,7-^{3}H oestradiol-17β) was given intravenously to 19 male patients with breast cancer. The urine was collected after oestrogen administration over a period of 48 hours. The metabolism of the tracer was examined by measuring total radioactivity, and the radioactive metabolites oestrone, 2-methoxyoestrone, oestradiol-17β and oestriol in the urine. Control examinations were made in 19 healthy men and in 5 men with other malignant diseases unrelated to the endocrine system, all in the same age group as the patients with breast cancer.

The metabolism of the tracer was compared in three groups, but no statistical difference was revealed. Total oestrogens were measured in the urine of the three groups, and here again no statistical difference was found. The results of this study do not confirm any specific oestrogen excretion pattern or any specific abnormality in the metabolism of intravenously administered oestradiol-17β in men with breast cancer.

Total urinary excretion of pituitary gonadrotrophins was determined according to the method of Johnsen (1958) in 25 of our patients with male breast cancer, and compared with normal values obtained in 60 healthy men of the same age (Johnsen, 1959). The men with breast cancer excreted a significantly lower amount of pituitary gonadotrophins ($p < 0.05$). The urinary excretion of fractionated 17-ketosteroids was determined in 22 patients and that of 17 ketogenic steroids was determined in 20 patients. Compared with the steroid excretion in healthy men of comparable age, no significant difference was observed.

The conclusions to be drawn from the above results is that men with breast cancer excrete a smaller quantity of pituitary gonadrotrophins, but that otherwise their urinary excretion of hormones does not differ from that found in healthy men of comparable age.

Hereditary factors

In the present series of male breast cancer patients, a total of 43 patients (i.e. 17% of the total) reported a history of cancer in the family (Scheike, unpublished results). Fifteen patients (i.e. 6% of the total) mentioned cases of breast cancer among their relatives. In one of these cases a brother had had breast cancer. Figure 1 shows the pedigree of this family. It will be seen that there is a high incidence of cancer (70%) among the patient's siblings.

Five cases of male breast cancer in relatives of patients with male breast cancer have been reported in the literature (Williams, 1889; Schottenfeld *et al.*, 1963: Schmitt and Scheffler, 1971; Haagensen, 1972). Two of the patients were brothers. Jacobsen (1946) is the only author who has made thorough hereditary studies in several patients with male breast cancer. In 6 of the cases there was a high incidence of cancer in the family, and in 5 of the families there had been cases of female breast cancer.

THE PROGNOSIS IN THE MALE WITH BREAST CANCER

The factors which influence prognosis in the male with developed breast cancer will be considered in relation to female breast cancer, duration of symptoms, clinical staging at presentation, histological grading and method of treatment.

Comparison with female breast cancer

The prognosis in males with breast cancer is generally believed to be much poorer than in females. A Danish series of 257 cases of male breast carcinoma and the series reported in the literature have been reviewed in order to test the above statement, and to investigate which factors most influence the prognosis (Scheike, 1974).

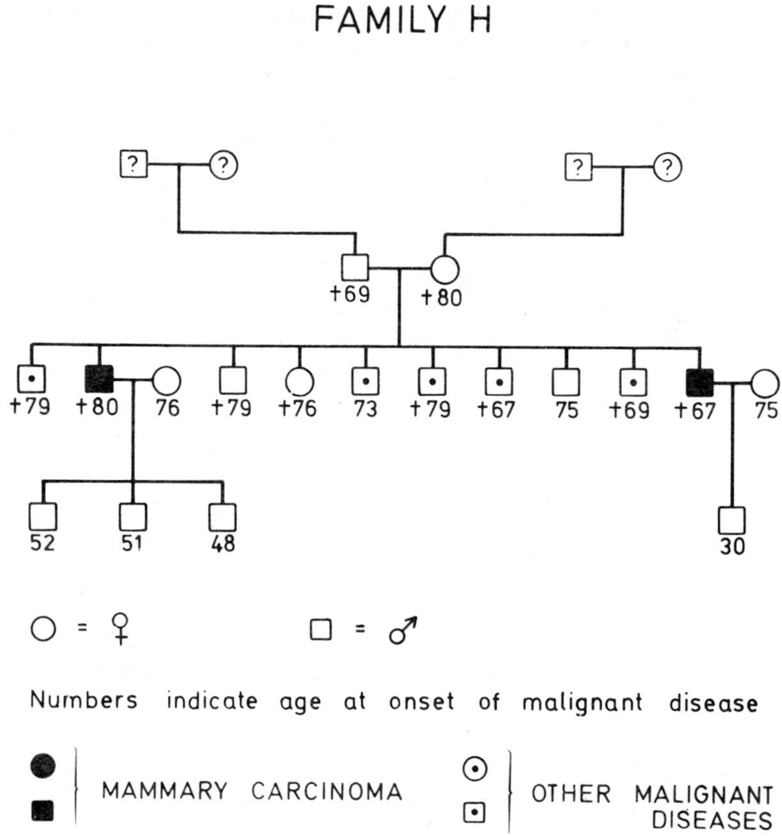

Fig. 1 Pedigree of family H, relatives of a male patient with mammary cancer.

The survival rates in 249 patients with a follow-up period of 1 year or more are shown in Fig. 2. The observed and corrected 5 year survival rates were 36% and 46% respectively. The observed 10 year survival rate was 17% and the corrected rate was 29%. Table 3 shows the 5 year survival rates in published series of male breast cancer, in which corrected survival rates have been calculated from the observations. It will be seen that the prognosis in the present material corresponds well with the prognosis found in most of these series.

Three published papers have compared the corrected 5 year survival rates in males with breast cancer, with the corrected 5 year survival rates in unselected series of females with breast cancer, treated in the same centres and over the same period as the males (Moss, 1964; MacKay and Sellers, 1965; Mausner *et al.*, 1969). The first two reports found the prognosis in

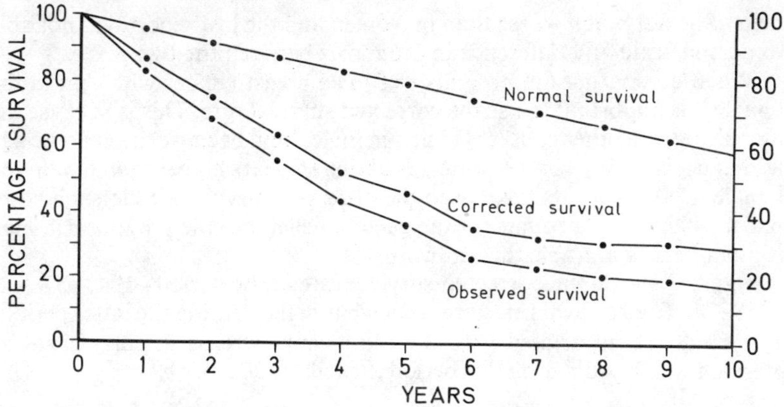

Fig. 2 Survival rates among 249 cases of male breast cancer with a follow-up of 1 year or more (from Scheike, 1974).

Table 3 The Prognosis of Male Breast Cancer in Reported Series (from Scheicke, 1974)

Author	*Number followed 5 years*	*5 year survival rate Observed*	*Corrected*
Moss (1964)	248	41%	43%
MacKay and Sellers (1965)	91	36%	44%
Norris and Taylor (1969)	111	41%	52%
Mausner *et al.*, (1969)	72	47%	60%
Present material	215	36%	46%

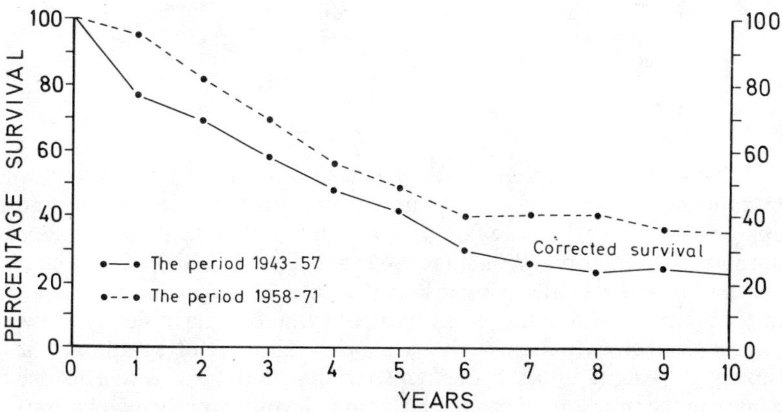

Fig. 3 Corrected survival among males with breast cancer during the period 1943–57 and the period 1958–71 (from Scheike, 1974).

men to be not much worse than in women and the last report was not able to demonstrate any difference in prognosis between the two sexes.

When comparing the prognosis of male breast cancer with that in the female it is important to use the corrected survival rate. This is because the mortality from other causes is higher in males, and because the average age at diagnosis of male breast cancer is about 15 years higher than that in the female. Many authors have used the observed survival rate in such comparisons and this accounts for the general belief that the prognosis in men is much less favourable than in women.

Figure 3 shows the corrected survival rate in the periods 1943–57 and 1958–71. The survival rates are somewhat higher during the latter period. This might be associated with the significant increase in early cases at presentation found during this period (Scheike, 1973d).

Duration of symptoms and prognosis

In males with breast cancer, the diagnosis is established much later than in women. In the present series, the mean duration of symptoms was 20.8 months, and in 16% of the cases it was 3 years or more (Scheike, 1973d).

Table 4 Influence of Duration of Symptoms on Survival (from Scheicke, 1974)

Duration of Symptoms	*Number patients*	*5 year survival Number*	*%*
Less than 3 months	63	24	38
3–5 months	13	4	31
6–11 months	35	8	23
12–23 months	36	13	36
24–35 months	27	12	44
36 months or more	32	13	41
Total	206	74	36

Table 4 shows the influence on prognosis of the duration of symptoms. In patients with a duration of symptoms of 1 year or more, the prognosis appears to be slightly more favourable than that in patients with a shorter duration of symptoms. Williams (1942) and Triska (1967) found a similar correlation in their series of male breast cancer. The explanation might well be that patients with a longer duration of symptoms have slowly growing tumours, whereas patients with a shorter duration of symptoms have rapidly growing tumours. It might also be that, in patients with a history of a lump in the breast for a prolonged period, the tumour is benign for part of the time, due for example to gynaecomastia.

Bloom (1950), Smithers *et al.* (1952), and Haagensen (1972) found that, in female breast cancer, the prognosis was no poorer in patients with a longer duration of symptoms than in patients with a shorter duration of symptoms. Hence, the duration of symptoms alone is not an accurate parameter for the evaluation of the prognosis in the *individual* patient, either in male or in female breast cancer. This does not mean, however, that the duration of symptoms has no influence on the prognosis in male breast cancer.

Table 5 Clinical Stage at Presentation and Duration of Symptoms (From Scheike, 1973d)

		Duration of Symptoms in months		
TNM Stage	*Cases*	*<5*	*6–23*	*>24*
I	87	58%	28%	14%
II	26	46%	31%	23%
III	100	25%	38%	37%
IV	29	27%	42%	31%

In the present series there was a significant correlation (P < 0.001) between the duration of symptoms and the clinical stage at presentation. Table 5 shows that 58% of the patients in clinical stage I had a duration of symptoms of less than 6 months, as against only 25% of the stage III patients and 27% of the stage IV patients. Only 14% of the patients in clinical stage I had a duration of symptoms of 2 years or more, as against 37% of stage III patients and 31% of stage IV patients.

Clinical stage at presentation and prognosis

On the basis of the data obtained from the case records it was possible to divide the 253 cases into stages according to the original version of the TNM classification (U.I.C.C. publication, 1968). Table 6 shows the in-

Table 6 Influence of Clinical Stage on Survival (from Scheike, 1974)

TNM–Stage	*No.*	*Number followed 5 Years*	*5 Year Crude Survival Rate*	*Number followed 10 Years*	*10 Year Crude Survival Rate*
I	89	72	58%	53	38%
II	28	26	38%	21	10%
III	107	91	29%	66	9%
IV	29	25	4%	24	0%
Total	253	214	36%	164	17%

fluence of the clinical stage on prognosis. There was a significant correlation between the clinical stage at presentation and the 5 and 10 year survival rates ($P < 0.001$).

Histological grade of malignancy and prognosis

It was possible to carry out histological grading in 150 cases in the present series (Visfeldt and Scheike, 1973). Grading was carried out according to the W.H.O. recommendation (Scarff and Torloni, 1968). Survival curves for the three grades are given in Fig. 4. There was a significant decrease in the 5 year and 10 year survival rates from grades I to II ($p < 0.05$ and < 0.01, respectively), and in the 5 year survival rate from Grade II to Grade III ($p < 0.01$).

Similar correlations in male breast cancer have been found by Greening and Aichroth (1965) and by Liechty *et al.* (1967), although these series compared only 28 and 40 cases respectively. Bloom and Richardson

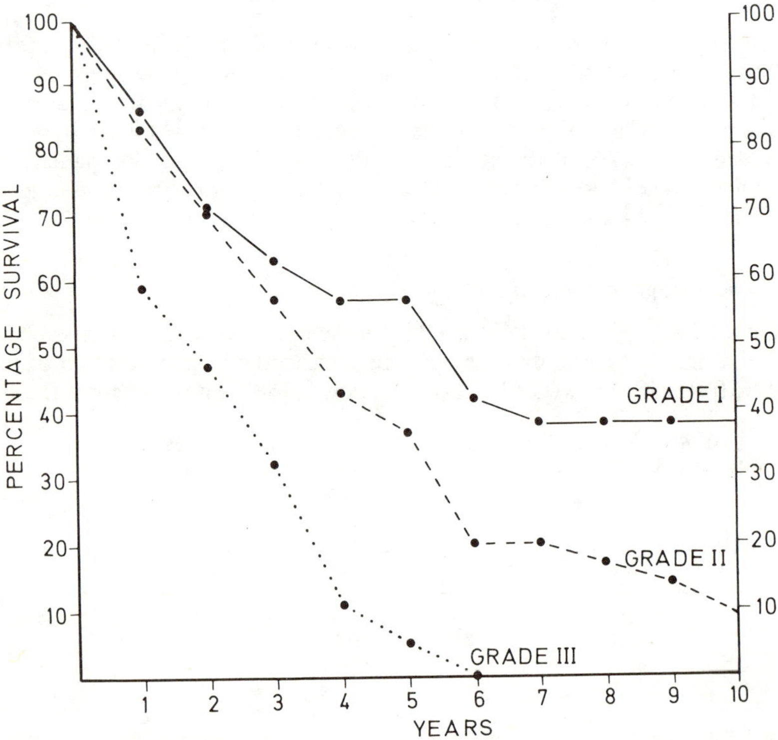

Fig. 4 Survival rates in relation to histological grade of malignancy (from Scheike 1974).

(1957) and Schiødt (1966) described similar correlations in series comprising 1409 and 579 patients, respectively in the case of female breast cancer. However, Schiødt concluded that only patients with grade III tumours had a diminished 5 year survival rate, as compared with the other groups.

Table 7 Influence of Histological Grade on Survival

	Total	*Reduced**	*Dead of breast carcinoma within 5 Years*	
	Number	*Number*	*No.*	*Per cent*
Grade I	44	23	3	13
Grade II	81	48	26	54
Grade III	25	17	16	94

*Patients followed for 5 years, and excluding those dying from causes other than breast cancer.

Table 7 illustrates the correlation between histological grade of malignancy and mortality excluding those patients dying from causes other than breast cancer. The correlation is even more pronounced than that found between histological grade of malignancy and survival rate (Fig. 4 above). Consequently, it is of particular importance to determine, as early as possible, the histological grade of malignancy of the tumour. This will affect choice of treatment and subsequent follow-up of the male patient with breast cancer.

A comparison between the present material and published series of female breast cancer showed that the present material had relatively fewer patients with grade III tumours (Visfeldt and Scheike, 1973). Hence, on the basis of this observation the somewhat poorer prognosis from breast cancer in men cannot be ascribed to a higher proportion of more malignant tumours.

Treatment and prognosis

Radical treatment

On the basis of data obtained from the hospital records it was possible to classify 253 cases according to the Columbia clinical classification (Haagensen, 1972). Of these, 197 cases (78%) were operable, and 56 cases (22%) inoperable. The surgical treatment of the operable patients was not uniform and included radical mastectomy, simple mastectomy and local excision. The indications for supplementing surgical treatment with

Table 8 Results of the Different Methods of Radical Treatment (from Scheike, 1974)

				Five-year results		
		Number	*Survival rate*	*Recurrence-free survival rate*	*Local/ regional recurrence*	*Distant metastases*
Simple mastectomy with or without radiotherapy	All cases	64	50%	36%	31%	28%
	Stage I cases	34	62%	53%	18%	24%
Radical mastectomy with or without radiotherapy	All cases	48	48%	31%	34%	48%
	Stage I cases	18	78%	67%	11%	28%

radiotherapy were not clear; and in most hospitals radiotherapy was given routinely, whether axillary node metastases were present or not.

Table 8 shows the results of the more common methods of treatment. A 5 year survival rate of 50% in patients treated with simple mastectomy, with or without radiotherapy corresponds well to the 53% found by Liechty *et al.* (1967). Radical mastectomy, with or without radiotherapy, resulted in a 5 year survival rate of 48% in the present material. In 143 patients who had undergone similar treatment, collected from the literature, the 5 year survival rate was 49% (Crichlow, 1972).

The cases were not randomized but there was no obvious improvement in the 5 year recurrence-free rate from the use of radical mastectomy. Until randomized series can show better results from radical mastectomy, the less traumatic simple mastectomy is recommended, because the average age of the patient is 65 (40% are 70 or more) and also because of the lesser likelihood of post-operative complications. In the literature some authors recommend radical mastectomy (Somerville, 1952; Holleb *et al.*, 1968b) while others recommend simple mastectomy (Greening and Aichroth, 1965; Liechty *et al.*, 1967). In the latter two reports simple mastectomy, with or without radiotherapy appeared to give just as good results as radical mastectomy with or without radiotherapy.

As the series was not randomized, it is impossible to state whether supplementary radiotherapy improved the results of treatment in the present material. It is interesting that the stage I patients presented a lower frequency of local/regional recurrences than of distant metastases (Table 8). It is possible that a high proportion of the patients, who received radical treatment had unrecognized distant metastases already at the time of treatment.

Palliative treatment

In cases with disseminated disease, oestrogen therapy was the method of treatment most frequently applied. In one third of the cases, or 20 patients, there was a good palliative effect from oestrogens for over 6 months, especially if the treatment was commenced at the first sign of dissemination (Table 9).

Orchiectomy was not used in the present series although most authors recommend it as the treatment of choice when the first sign of dissemination is observed. The results claimed are much better than those obtained in our series using hormonal therapy. Treves (1959) reported an average period of remission of 29.6 months in 28 out of 42 orchiectomized patients.

Male breast cancer is such a rare disease that it would be useful to centralize treatment of such cases. By this means it would be possible to apply scientifically randomized methods of treatment and thus obtain more significant assessment of the results. In addition, it would be useful if the

Table 9 Results of Primary or Secondary Hormonal Treatment (from Scheike 1974)

Treatment	*Number*	*Palliation* ⩾ *6 Months*	*Palliation* < *6 Months*
Stilboestrol	63		
Primary	13	6	7
Secondary	50	14	36
Corticosteroids	24		
Primary	1	1	
Secondary	23	4	19
Anabolic steroids	5		
Secondary	5		5

general public were educated about the existence of this disease and about the value of early diagnosis and treatment. As a result, the prognosis could no doubt be improved.

CONCLUSION

It is possible to recognise certain factors putting the male at risk to the development of breast cancer. Calculated on the basis of personal findings and the results reported by others, the incidence of breast cancer in men with the Klinefelter syndrome is found to be about 20 times higher than in normal men and about one fifth of the incidence in females. It is also concluded that several features support the theory that gynaecomastia may be a premalignant state.

Comparison of the 5 year corrected survival rates in series of male and female breast cancer shows that the prognosis in male breast cancer is not much worse than the prognosis in females. The duration of symptoms has a significant influence on the clinical stage found at presentation. The duration of symptoms, the clinical staging at presentation and the histological grade of malignancy influence the prognosis considerably.

No evidence has been found to favour radical mastectomy rather than simple mastectomy in the treatment of male breast cancer. It is concluded that if the general public was better educated about the existence of this disease, and if treatment of this rare disease was more centralized, the prognosis could be improved.

REFERENCES

Bauer, D. F. and Erickson, R. L. (1955): Male breast cancer. Klinefelter syndrome with prostatic, adrenal and mammary tumors. *Northw. Med.,* **54,** 472.

Berge, T. (1971): Metastases to the male breast. *Acta path. microbiol. scand,* **79A,** 491.

Bhagwandeen, S. B. (1972): Carcinoma of the male breast in Zambia. *E. Afr. med. J.,* **49,** 89.

Bloom, H. J. G. (1950): Further studies on prognosis of breast carcinoma. *Br. J. Cancer,* **4,** 347.

Bloom. H. J. G. and Richardson, W. W. (1957): Histological grading and prognosis in breast cancer. *Br. J. Cancer,* **11,** 359.

Campbell, J. H., Cummins, S. D., Kirk, D. L. and Mathews, W. R. (1962): Secondary breast cancer of prostatic origin. *J.A.M.A.,* **179,** 158.

Crichlow, R. W. (1972): Carcinoma of the male breast. *Surgery Gynec. Obstet.,* **134,** 1011.

Court Brown, W. M. (1969): Sex chromosome aneuploidy in man and its frequency with special reference to mental subnormality and criminal behaviour. *Int. Rev. exp. Path.,* **7,** 31.

Cuenca, C. R. and Becker, K. L. (1968): Klinefelter's syndrome and cancer of the breast. *Arch. intern. Med.,* **121,** 159.

Davies, J. N. P. (1949): Sex hormone upset in Africans. *Brit. Med. J.,* **2,** 676.

Dodge, O. G., Jackson, A. W. and Muldal, S. (1969): Breast cancer and interstitial-cell tumor in a patient with Klinefelter's syndrome. *Cancer, N.Y.,* **24,** 1027.

El-Gazayerli, M. M. and Abdel-Aziz, A. S. (1963): On bilharziasis and male breast cancer in Egypt: A preliminary report and review of the literature. *Brit. J. Cancer,* **17,** 566.

Gilbert, J. B. (1933): Carcinoma of the male breast. *Surg. Gynec. Obstet.,* **57,** 451.

Gleichman, H. G. (1953): Die beziehungen zwischen gynäkomastie und karzinom der mamma. *Z. ges. inn. Med.,* **8,** 567.

Greening, W. P. and Aichroth, P. M. (1965): Cancer of the male breast. *Brit. J. Cancer,* **19,** 92.

Gupta, R. L. (1966): Carcinoma of the breast in a case of Klinefelter syndrome. *Indian J. Cancer,* **3,** 184.

Haagensen, C. D. (1972): *Diseases of the breast.* 2nd. ed. p. 358, 470 ff, 779 f. Saunders, Philadelphia.

Hambert, G. (1966): *Males with positive sex chromatin.* Thesis. Akademiförlaget. Gothenburg.

Harnden, D. G., Maclean, N. and Langlands, A. O. (1971): Carcinoma of the breast and Klinefelter's syndrome. *J. med. Genet.,* **8,** 460.

Holleb, A. I., Freeman, H. P. and Farrow, J. H. (1968a): Cancer of male breast – I. *N.Y. St. J. Med.*, **68,** 544.
Holleb, A. I., Freeman, H. P. and Farrow, J. H. (1968b): Cancer of the male breast – II. *N.Y. St. J. Med.*, **68,** 656.
Huggins, C. and Taylor, G. W. (1955): Carcinoma of male breast. *Arch. Surg.*, **70,** 303.
International Union Against Cancer (1968): *TNM Classification of Malignant Tumors.* Geneva.
Jackson, A. W., Muldal, S., Ockey, C. H. and O'Connor, P. J. (1965): Carcinoma of male breast in association with the Klinefelter syndrome. *Brit. med. J.*, **1,** 223.
Jacobsen, O. (1946): *Heredity in breast cancer.* Thesis, p. 65 ff, 106, 128, 157. Nyt Nordisk Forlag, Copenhagen.
Johnsen, S. G. (1958): A clinical routine method for the quantitative determination of gonadotrophine in 24 hour urine samples. *Acta endocr.* (Kbh.), **28,** 69.
Johnsen, S. G. (1959): A clinical routine method for the quantitative determination of gonadotrophine in 24 hour urine samples. II. Normal values for men and women at all age groups from pre-puberty to senescense. *Acta endocr.* (Kbh.), **31,** 209.
Johnsen, S. G.: To be published.
Krückemeyer, K. (1968): Dysplasien des drüsenepithels bei fibrosis mammae virilis. Beziehungen zum karzinom. *Münch. med. Wschr.*, **110,** 2798.
Lacassagne, A. (1932): Apparition de cancers de la mamelle chez la souris mâle, soumise à des injections de folliculine. *CR. Acad. Sci.* (Paris), **195,** 630.
Liechty, R. D., Davis, J. and Gleysteen, J. (1967): Cancer of the male breast. *Cancer, N.Y.*, **20,** 1617.
Lyall, A. (1947): Chorioncarcinoma of the testis with gynecomastia. Report of case with early breast cancer. *Brit. J. Surg.*, **34,** 278.
MacKay, E. N. and Sellers, A. H. (1965): Breast cancer at the Ontario Cancer Clinics, 1938–1956: A statistical review. *Canad. Med. Ass. J.*, **92,** 647.
Marsden, A. T. H. (1955): The aetiology of carcinoma of the male breast. *Schweiz Z. allg. Path. Bakt.*, **18,** 728.
Mausner, J. S., Shimkin, M. B., Moss, N. H. and Rosemund, G. P. (1969): Cancer of the breast in Philadelphia hospitals 1951–1964. *Cancer, N.Y.*, **23,** 260.
Moss, N. H. (1964): Cancer of the male breast. *Ann. N.Y. Acad. Sci.*, **114,** 937.
Nadel, M. and Koss, L. G. (1967): Klinefelter's syndrome and male breast cancer. *Lancet,* **2,** 366.

Nicolis, G. L., Modlinger, R. S. and Gabrilove, J. L. (1971): A study of the histopathology of human gynecomastia. *J. clin. Endocr.*, **32**, 173.

Norris, H. J. and Taylor, H. B. (1969): Carcinoma of the male breast. *Cancer, N.Y.*, **23**, 1428.

Nydick, M., Bustos, J., Dale, J. H. and Rawson, R. W. (1961): Gynecomastia in adolescent boys. *J. Amer. med. Ass.*, **178**, 449.

Robson, M. C., Santiago, Q. and Huang, T. W. (1968): Bilateral carcinoma of the breast in a patient with Klinefelter's syndrome. *J. Clin. Endocrin.*, **28**, 897.

Scarff, R. W. and Torloni, H. (1968): *Histological Typing of Breast Tumours.* International Histological Classification of Tumours. No. 2, W.H.O., Geneva.

Scheike, O., Svenstrup, B. and Frandsen, V. A. (1973a): Male breast cancer. 2. Metabolism of oestradiol-17β in men with breast cancer. *J. steroid. Biochem*, **4**, 489.

Scheike, O., Visfeldt, J. and Petersen, B. (1973b): Male breast cancer. 3. Breast carcinoma in association with the Klinefelter syndrome. *Acta path. microbiol. scand.*, **81 A**, 352.

Scheike, O. and Visfeldt, J. (1973c): Male breast cancer. 4. Gynecomastia in patients with breast cancer. *Acta path. microbiol. scand.*, **81 A**, 359.

Scheike, O. (1973d): Male breast cancer. 5. Clinical manifestations in 257 cases in Denmark. *Br. J. Cancer*, **28**, 552.

Scheike, O. (1974): Male breast cancer. 6. Factors influencing prognosis. *Br. J. Cancer*, **30**, 261.

Scheike, O.: Unpublished results.

Schiødt, T. (1966): Breast carcinoma. A histologic and prognostic study of 650 followed-up cases. Thesis, p. 72 f., 96 ff. Munksgaard, Copenhagen.

Schmitt, G. and Scheffler, J. (1971): Das karzinom der männlichen brustdrüse. *Dtsch. Med. Wschr.*, **96**, 931.

Schottenfeld, D., Lilienfeld, A. M. and Diamond, H. (1963): Some observations on the epidemiology of breast cancer among males. *Amer. J. publ. Hlth.*, **53**, 890.

Sirtori, C. and Veronesi, U. (1957): Gynecomastia. A review of 218 cases. *Cancer*, **10**,645.

Smithers, D. W., Rigby-Jones, P., Galton, D. A. G. and Payne, P. M. (1952): Cancer of the breast. *Br. J. Radiol.* Suppl. 4.

Somerville, P. (1952): Carcinoma of the male breast. A report of 19 cases and a review of the literature. *Br. J. Surg.*, **39**, 296.

Stewart, J. S. S., Mack, W. S., Govan, A. D. T., Ferguson-Smith, M. A. and Lennox, B. (1959): Klinefelter's syndrome. Clinical and hormonal aspects. *Quart. J. Med.*, **28**, 561.

Symmers, W. St. C. (1968): Carcinoma of breast in trans-sexual individuals after surgical and hormonal interference with the primary and secondary sex characteristics. *Brit. med. J.*, **2**, 83.

Treves, N. (1959): The treatment of cancer, especially inoperable cases of the male breast by ablative surgery (orchiectomy, adrenalectomy and hypophysectomy) and hormone therapy (estrogens and corticosteroids). An analysis of 42 patients. *Cancer, N.Y.*, **12,** 820.

Triska, H. (1967): Das brustdrusenkarzinom beim manne. *Mitteilungsdienst G.B.K. NWR e. V.*, **4,** 535.

Visfeldt, J. and Scheike, O. (1973): Male breast cancer. 1. Histologic typing and grading of 187 Danish cases. *Cancer, N.Y.*, **32,** 985.

Williams, W. R. (1889): Cancer of the male breast, based on the records of one hundred cases; with remarks. *Lancet*, **2,** 261.

Williams, I. G. (1942): Carcinoma of the male breast. *Lancet,* **2,** 701.

Williams, M. J. (1963): Gynecomastia. Its incidence, recognition and host characterization in 447 autopsy cases. *Amer. J. Med.*, **34,** 103.

Zumoff, G., Fischmann, J., Cassouto, J., Hellman, L. and Gallagher, T. F. (1966): Estradiol transformation in men with breast cancer. *J. clin. Endocr.*, **26,** 960.

12

Psychosomatic Factors and Tumour Growth

Basil A. Stoll

There have recently been a number of reports suggesting that emotional stress in women may influence the development and growth of breast cancer. It has been suggested that a tendency to breast cancer may be associated with specific personality traits or behaviour patterns (Pauli and Schmid, 1972; Greer and Morris, 1975), or is more common in women who have received treatment in mental hospitals (Ettigi, Lal and Friesen, 1973). Some observers have examined the possibility that episodes of mental stress may precede the appearance of breast cancer (Katz *et al.*, 1969; Snell and Graham, 1971).

The hypothalamo-pituitary pathway could mediate a cerebral influence on breast cancer growth. The results of hypophyseal ablation suggest that the growth of breast cancer in some patients is influenced through the trophic hormones of the anterior pituitary gland. A change in the level of prolactin, growth hormone, gonadotrophin or corticotrophin is capable of modifying the growth of experimental mammary cancer (Kim, 1965).

The hypothalamus is likely to be a key controller in the growth of human mammary cancer, as well as in the case of the experimental tumour. Lesioning of the hypothalmus in rats has been shown to modify the growth of experimental mammary cancer (Clemens, Welsch and Meites, 1968; Klaiber *et al.*, 1969). Recent reports confirm that levodopa, a precursor of brain amines, can cause temporary regression of mammary cancer not only in experimental animals, but also in the human (Stoll, 1972; Friesen, 1972; Pearson, 1972; Meites *et al.*, 1972).

STRESS AND PITUITARY SECRETION

A great deal of recent work has shown that emotional as well as somatic stress can affect the circulating levels of pituitary trophic hormones such as prolactin, growth hormone, gonadotrophin and corticotrophin (Beumont, 1972). It is possible therefore that a psychosomatic influence on the growth of breast cancer could be exerted by emotional stress. The growth pattern of breast cancer shows a remarkable diversity and this is thought to result from interaction between the aggressive potential of the tumour cells on the one hand and host factors on the other (see Chapters 7 and 8). The latter may well include psychosomatic factors in addition to the more commonly recognized endocrinological and immunological factors.

The hypothalamic neurohormones permit the anterior pituitary gland to be influenced by stimuli from the forebrain and limbic system. The effect is to modify the normally regular diurnal variation characteristic of most pituitary secretion. Continuous interaction between the endocrine system and the brain is obviously necessary in the human in regulating hormonal secretion in response to emotional and other environmental stimuli.

Of the pituitary trophic hormones which affect the growth of established mammary cancer in the human, prolactin is considered the most important. The evidence is mainly from analogy with experimental mammary carcinoma (Pearson *et al.*, 1969), but in addition, prolactin dependence of some breast cancers has been shown in organ cultures (Mioduszewska, 1968; Salih *et al.*, 1972). It is well established that emotional stress can markedly increase the release of prolactin from the human pituitary (Noel *et al.*, 1972; Stearns *et al.*, 1973). There may even be a cerebral centre controlling prolcatin secretion, and in the case of the rabbit, such a centre is found to be located in the orbitofrontal region (Tindal and Knaggs, 1972).

Growth hormone dependence has been suggested in breast cancer for many years but has only recently been demonstrated in organ culture (De Souza *et al.*, 1974). Stimulation of growth hormone secretion has been shown to follow not only emotional stress, but also other neural stimuli such as fear and noise (Catt, 1971).

Gonadotrophin secretion in the human is well known to be influenced by emotional stress and, in turn, regulates oestrogen secretion both in the premenopausal and in the postmenopausal woman (Dilman, 1974). Oestrogen dependence of breast cancer is claimed by some to explain the benefits of endocrine ablative therapy in this disease (Dao, 1972).

Of all the pituitary hormones, it is the pituitary adrenal axis which has received the most intensive study in patients with breast cancer. Increased corticosteroid production is common in breast cancer patients (Bulbrook, Hayward and Thomas, 1964), and was originally suspected to be evidence of adrenal dysfunction related to the development of breast cancer. It is now believed more likely that the increased corticosteroid production results from the somatic stress accompanying the presence of breast cancer (Durant and Miller, 1973; Saez, 1974). It has been reported that raised excretion of 17-hydroxycorticosteroids in breast cancer patients can be associated with evidence of depression of the immune mechanism (Mackay *et al.*, 1971), and both may be evidence that the host defence against breast cancer is breaking down.

Increased adrenocortical activity is also associated with mood disturbance such as anxiety or depression (Beumont, 1972). It is therefore not surprising that a higher corticosteroid production has been noted in breast cancer patients who are apprehensive or depressed than in those who are more fatalistic or stoic (Katz *et al.*, 1970). It may, however, be relevant to an investigation of the effects of emotional stress on the growth of breast cancer, as Saez (1974) has noted that increased cortiscosteroid production in breast cancer patients is associated with a high ACTH secretion. If this stimulates oestrogen secretion by the adrenal, it might possibly stimulate the growth of hormone sensitive breast cancer.

Androgen excretion in breast cancer patients has also been related to the course of the disease. It has been suggested that women with breast cancer who have a lowered androgen excretion have a relatively poor prognosis (Bulbrook, Hayward and Thomas, 1964). A similar observation has been made in patients with lung cancer (Rao and Hewit, 1970), and it has recently been established that a lowered androgen excretion is found following somatic stress or associated with general debility in non malignant disease (Durant and Miller, 1973). A lowered androgen excretion, like a raised corticosteroid excretion, may therefore be evidence of a failing host defence in patients with breast cancer.

EMOTIONAL DISTRESS AND BREAST CANCER

In assessing the role of psychosomatic influences on the development of breast cancer, the authors mentioned at the beginning of this chapter used one of two approaches. Either the personality traits or behaviour pattern of the patient were explored (Katz *et al.*, 1970; Pauli and Schmid, 1972), or else a history of stressful psychological events involving the patient (Katz *et al.*, 1969; Snell and Graham, 1971). These two psychometric procedures are essentially the soil and the seed of emotional stress, while the psychoendocrine effects of emotional stress must be related to the patient's *response* to that stress.

We have so far used the non specific term of "emotional stress" to describe the mental effect of a change in life's circumstances but it might be better to define the terms used. Stressful psychological events endured by a patient with certain personality traits can lead to mood disturbance such as anxiety or depression and the effect on the patient can better be described as "emotional distress" (Aitken, 1975). In order to investigate the possible effect of prolonged emotional distress on the rate of growth of breast cancer, we need to define it in each individual in terms of "when" and "how much".

By the time breast cancer is diagnosed, several years of subclinical tumour growth have already occurred and the pattern of the disease established in three quarters of all cases (Macdonald, 1965). In attempting to establish a psychosomatic pointer to the prognosis, the approach can therefore be either retrospective or prospective. The first approach is to relate the degree of advancement of breast cancer at its presentation to the record of the patient's emotional distress over the preceding years. The second approach is to relate the progress of the disease *after* the diagnosis to the patient's personality traits or mood disturbance estimated at the time of primary treatment (see Chapter 5).

The second approach has the advantage that there are several psychological tests which will reflect personality traits or mood disturbance at the time of examination. However, the approach has the disadvantage that it introduces additional variables including the psychological response of the patient to the diagnosis of cancer and to the mutilation from treatment.

The first approach has the advantage that it investigates the existence of long term emotional distress during the major part of the tumour's life history *before* it manifests clinically. However, the approach presents a problem in psychological assessment. How does one assess emotional distress retrospectively except in a very approximate manner? In any group of women there are likely to be infinite gradations from the phlegmatic to the psychiatrically disturbed. Depending on the criteria used, it has been calculated that the incidence of mood disturbance in general medical practice can be assessed at any level between 5% and 50% (Kessel, 1960).

Because of the obvious difficulties in measuring retrospectively a patient's reaction to stressful psychological events, it was decided to use an indirect measure of emotional distress.

An approximate method of comparing one patient with another may be the patient's need for medical help in the preceding years for the treatment of anxiety/depression. This information can be derived from the patient's usage of tranquillisers, antidepressants, sedatives or hypnotics. It is reasonable to assume that the daily use of such drugs for periods of one month or longer indicates a degree of emotional distress beyond the average.

RETROSPECTIVE INVESTIGATION OF EMOTIONAL DISTRESS

The following account is of an investigation aiming to establish whether patients' emotional distress over the years preceding the diagnosis of breast cancer was related to the degree of advancement of the disease at its presentation.

A consecutive series of 250 women attending for periodic follow-up at two general hospitals was asked to complete a questionnaire at least 12 months after the diagnosis of their breast cancer. A retrospective survey was made of the regular use by the patient of tranquillisers, antidepressants, hypnotics or sedatives for periods of one month or longer.

Separate assessment was made of the 10 years preceding the diagnosis and of the period subsequent to the diagnosis.

Drugs mentioned by the patient were classified in the following groups: hypnotics (mainly barbiturates and Diazepam), minor tranquilisers (mainly Diazepam and Chlordiazepoxide), sedatives (barbiturates or non barbiturates) and antidepressants (tricyclic agents or MAO inhibitors). Drugs which did not fall into these categories were not included in the assessment. Some patients used different drugs at different times, some used tranquillisers as hypnotics and some took barbiturates for the prevention of epilepsy – but all were included in the assessment.

No attempt was made to go beyond this in establishing a psychiatric diagnosis in the cases where the drugs had been taken. There is considerable difficulty in distinguishing anxiety from depression outside the psychiatric clinic, especially in the menopausal woman (Blackwell, 1973). The true incidence of anxiety/depression in the community may well be higher than that indicated by our figures, but it should be stated that the mood disturbances seen in our patients were almost entirely of a neurotic type. In only 3 of the 250 patients questioned had symptoms been severe enough to warrant referral to a psychiatrist.

Table 1 Drug usage in breast cancer patients for one month or more in the 12 months prior to diagnosis and in the 12 months prior to the questionnaire, according to age group.

	Number and % using drugs			
Age Group	*Prior to diagnosis*		*Prior to questionnaire*	
Under 44	9/50	18%	11/26	42%
45–54	7/85	8%	13/57	23%
55–64	11/62	18%	26/81	32%
65–74	7/41	17%	17/60	28%
Over 75	2/12	17%	13/26	50%
Total	36/250	14%	80/250	32%

Table 1 shows the use of tranquillisers, antidepressants, hypnotics or sedatives (from now on to be referred to as "drug usage") for a month or more in the 12 months prior to diagnosis of breast cancer. Also noted is the drug usage in the 12 months prior to the questionnaire, which in all cases took place more than one year after diagnosis. The 250 women are subdivided according to age group so that they can be compared with Table 2 which is a survey of the drug usage recently reported in the general population of the United Kingdom (Balter, Levine and Mannheimer, 1974).

We find that the drug usage of the patients in the 12 months prior to diagnosis is very similar to that of women in the general population.

However, after diagnosis, the overall drug usage is two to three times higher among breast cancer patients than it is in the general population. This is presumably due to the anxiety incidental to the recognition and treatment of the disease. These observations emphasise that evidence of emotional distress in a patient *after* the diagnosis of breast cancer cannot be assumed to reflect pre-existing emotional distress. Yet, it is only the *latter* factor which could have influenced the preclinical growth of her breast cancer, and set the pattern which decides prognosis.

Table 2 Use of antianxiety or sedative drugs by the general population in the U.K. for one month or more in the 12 months prior to questionnaire, according to age and sex (Balter, Levine and Mannheimer, 1974).

	% using drugs	
Age Group	*Males*	*Females*
25–34	2.5%	10.4%
35–44	4.9%	6.4%
45–54	4.2%	15.2%
Over 55	9.3%	12.9%

Table 3 shows the incidence of drug usage before the diagnosis in relation to the staging of the disease found at presentation, and to the clinical appearance of recurrence or metastases within 12 months of diagnosis. (The latter indicates the almost certain presence of occult metastases at the time of diagnosis). It is interesting to note that of the five groups of patients distinguished, those with evidence of metastases beyond the axilla at the time of diagnosis and those showing evidence of recurrence or metastases

Table 3 Drug usage prior to diagnosis of breast cancer in relation to the stage of disease found at presentation and to the appearance of recurrence after radical treatment.

	Number and % using drugs		
Locally advanced at presentation	5/45	11%	
Metastases at presentation or recurrence within 12 months	13/59	22%	$p<0.03$
Recurrence after 12 months	7/44	16%	
Recurrence-free 1 to 5 years	6/40	15%	
Recurrence-free over 5 years	5/52	8%	
Total	36/250	14%	

within 12 months of radical treatment, include the highest proportion of drug users. There is a statistically significant difference ($p < 0.03$) between this group and the other groups of patients, all of whom have been followed up for 12 months or longer.

It is interesting to note also that the patients with locally advanced tumours at presentation do not show a high level of drug usage. It has been pointed out by several authors that these tumours are often of slow growth (Bloom, 1965). It is recognized by the writer that the significance of a retrospective study of drug usage based on a questionnaire must be accepted with caution. Nevertheless, indirect assessment of the individual's reaction to stress in her past history is found to be useful, expecially in combination with psychological testing (Chapter 5).

ANXIETY/DEPRESSION SYNDROME AND HYPOTHALAMIC DYSFUNCTION

Even if a relationship should be confirmed between the presence of persistent emotional distress on the one hand and an increased rate of breast cancer growth on the other, it does not follow that the relationship is one of cause and effect. It is possible that both may arise from a common basis. It has been postulated that changes in brain amine metabolism may play a part both in the development of mood disturbance (Schildkraut, 1965; Janowsky *et al.*, 1972), and in the regulation of pituitary secretion (Stoll, 1972).

A rise in the hypothalamic threshold to feedback suppression has been found in patients with advanced breast cancer (Dilman, 1974; Saez, 1974), in patients with endogenous depression (Prange *et al.*, 1972), and with increasing age (Dilman, 1974). Since abnormal metabolism of biogenic amines at receptor sites in the brain is found to be associated with depression (van Praag and Korf, 1973) and with increasing age (Robinson *et al.*, 1972; Gottfries *et al.*, 1974), it is possible that changes in brain amine metabolism may play a part in the growth of breast cancer also. Supporting evidence is the observation that the administration of levodopa may be followed by tumour response to oestrogen in women previously not responding to such treatment (Stoll, 1972).

ROLE OF PSYCHOTROPIC AGENTS IN BREAST CANCER

It has been suggested that breast cancer may be more frequent among women who have received treatment in mental hospitals (Ettigi, Lal and Friesen, 1973), or in women who have received long term Rauwolfia therapy for hypertension (Boston C.D.S.P., 1973). Neuroleptic agents such as reserpine, and phenothiazines such as chlorpromazine can depress dopamine transmission in the hypothalamus and thus lead to elevation of serum prolactin levels both in animals and in the human (Sherman and

Kolodny, 1974). By analogy with experimental mammary cancer, it has been suggested that this may cause an increased incidence of breast cancer (Boston C.D.S.P., 1973) or stimulation of existing breast cancer growth (Palmer and Maurer, 1972).

It should be taken into account, however, that the psychotropic agents which cause a rise in the serum prolactin levels will tend to depress both gonadotrophin and ACTH levels at the same time (McCann *et al.*, 1971), and this should lead to a decrease in the secretion of oestrogen both from the ovary and from the adrenal cortex. A rise in the serum prolactin level and fall in the gonadotrophin and ACTH levels have been shown to accompany regression of breast cancer following pituitary stalk section (Antony *et al.*, 1969). It is therefore a matter for conjecture whether a rise in serum prolactin levels in the patient taking psychotropic agents is likely to stimulate the growth of human mammary cancer as has been suggested.

It should also be stressed that in the case of experimental rat mammary cancer, elevation of prolactin levels acts as a stimulant of tumour growth only when it occurs in the presence of established tumour. If prolactin levels are elevated *before* the carcinogen operates, the rat is *protected* from the development of cancer (Welsch and Meites, 1974). If this latter observation applies also to the human, it may explain the protective effect exerted by pregnancy at a young age against the development of breast cancer (Cole and MacMahon, 1969). It is also possible that the administration at an early age of agents causing increase in prolactin levels might *protect* the breast from, rather than predispose it to, the development, of breast cancer. Such agents include not only psychotropic agents but also many types of oral contraceptive.

CONCLUSION

The hypothalamo-pituitary pathway could mediate a cerebral influence on breast cancer growth. Emotional stress can affect the circulating levels of prolactin, growth hormone, gonadotrophin and corticotrophin. The possible effects of psychosomatic factors on the growth of breast cancer have been investigated by relating the degree of advancement of breast cancer at its presentation to the patients' history of emotional distress over the preceding years.

In a retrospective survey, 250 patients with breast cancer were questioned as to the treatment of emotional distress by the use of tranquillisers, antidepressants, sedatives or hypnotics in the 10 years prior to diagnosis. The results suggest that the group of patients with evidence of metastases beyond the axilla at the *time of presentation*, and those showing evidence of recurrence or metastases within 12 months of treatment, include the highest proportion of those who, in the past, required medication for emotional distress.

REFERENCES

Antony, G. J., van Wyk, J. J., French, F. S. *et al.* (1969): Influence of pituitary stalk section on growth hormone, insulin and TSH secretion in women with metastatic breast cancer. *Journal Clin, Endoc.,* **29,** 1238.

Balter, M. B., Levine, J., and Mannheimer, D. I. (1974): Cross national study of the extent of anti-anxiety/sedative drug use. *New Engl. J. Med.,* **290,** 769.

Beumont, P. J. V. (1972): Endocrines and Psychiatry, *Brit. J. Hosp. Med.,* **8,** 458.

Blackwell, B. (1973): Psychotropic drugs in use today. *J. Amer. Med. Assoc.,* **225,** 1537.

Bloom, H. J. G. (1965): The influence of delay on the natural history and prognosis of breast cancer. *Brit. J. Cancer,* **19,** 228.

Boston Collaborative Drug Surveillance Program (1973): *Lancet,* **1,** 1399.

Bulbrook, R. D., Hayward, J. L. and Thomas, B. S. (1964): The relation between the urinary 17-hydroxycorticosteroids and 11 deoxy 17 oxosteroids and the fate of patients after mastectomy. *Lancet,* **1,** 945.

Catt, K. J. (1971): Growth Hormone in *Endocrinology,* Lancet Press, London, p. 29.

Clemens, J. A., Welsch, C. W. and Meites, J. (1968): Effect of hypothalamic lesions on incidence and growth of mammary tumours in carcinogen treated rats. *Proc. Soc. Exper. Biol. Med.,* **127,** 969.

Cole, P. and MacMahon, B. (1969): Oestrogen fractions during early reproductive life in the aetiology of breast cancer. *Lancet,* **1,** 604.

Dao, T. L. (1972): Ablation therapy for hormone dependent tumours. *Ann. Rev. Med.,* **23,** 1.

De Souza, I., Morgan, L., Lewis, U. J. *et al.* (1974): Growth hormone dependency among human breast cancers. *Lancet,* **2,** 182.

Dilman, V. M. (1974): In *Mammary Cancer and Neuroendocrine Therapy,* Ed. B. A. Stoll, Butterworth, London, p. 197.

Durant, J. A. and Miller, H. (1973): Non specific factors that may influence the significance of urinary steroid excretion in breast cancer. *Brit. Med. J.,* **4,** 767.

Ettigi, P., Lal, S. and Friesen, H. G. (1973): Prolactin, phenothiazines, admission to mental hospitals and carcinoma of the breast. *Lancet,* **2,** 266.

Friesen. H. G. (1972): In *Prolactin and Carcinogenesis,* Ed. A. R. Boyns and K. Griffiths, Alpha Omega Alpha, Cardiff, p. 64.

Gottfries, C. G., Oreland, L., Wiberg, A. and Winblad, B. (1974): Brain levels of MAO in depression. *Lancet,* **2,** 360.

Janowsky, D. S., Davis, J. M. El-Yousef, E. K. and Sekerke, H. J. (1972): Cholinergic reversal of manic symptoms, *Lancet,* **1,** 1236.

Katz, J. L., Ackman, P., Rothwax, Y. *et al.* (1970): Psychoendocrine aspects of cancer of the breast. *Psychosom. Med.,* **32,** 1.

Katz, J., Gallagher, T., Hellman. L. *et al.* (1969): Psychoendocrine considerations in cancer of the breast. *Ann. N.Y. Acad. Sci.,* **164,** 509.

Kessel, N. (1960): Psychiatry in general practice. *Brit. J. Prev. Soc. Med.,* **14,** 16.

Kim, U. (1965): Pituitary function and hormonal therapy of experimental breast cancer. *Cancer Res.,* **25,** 1146.

Klaiber, M. S., Gruenstein, M., Meranze, D. R. and Shimkin, M. B. (1969): Influence of hypothalamic lesions on induction and growth of mammary cancer in Sprague Dawley rats receiving DMBA. *Cancer Res.*, **29,** 999.

MacDonald, I. (1965): Indicators of the fundamental biology of mammary carcinoma. *Proc. 3rd Nat. Cancer Conf.,* Lippincott, Philadelphia, p. 87.

Mackay, W. D., Edwards, M. H., Bulbrook, R. D. and Wang, D. Y. (1971): Relation between plasma androgen sulphates and immune response in women with breast cancer. *Lancet,* **2,** 1001.

McCann, S. M. *et al.* (1971): In *Brain-Endocrine Interaction.* Eds. K. M. Knigge, D. E. Scott and A. Weindl, Karger, Basel, p. 224.

Meites, J., Lu, K. H., Wuttke, W. *et al.* (1972): Recent studies in function and control of prolactin secretion in rats. *Rec. Prog. Horm. Res.,* **28,** 471.

Mioduszewska, O. (1968): In Prognostic Factors in Breast Cancer. Eds. A. P. M. Forrest and P. B. Kunkler. E. & S. Livingstone, Edinburgh, p. 347.

Noel, G. L. Suh, S. K., Stone, J. G. *et al.* (1972): Human prolactin and growth hormone release during surgery and other conditions of stress. *J. Clin. Endoc.,* **35,** 840.

Palmer, J. and Maurer, L. H. (1972): Prolactin and breast cancer. *Lancet,* **2,** 1036.

Pauli, H. K. and Schmid, V. (1972): Psychosomatic aspects in the clinical manifestation of breast cancer. *Z. Psychother. Med. Psychol.,* **22,** 76.

Pearson, O. H. (1972): In *Prolactin and Carcinogenesis.* Eds. A. R. Boyns and K. Griffiths, Alpha Omega Alpha, Cardiff, p. 154.

Pearson, O. H. Llerena, O. Llerena, L. *et al.* (1969): Prolactin dependent rat mammary cancer, a model for man? *Trans Amer. Assoc. Phys.*, **82,** 225.

Prange, A. J., Wilson, L. C., Lara, P. P. *et al.* (1972): Effect of TRH on depression. *Lancet,* **2,** 999.

Rao, L. G. S., and Hewit, M. L. (1970): Prognostic significance of a steroid discriminant function in patients with inoperable lung cancer. *Lancet,* **2,** 1063.

Robinson, D. S., Davis, I. M., Nies, J. *et al.* (1972): Ageing, monoamines and monoamine oxidase levels. *Lancet*, **1,** 290.

Saez, S. (1974): In *Mammary Cancer and Neuroendocrine Therapy*. Ed. B. A. Stoll, Butterworths, London, p. 101.

Salih, H., Brander, W., Flax, H. and Hobbs, J. R. (1972): Prolactin dependence in human breast cancers. *Lancet,* **2,** 1103.

Sherman, L. and Kolodny, H. D. (1974): In *Mammary Cancer and Neuroendocrine Therapy*. Ed. B. A. Stoll, p. 369.

Schildkraut, J. J. (1965): The catecholamine hypothesis of affective disorders. *Amer. J. Psychiat.*, **122,** 509.

Snell, L. and Graham, S. (1971): Social trauma as related to cancer of the breast. *Brit. J. Cancer,* **25,** 720.

Stearns. E. L. Winter, J. R. D. and Faiman, C. (1973): Effect of coitus on gonadotrophin, prolactin and sex steroid levels in man. *J. Clin. Endoc.,* **37,** 687.

Stoll, B. A. (1972): Breast cancer and brain catecholamines. A hypothesis. *Lancet,* **1,** 431.

Stoll, B. A. (1974): In *Mammary Cancer and Neuroendocrine Therapy,* Ed. B. A. Stoll, Butterworths, p. 326.

Tindal, J. S. and Knaggs, G. S. (1972): Pathways in the forebrain of the rabbit concerned with the release of prolactin. *J. Endoc.,* **52,** 253.

Van Praag, H. M. and Kroff, J. (1973): Cerebral monoamines and depression. *Arch. Gen. Psychiat.,* **28,** 827.

Welsch, C. W. and Meites, J. (1974): In *Mammary Cancer and Neuroendocrine Therapy*. Ed. B. A. Stoll, Butterworths, London, p. 25.

Late references

Aitkin, R. C. B. (1975): Stress and distress. *Brit. Med. J.*, **1,** 611.

Greer, S. and Morris, T. (1975): Psychological attributes of women who develop breast cancer. *J. Psychosom. Med.,* **19,** 147.

Section 3
SELECTIVE SCREENING

13

The Search for Women at High Risk

Henry P. Leis, Jr., and Alfio Raciti

In the search for the patient with a high risk of developing breast cancer one must recognize that both experimental and and clinical observations indicate that development of breast cancer is not a chance event that occurs randomly throughout the population. There are certain women who are in a high risk group.

Carcinogenesis seems to be a multiphase process involving a number of risk factors, and the development of breast cancer depends on a dynamic interplay between genetic, viral, hormonal and immunologic factors. The progression from a normal cell pattern through hyperplasia, atypia and *in situ* carcinoma, to invasive carcinoma is not inevitable but can be arrested or reversed at any time by alterations in the interplay of these factors (Gallagher and Martin, 1969).

Numerous factors have been credited with a role in the epidemiology of breast cancer. Some of these play the major role while others have a prominent influence. There is a third group which may have a possible role but whose relative importance is small.

MAJOR FACTORS

The major predictors of high risk include: sex, age, familial history of breast cancer, parity, previous cancer in one breast and the precancerous type of fibrocystic disease.

Age and sex

Over 99% of breast cancers occur in the female and less than 1% in the male. The majority of breast cancers manifest after the menopause and the incidence progressively increases to reach its highest level in the over 85 age group (Haagensen, 1971; Leis, 1971; Seidman, 1972). Around the usual age of the menopause between 45 and 54, there is a "break" in the constantly rising incidence curve in women, presumably due to the physiological hormonal change (Clemmesen, 1965).

Over 75% of breast cancers occur over the age of 40 and over half occur between 45 and 59. Only about 1.5% occur below the age of 30, and under 21 years of age, breast cancer is a medical curiosity (Haagensen, 1971; Leis, 1970; O'Donnell, Day and Venet, 1962; Seidman, 1972). Breast cancer tends to occur later in the male than in the female, the median age for males being 64 and for females 58 (Moss, 1965).

From the high risk standpoint, it would therefore, seem logical to concentrate on women over the age of 40 with increasing emphasis as women become older. However, breast cancer is likely to be present in a preclinical stage for an average of six years before it reaches the clinically palpable size of 1 cm (MacDonald, 1966). Since diagnostic aids can detect some breast cancers before they are detectable by palpation, patients with several high risk factors should start regular mammogram, thermogram and physical examination at the age of 35 rather than 40 (Leis, 1971).

Familial history

Anderson (1974) states that the hereditary forms of breast cancer are more frequent than is generally suspected. They have an early age of onset, tend to be bilateral or multiple and they seem to fit the two step mutational concept of Knudson (1971). Genetic factors seem to be most important in patients in whom the disease is bilateral and develops before the menopause.

Female relatives of women with breast cancer have an increased risk of developing the disease as compared with the general population. The studies of Lilienfeld (1963) showed double the risk of breast cancer for daughters of mothers with breast cancer as compared to the general population, and for sisters of patients with breast cancer, the risk was even greater than this. Macklin (1959) reported an increased familial risk of mammary cancer not only in relation to mothers and sisters but also in relation to grandmothers, aunts and female cousins. The risk is highest in women who have never been pregnant.

Anderson (1972) in a large study of the familial incidence of breast cancer noted that the increased risk of developing cancer of the breast was most marked in those women with relatives in whom the disease appeared before the menopause. For patients in whom the disease was bilateral, the risk for relatives was 5.4 times greater than that for age matched controls, but 8.5 times greater if the patient was also premenopausal. The risk for relatives of patients with unilateral disease either before or after the menopause, however, was only 1.2 to 1.8 times greater than the risk for controls. Thus among the relatives of patients with bilateral disease, the risk was five times higher than it was for relatives of patients with unilateral disease. Relatives of patients with bilateral cancers also had a nine times greater risk of developing bilateral disease themselves, when compared with relatives of patients with unilateral involvement.

Parity (marriage–fertility–nursing)

Parity is a most important factor in breast cancer risk. The protective influence of parity has been emphasized by Dunn (1969), the risk of breast cancer in women with one or two children being 1.5 to 2.0 times that of women with three or more children. New studies show that the association between the risk of developing breast cancer and parity is related to a woman's age at her first full term pregnancy. Those with first births after the age of 35 have three times the risk of those with first births before the age of 18 (MacMahon *et al.*, 1970). While this study indicates that parity before the age of 25 exerts a definite protective influence against breast cancer, it also suggests that pregnancy after 35 may well carry a breast cancer risk greater even than that for nulliparous women. The very low incidence rate of breast cancer among the Ishans of Nigeria who belong to the Negro race is probably related to their becoming pregnant at an early age rather than to racial factors or to their low fat diet (Okojie, 1974).

The highest incidence of breast cancer is in nuns (Fraumeni *et al.*, 1969), while single women have a relative risk of breast cancer 1.35 to 2.3 times that of women who have been married (Dunn, 1969). The risk for infertile married women is 1.15 to 1.6 times that of the fertile (Dunn, 1969). International collaborative case controlled studies in progress in seven areas since 1965 are in general agreement with these findings (Seidman, 1972). They include two high risk areas – Boston, Massachusetts and Glamorgan, Wales; three intermediate risk areas – Slovina, Yugoslavia, Greater Athens, Greece and Sao Paulo, Brazil, and two low risk areas – Tokyo, Japan and Taipei, Taiwan.

Breast feeding especially if prolonged has, in the past, been assumed to reduce breast cancer risk, In the United States, little correlation has been shown except in one study (Levin *et al.*, 1964) which showed a protective influence if nursing was for 36 months or more. Wynder, Bross and Hirayama (1960) quoting data from New York, England, India and Japan, indicated that there might be some decrease in the risk following long term nursing, but the recent collaborative studies reported by MacMahon *et al.* (1970) show little or no correlation.

Previous cancer in one breast

The risk of developing cancer in the second breast after the first has been removed for cancer, is about five times greater than the risk of initial breast cancer in the general population (Robbins and Berg, 1964; Leis *et al.*,

1965; Urban, 1969: Leis, 1971, 1974). Some in this group of patients have an even higher risk of developing cancer in the second breast. This group includes patients with a good expectation of long term survival including those with non-invasive cancers, those with invasive cancers that are not prone to metastasize (adenoid cystic, tubular, medullary with lymphoid infiltrate, colloid, comedo with minimal stromal invasion and papillary types), and those whose cancers are Stage O or 1. It also includes patients with a familial history of breast cancer, those with multicentric primary cancers in the first breast, those with precancerous mastopathy shown in random biopsy of the other breast, and patients under 50 years of age (Leis, 1971, 1974, 1975).

Precancerous type of fibrocystic disease

Davis, Simons and Davis (1964) in a review of the world literature found that the presence of fibrocystic disease of the breast increased the risk of developing cancer of the breast by 2.64 times. Cole and MacMahon (1969) noted certain similarities between breast cancer and cystic mastopathy which suggest a common hormonal predisposition.

The term fibrocystic disease has been a common dumping ground for many types of lesion. Certainly not all of its forms are related to the subsequent development of mammary carcinoma because it is so common, and if this were the case, the incidence of breast cancer would be much higher than it actually is. The two types of fibrocystic disease that seem to play a role in the development of breast cancer are duct epithelial hyperplasia with atypia and apocrine metaplasia with atypia (Black *et al.*, 1972; Leis, 1973). Black recommended the term precancerous mastopathy for these lesions and reported that a woman with ductular atypia in a benign lesion has a risk of developing breast cancer five times greater than that of a woman without evidence of atypia. If apocrine metaplasia with atypia was included, however, the risk was somewhat smaller.

PROMINENT FACTORS

Prominent predictors of high risk include: viral factors, immunologic factors, genetic factors, radiation exposure, cancer in other organs, alteration in hormonal milieu including estrogen, castration and menstrual activity, aetiocholanolone and/or androsterone excretions.

Viral factors

It has been suggested that viruses may be involved in the development of leukemia, osteosarcoma, Burkitt's lymphoma and cancers of the uterine cervix and postnasal space. Breast cancer may also be included in this group (Feller and Chopra, 1971).

Bittner (1939) demonstrated that breast cancer in the mouse required the transmission of a carcinogenic agent through the milk. This has been identified as a ribonucleic acid virus characterized as B particle, with a characteristic size, structure and property for inducing breast tumors (Moore, 1965).

Squartini (1974) has collated the observations which indicate that a viral agent, like the mouse tumor virus (MTV), might be involved in the aetiology of human breast cancer. B particles (the morphologic expression of murine MTV) have been found in the milk of women with breast cancer and also in malignant tumors of the breast in humans (Dmochowski, Seman, Gallagher, 1969). They have also been found in about 5% of samples of milk from healthy women (Moore, Sarkar and Kelly, 1969). An identical RNA reverse transcriptase (biochemical marker of oncogenic ribonucleic acid virus) to that found in the milk of mice with breast cancer, has also been observed in the milk of women with breast cancer and in those with a familial history of breast cancer (Axel, Schlom and Spiegelman, 1972; Schlom, Spiegelman and Moore, 1972). Finally, antibodies neutralizing murine MTV have been detected in the sera of breast cancer patients (Charney and Moore, 1971), and it has been reported that patients with breast cancer exhibit cellular hypersensitivity responses to MTV-containing milk from RIII mice by the leukocyte migration index procedure (Black *et al.*, 1974).

It is suggested that virus transmission may be through the milk, ovum or sperm. Bentvelzen, Daams and Hageman (1972) postulate that viruses indigenous to a strain are transmitted genetically while those introduced in other strains are transferred through the milk.

If milk may be one route of transmission of human ribonucleic acid type oncogenic viruses, then there should be complete abstinence from breast feeding of infants in families with a history of breast cancer. Not only does the familial tendency increase the risk of breast cancer in these infants, but nursing could further increase the risk if the virus is transmitted through the milk.

Immunologic factors

There is an increasing body of evidence, mainly in animals but lately also in humans, which suggests that immunological mechanisms are important in the development of human breast cancers. It is possible that any breakdown in the normal immune mechanism may facilitate the development of malignant tumours (Leis, 1975); Papaioannou, 1974).

Immunological factors may play a major role in breast carcinogenesis either alone or more commonly in combination with genetic, viral, chemical or hormonal factors (Papaioannou, 1974). Immunodepression or deficiency can be caused by a virus or other carcinogen, by thymectomy and by thymus atrophy, by ageing (spontaneous immunodepression), by x-ray therapy, by chemotherapy and by immunosuppressant drugs used in transplants (Serrou *et al.*, 1974).

Women with immunodepression or deficiency may have an increased risk of developing breast cancer and this would include women with decreased thymus – dependent T lymphocytes, those who have had radiotherapy or chemotherapy, and those who have received immunosuppressant drugs.

Genetic factors

Genetic predisposition plays a very important role in the development of breast cancer and it is doubtful if the other factors could induce breast cancer without a proper genetic setting. Among the risk factors in breast cancer, the one that holds most interest for geneticists, apart from familial history, is the possibility that genetic variations in the apocrine glands may also influence susceptibility to breast cancer. Petrakis in 1971 reported an association between the type of cerumen or ear wax (wet or dry) and breast cancer mortality in various ethnic groups. He showed the existence of a strong correlation between breast cancer mortality and the presence of wet cerumen.

Hems (1970) demonstrated a positive association between breast cancer and ABO blood, group A, but this was not confirmed later by other observers. The Boston Collaborative Drug Surveillance Programme documented an excess of the ss blood phenotype in patients with breast cancer but again this was not confirmed by other groups later.

A new concept has recently been introduced, namely that of genetic control of susceptibility and resistance to viruses. Support for this theory in the experimental field has been given by Huebner and Todaro (1969), with the oncogene concept as a prerequisite for the development of breast cancer.

Turkington (1970) demonstrated a biochemical difference between normal and neoplastic mammary cells which he believed to be related to specific genes actively transcribed. Neoplastic mammary cells possess a specific enzyme which is absent in normal cells, the transfer ribonucleic acid guanine 7-methylase. On this basis the author suggested that altered regulation of gene expression may be a basic property of neoplastic mammary cells.

Radiation exposure

Nohrmann (1949) was the first to call attention to the fact that ionizing radiation was a possible carcinogen to the breast. Since then there have been numerous other reports incriminating radiation exposure as an etiological agent in mammary carcinoma. Five cases of cancer of the male breast have been reported as developing up to 35 years after radiation exposure (Guthorn, 1951; Lowell, Martinean and Luria, 1968; Peck, 1944; Schottenfeld, Lilienfeld and Diamond, 1963).

Women who have had repeated fluoroscopies during pneumothorax treatment for tuberculosis have been reported as having a considerably increased incidence of breast cancer on the treated side (MacKenzie, 1965; Myrden and Hiltz, 1969). An increased incidence of breast cancer has also been reported in women receiving radiation for puerperal mastitis (Mettler, Hempelmann and Dutton, 1969) and among survivors of the atomic bombings in Hiroshima and Nagasaki (Wanebo *et al.*, 1968).

Postoperative radiotherapy following mastectomy consistently reduces peripheral lymphocyte counts and host resistance (immunocompetence) over long periods of time. (Meyer, 1970; Black and Leis, 1973; Leis, 1975). Stjernsward, Jondal and Vansky (1972) have shown that post-mastectomy radiotherapy selectively destroys thymus-dependent lymphocytes, changing the ratio between circulating thymus-dependent (T) lymphocytes and bone marrow-dependent (B) lymphocytes. This reduces cell mediated immune response and might permit the elaboration of antibiodies that enhance tumor growth.

In view of the fact that ionizing radiation can be carcinogenic to the breast and that it can reduce host resistance, its use in potentially curable breast cancer either alone (Atkins *et al.*, 1972), or combined with simple mastectomy (McWhirter, 1955), is open to serious question. In our opinion, it should not be used routinely after modified or radical mastectomy but only where specifically indicated (Leis and Pilnik, 1974). Methods are now available whereby one can measure the degree of host resistance to breast cancer at the time of surgery and subsequently (Black, 1973; Black and Leis, 1971, 1973; Black *et al.*, 1974; Leis, 1975). Patients who have had modified or radical mastectomy for potentially curable breast cancer and who show evidence of good host resistance should not receive routine postoperative radiotherapy.

The widespread use of mammography and xerography in high risk patients and in screening techniques for the early detection of breast cancer is also open to some question (Papaioannou, 1974). However, its usefulness in the diagnosis of the presymptomatic type of breast cancer where the prognosis for cure is excellent, would seem to far outweigh its disadvantage (Chamberlain, Egan and Harvey, 1970; Leis, 1970; 1971).

The increased incidence of breast cancer reported among the survivors of the atomic bombings in Hiroshima and Nagasaki exposed to more than 90 rads (Wanebo *et al.*, 1968) has been used as a basis for advising that the total accumulated dose of radiation in mammography be kept below 90 rads. According to the report six women developed breast cancer compared with the expected number of 1.55. The number of cases was very small and a dose-response relationship was not demonstrated, so that this evidence cannot be considered conclusive. However, attempts should be made to keep the accumulated dose to a minimum. The low dose technique with vacuum cassettes, involving doses of 1 to 2 rads per examination, would seem an advantage if it offers satisfactory accuracy (Strax, 1974).

Cancer in other organs

There is an increased risk of developing cancer of the breast as a second primary neoplasm, in patients who have had either previous carcinoma of the ovary (Lynch *et al.*, 1974), carcinoma of the endomentrium (MacMahon and Austin, 1969; Schottenfeld and Berg, 1971), carcinoma of the colon (Schoenberg, Greenberg and Eisenberg, 1969), or carcinoma of a major salivary gland (Dunn *et al.*, 1972).

MacMahon and Austin (1969) in a study of 869 women with endometrial cancer reported a 30% increase in breast cancer over the expected number. Haagensen (1971) suggests that this is the main second primary cancer associated with breast cancer.

Alteration in hormonal milieu including estrogen

There is ample evidence that estrogens are involved in mammary carcinogenesis. However, while they used to be considered the main carcinogenic factor, they are now believed to act primarily as powerful promoters in carcinogenesis. It is not known whether their action is directly on the cell, or indirectly by affecting metabolic processes or the immune response of the host (Papaioannou, 1974).

It has been postulated that there are two main etiological types of breast cancer with different age peaks and hormonal relationships. The first peak occurs in premenopausal women aged 45 to 49 and this type of breast cancer is presumed to be related to ovarian dysfunction. The second peak occurs about the age of 65 and is presumed to be related to imbalance of adrenal estrogens. Adrenal insufficiency is suggested by the increased frequency of breast cancer in patients who are obese, hypertensive and diabetic (De Waard, Baanders-Van Halewijn and Huizinga, 1964).

There are many observations suggesting that ovarian hormones play a role in mammary carcinogenesis. Cancer of the breast occurs predominantly in women and is a medical curiosity before puberty. There is a dramatic decrease in the risk of developing breast cancer in women castrated before the age of 37, and in those with decreased over-all menstrual activity.

There are three main estrogen fractions – estrone, estradiol and estriol.

Estradiol is a stronger estrogen and a weaker carcinogen than estrone, whereas estriol has minimal if any estrogenic action and no carcinogenic potential (Shubik and Hartwell, 1957). Estriol seems to serve as an impeding or blocking agent against the potential carcinogenic effects of estrone and estradiol, possibly by competing with them for intracellular receptor sites (Lemon *et al.*, 1966; Lemon, 1970). Progesterone has a direct antagonistic effect against estrogens (Lerner and Hilf, 1967).

Cole and MacMahon (1969) and MacMahon, Cole and Brown (1971) have emphasized the importance of the proportion of the various estrogen fractions in a woman's risk of developing breast cancer. Estrogen fractions in women 15 to 19 and 35 to 39 years of age were studied, and the proportion of estriol excreted in the urine was found to be considerably higher in women from low breast cancer incidence areas as compared to those from high incidence areas. The difference was significant in the young women, but only slight in women in the older group. Thus, it may be possible by estimating estriol fractions to recognize young women who have an increased subsequent risk of developing breast cancer.

This might also explain why early pregnancy offers a protection against subsequent development of breast cancer, since during pregnancy estriol production is increased to a much greater degree than that of the other two estrogen fractions. Pregnancy may alter the estrogen binding sites of mammary parenchymal cells making for more binding of estriol and less of estradiol and estrone. Alternatively, it might be that hormonal homeostatic mechanisms in normal parous women inactivate or compensate for exogenous estrogens (Black and Leis, 1972).

Castration and menstrual activity

The induction of an artificial menopause, whether by surgery or by irradiation, dramatically reduces the risk of breast cancer. Dunn (1969) from three studies concluded that an artificial menopause reduced the risk of breast cancer between 50–60%. Similar findings were reported by Hirayama and Wynder (1962) who emphasized that the greatest reduction in the risk occurs in those castrated before the age of 37. Trichopoulos, MacMahon and Cole (1972) reported that in women castrated before the age of 35 years the subsequent risk of breast cancer development was one third of that expected.

Shapiro *et al.* (1968) reported a slightly increased risk of breast cancer in women under 12 years of age at the time of menarche, as compared with those who were 15 or older at the time of menarche. A similarly increased risk was present in women with 30 or more years of menstrual activity as compared with those with less than 30 years of active menstrual history. Trichopoulos *et al.* (1972) noted that the risk of breast cancer in women undergoing the menopause at 55 or later was twice as great as for those whose menopause occurred before the age of 45, while Seidman (1972) states that women undergoing the menopause at 50 or later have 1.4 to 1.7 times the risk of those with a natural menopause before the age of 45.

It would seem that early onset of menopause, whether natural or artificial, provides the same kind of protection against breast cancer for older women, that early pregnancy does for younger women.

Aetiocholanolone and/or androsterone excretion

The type of breast cancer that has its age peak at 65 rather than at 45 to 49 is thought more likely to be related to adrenal gland dysfunction than to ovarian dysfunction. In the course of the Guernsey Island prospective endocrine studies, samples of urine are being examined in a large number of presumably normal women. Those women who later developed breast cancer have been found to excrete subnormal amounts of urinary aetiocholanolone and/or androsterone as compared to controls (Bulbrook, Hayward and Spicer, 1971). A similar pattern of abnormal urinary steroid metabolite excretion was observed also in the sisters of the patients with cancer of the breast (Bulbrook, Hayward and Allen, 1969). This suggests a familial predisposition associated with an abnormal hormonal milieu (genetic predisposition). Other women with similarly abnormal urinary hormonal discriminants may also have an increased risk of developing breast cancer.

POSSIBLE RISK FACTORS

The "possible" predictors of high risk of breast cancer have varied statistical significance. They include: high dietary fat, chronic psychogenic stress, hormone administration, trauma, chemical agents, hypothyroidism, living in the Western Hemisphere, upper socio-economic status, living in a cold climate, the white race and Jewish women.

High dietary fat

There is considerable epidemiological evidence of an increased tendency to develop breast cancer associated with the consumption of a diet high in fat (Carroll, Gammel and Plunkett, 1968; Hems, 1970; Lea, 1966; Wynder, 1969). This relationship was found in many countries, with Denmark, New Zealand, Great Britain, Canada and the United States showing the highest degree of correlation (Papaioannou, 1974).

Chronic psychogenic stress

Pituitary and adrenal hormone secretion as well as catecholamines may be the link between chronic psychologic stress and breast cancer induction.

Excess corticosteroids produced under stress have a marked immunosuppressive effect and may overcome possible immunostimulatory effects of growth hormone, thyroxin and catecholamines which are also prominent in stress (Papaioannou, 1974). The chronic psychological stress which is so commonly a feature of the woman developing breast cancer, may also affect growth of the tumor, possibly by mobilizing fats (Feldman and Carter, 1971).

Hormone administration

One of the most commonly raised questions in breast cancer risk is whether hormone administration increases the incidence of breast cancer. Since the first reports of Lacassagne (1939) and Lipschutz and Varga (1940) that estrogens administered to mice resulted in cancerous growths of the breast, there have been ample studies to show that estradiol administered for prolonged periods and in large doses to rodents and other laboratory animals can produce mammary hyperplasia and cancer. However, all of these studies involved administration of estrogen not containing the estriol fraction, and were given in doses well above physiological levels thus causing an unnatural response in the target organ (Leis, 1970).

Estrogens can also induce breast and endometrial hyperplasia in human beings. However, despite the extensive use of estrongens at the menopause for over 35 years, and the large number of women who have taken estrogen-progesterone contraceptive pills for nearly 15 years, there is no statistically significant evidence to date to show that their administration has caused a deleterious effect on the human breast (Taylor, 1971), or an increase in the incidence of breast cancer (Leis, 1970; Papaioannou, 1974).

In the male most carcinomas of the breast which have developed while receiving large doses of estrogen for carcinoma of the prostate have been shown to be metastatic. Occasionally however, breast cancers were induced when large doses of estrogen were given for other reasons (Papaioannou, 1974).

While there is no evidence to date that estrogen administration increases the overall incidence of mammary carcinoma, there may be different responses in certain groups of women. Black and Leis (1972) have reported that estrogen seemed to accentuate the risk of breast cancer in nulliparous or late parous women but that in early parous women the reverse seemed to be true. This would account for the absence of any change in breast cancer incidence in the total population who received estrogens, since no division as to parity or age at first pregnancy was made. One must await the results of the prospective randomized studies now in progress for a more accurate evaluation of the breast cancer risks from estrogen administration in humans.

Meanwhile it is recommended that the dosage of estrogen administration be within physiological levels and cyclic rather than continuous. Also that administered estrogen should contain the estriol fraction for its blocking effect on estrone and estradiol, and that progesterone should be added for its antagonistic effect to estrogens (Leis, 1970).

Trauma

No definite relationship can be established between single injury and the inception of breast cancer in humans, but it is possible that trauma may aggravate pre-existing carcinoma (Donegan, 1967; Leis, 1970; Pelner, 1961; Wynder, Bross and Hirayama, 1960).

Chemical agents

Polycyclic hydrocarbons have been shown to induce breast cancer in small laboratory animals. These agents have a structural similarity to the steroid hormones, and some have physiologic effects in animals similar to those produced by hormones. Much more work needs to be done before any conclusions can be drawn regarding their possible role in human breast cancer (Bonser, Dossett and Jull, 1961).

Hypothyroidism

Hypothyroidism has been shown to be associated with an increased risk of breast cancer (Blackwinkel and Jackson, 1964). It has been observed that patients with localized breast cancers show normal thyroid function whereas those with metastatic cancer show evidence of hypothyroidism (Edelstyn, Lyons and Welbourn, 1958). Thyroid hormones may well have an indirect role on breast carcinogenesis but the mechanism is not clear at present.

Other factors

The increased risk of breast cancer in certain geographic locations (Western Hemisphere), in certain races and ethnic groups (white race and Jewish women), in cold climates and in patients in the upper socioeconomic group, are probably related to genetic predisposition, parity, diet, viruses, hormones, chronic psychogenic stress or other factors which have been previously discussed (Leis, 1970; Ketcham, 1974; Papaioannou, 1974).

CONCLUSION

In the search for the high risk patient it is important to realize that the development of breast cancer is not a chance event that occurs randomly throughout the population, but that there are certain patients who have an increased risk of developing it, and that it seems to be a multiphase process involving a number of risk factors. The most significant of these would seem to be: genetic, viral, hormonal and immunologic.

The major risk factors are: sex, with over 99% of breast cancers occurring in the female; age, with 75% occurring over the age of 40, familial history of breast cancer with emphasis on mothers and sisters and premenopausal bilateral cancers, partiy with stress on the age at the first birth, previous cancer in one breast and the precancerous type of fibrocystic disease.

Prominent risk factors include: viral factors, immunologic factors, dominant gene for wet type cerumen and possibly some other genetic factors, radiation exposure, cancers in other organs, alterations in hormonal milieu including estriol fractions, castration (artificial menopause), total menstrual activity and aetiocholanolone and/or androsterone excretion.

Possible risk factors with varied statistical significance are: high dietary fat intake, chronic psychogenic stress, hormone administration, trauma, chemical agents, hypothyroidism, living in the Western hemisphere, upper socio-economic status, living in a cold climate, the white race and Jewish women.

The search for the patient with the highest risk of developing breast cancer would culminate in the finding of a 51 year old, fat, hypothyroid, Caucasian nun, living in a cold climate in the Western hemisphere, with a wet type of cerumen and a prolonged menstrual history, whose mother and sister had premenopausal bilateral breast cancer, who was nursed by a mother who had B viral particles in her milk, who has had endometrial cancer and a cancer in one breast, whose random biopsy of the other breast showed a precancerous mastopathy, who has a low estriol fraction and an abnormal Bulbrook discriminant, who is immunodeficient, who received heavy radiation exposure during treatment for tuberculosis by repeated fluoroscopies and who has a high dietary fat intake.

REFERENCES

Anderson, D. E. (1972): A genetic study of human breast cancer. *J. Natl. Cancer Inst.*, **48,** 1029.

Anderson, D. E. (1974): The role of genetics in human cancer. *Ca.*, **24,** 130.

Atkins, H., Hayward, D. L. Klugman, D. J. and Wayte, A. B. (1972): Treatment of early breast cancer: A report after 10 years of clinical trial. *British Med. J.*, **2,** 423.

Axel, R., Schlom, J. and Spiegelman, S. (1972): Presence in human breast cancer of RNA homologous to mouse mammary tumor virus RNA. *Nature,* **235**, 32.

Bentvelzen, P., Daams, J. H. and Hageman, P. (1972): Interactions between viral and genetic factors in the origin of mammary tumors in mice. *J. Nat. Cancer Inst.,* **48,** 1089.

Bittner, J. J. (1939): Relation of nursing to the extra chromosomal theory of breast cancer in mice. *Amer. J. Cancer,* **35**, 90.

Black, M. M. (1973): Human breast cancer. A model for cancer immunology. *Israel J. Med. Sc.,* **9,** 284.

Black, M. M., Barclay, T. H. C., Cutler, S. J. Hankey, B. F. and Asire, A. J. (1972): Association of atypical characteristics of benign breast lesions with subsequent risk of breast cancer. *Cancer,* **29,** 338.

Black, M. M. and Leis, H. P. Jr. (1972): Mammary carcinogenesis. *N.Y.S. Jour. Med.,* **72,** 1601.

Black, M. M. and Leis, H. P., Jr. (1973): Cellular responses to autologous breast cancer tissue – Sequential observations. *Cancer,* **32,** 384.

Black, M. M. Leis, H. P., Jr., Shore, B. and Zachrau, R. (1974): Cellular hypersensitivity to breast cancer; Assessment by a leukocyte migration procedure. *Cancer,* **33,** 952.

Black, M. M., Moore, D. H. Shore, B., Zachrau, R. E. and Leis, H. P., Jr. (1974): Effect of murine milk samples and human breast tissues on human leukocyte migration indices. *Cancer Research,* **34,** 1054.

Blackwinkel, K. and Jackson, A. S. (1964): Some features of breast cancer and thyroid deficiency. *Cancer,* **17,** 1174.

Bonser, G. M., Dossett, J. A. and Jull, J. W. (1961): Human and Experimental Breast Cancer. Pitman Med. Pub. Co., London.

Boston Collaborative Drug Surveillance Programme (1971): Relation between breast cancer and S Blood-Antigen System. *Lancet,* **1,** 301.

Bulbrook, R. D., Hayward, J. L. and Allen, D. S. (1969): Further observations on steroid excretion and subsequent breast cancer in Guernsey. In: Hormonal Aspects in the Epidemiology of Human Breast Cancer (J. H. De Bussy, Ed.) Amsterdam, p. 163.

Bulbrook, R. D., Hayward, J. L. and Spicer, C. C. (1971): Relation between urinary androgen and corticoid excretion and subsequent breast cancer. *Lancet,* **21,** 395.

Carroll, K. K., Gammel, E. B. and Plunkett, E. R. (1968): Dietary fat and mammary cancer. *Can. Med. Assoc.,* **98,** 590.

Chamberlain, R. H., Egan and R. L. and Harvey, R. A. (1970): Report and commentary: the carcinogenic hazard of radiation to the breasts. *Ca.,* **20,** 24.

Charney, J. and Moore, D. H. (1971): Neutralization of murine mammary tumor virus by sera of women with breast cancer. *Nature,* **229,** 627.

Clemmesen, J. (1965): Statistical Studies in the Aetiology of Malignant Neoplasms, p. 249, I. Review and Results, Copenhagen, Munksgaard.

Cole, P. and MacMahon, B. (1969): Hypothesis: Oestrogen fractions during early reproductive life in the etiology of breast cancer. *Lancet,* **1,** 604.

Davis, H. H., Simons, M. and Davis, J. B. (1964): Cystic disease and carcinoma of the breast; relationship to carcinoma. *Cancer,* **17,** 957.

De Waard, F., Baanders-Van Halewijn, E. D. and Huizinga, J. (1964): The bimodal age distribution of patients with mammary carcinoma; evidence for the existence of two types of human breast cancer. *Cancer,* **17,** 141.

Dmochowski, L., Seman, G. and Gallagher, H. S. (1969): Viruses as possible etiologic factors in human breast cancer. *Cancer,* **24,** 1241.

Donegan, W. L. (1967): Epidemiology of mammary cancer. In: Cancer of the Breast by J. S. Spratt, Jr. and W. L. Donegan. W. B. Saunders Co.

Dunn, J. E., Jr. (1969): Epidemiology and possible identification of high-risk group that could develop cancer of the breast. *Cancer,* **23,** 775.

Dunn, J. E., Bragg, K. O., Sautter, C. and Cardipee, C. (1972): Breast cancer risk following a major salivary gland carcinoma. *Cancer,* **29,** 1343.

Edelstyn, G. A., Lyons, A. R. and Welbourn, R. B. (1958): Thyroid function in patients with mammary cancer. *Lancet,* **1,** 670.

Feldman, E. B. and Carter, A. C. (1971): Circulatory lipids and lipoproteins in women with metastatic breast carcinoma. *J. Clin. Endocrinol. Metab.,* **33,** 8.

Feller, W. F. and Chopra, H. C. (1969): Studies of human milk in relation to possible viral etiology of breast cancer. *Cancer,* **24,** 1250.

Fraumeni, J. F., Jr., Lloyd, J. W., Smith, E. M. and Wagover, J. K. (1969): Cancer mortality among nuns. *J. Natl. Cancer Inst.,* **42,** 455.

Gallagher, H. S. and Martin, J. E. (1969): Early phases in the development of breast cancer. *Cancer,* **24,** 1170.

Guthorn, P. J. (1951): Carcinoma of the male breast. *Milit. Surg.,* **109,** 110.

Haagensen, C. D. (1971): Diseases of the Breast. W. B. Saunders Co., Philadelphia–London–Toronto.

Hems, G. (1970): Epidemiological characteristics of breast cancer in middle and late age. *Br. J. Cancer,* **24,** 226.

Hirayama, T. and Wynder, E. L. (1962): A study of the epidemiology of cancer of the breast. The influence of hysterectomy. *Cancer,* **15,** 28.

Huebner, R. J. and Todaro, G. J. (1969): Oncogenesis of RNA-tumor viruses as determinants of cancer. *Proc. Natl. Acad. Sci.,* **64,** 1087.

Karpas, C. M., Leis, H. P., Jr., Oppenheim, A. and Mersheimer, W. L. (1965): Relationship of fibrocystic disease to carcinoma of the breast. *Ann. Sung.,* **162,** 1.

Ketcham, A. S. (1974): Predictable categories of increased risk to breast cancer. *A.O.R.N. Jour.,* **19,** 852.

Knudson, A. G., Jr. (1971): Mutation and cancer. *Proc. Nat. Acad. Sci.,* **68,** 820.

Lacassagne, A. (1939): Essai d'une hormone thyreotrope en vue to modifier l'apparition de l'adenocarcinome mammaire chez la souris. *Compt. Rend. Soc. de biol.,* **130,** 591.

Lea, A. J. (1966): Dietary factors associated with death rates from certain neoplasms in man. *Lancet,* **2,** 332.

Leis, H. P., Jr. (1970): Diagnosis and Treatment of Breast Lesions. Medical Examination Publishing Co., Inc., Flushing, New York.

Leis, H. P., Jr. (1970): The pill and the breast. *N.Y.S. Jour. Med.,* **70,** 2911.

Leis, H. P., Jr. (1971): Selective, elective, prophylactic, contralateral simple mastectomy. *Cancer,* **28,** 956.

Leis, H. P., Jr. (1971): Multidisciplinary approach to the early diagnosis of breast cancer. *Intern. Surgery,* **56,** 135.

Leis, H. P., Jr. (1973): Premalignant Breast Lesions. In: Symposium on Neoplastic and Reconstructive Problems of the Female Breast. (Ed. R. Snyderman), C. V. Mosby Co., St. Louis, p. 11.

Leis, H. P., Jr. (1974): Primary Cancer in the Second Breast. In: Multiple Primary Malignant Tumors. (Ed. I. Severi), Perugia University Medical School Press, Monteluce, Italy.

Leis, H. P., Jr. (1975): Prophylactic, Immunologic and Prognostic Factors in Breast Cancer. Proceedings of the 19th World Congress of the International College of Surgeons (1974): Lima, Peru. (Eds. E. Rocca, E. Sabogal and U. Rocca). Excerpta Medica, Amsterdam.

Leis, H. P., Jr. (1975): Management of the Second Breast. Proceedings of the 19th World Congress of the International College of Surgeons (1974). Lima, Peru. (Eds. E. Rocca, E. Sabogal and U. Rocca). Excerpta Medica, Amsterdam.

Leis, H. P., Jr., Mersheimer, W. L., Black, M. M. and de Chabon, A. (1965): The second breast. *N.Y.S. Jour. Med.,* **65,** 2460.

Leis, H. P., Jr. and Pilnik, S. (1974): Breast cancer – A therapeutic dilemma. *A.O.R.N. Jour.,* **19,** 813.

Lemon, H. M. (1970): Abnormal estrogen metabolism and tissue estrogen receptor proteins in breast cancer. *Cancer,* **25,** 423.

Lemon, H. M., Wotiz, H. H., Parsons, L. and Mozden, P. J. (1966): Reduced estriol excretion in patients with breast cancer prior to endocrine therapy. *J.A.M.A.,* **196,** 1128.

Lerner, L. J. and Hilf, R. (1967): Biological Activities of Steroids and their Relationship to Breast Cancer Therapy. In: Current Concepts of Breast Cancer (Eds. A. Segaloff, K. K. Meyer and S. De Bakey). Williams and Wilkins Co., Baltimore, p. 80.

Levin, M. L., Sheehe, P. R., Graham, S. and Glidewell (1964): Lactation and menstrual function as related to cancer of the breast. *A.J.P.H.,* **54,** 580.

Lilienfeld, A. M. (1963): The epidemiology of breast cancer. *Cancer Res.* **23,** 1503.

Lipschutz, A. and Varga, L., Jr. (1940): Tumorigenic powers of stilbestrol and follicular hormones. *Lancet,* **1,** 541.

Lowell, D. M., Martinean, R. G. and Luria. S. B. (1969): Carcinoma of the male breast; report of a case occurring 35 years after radiation therapy of unilateral prepubertal gynecomastia. *Cancer,* **22,** 585.

Lynch, H. T., Guirgis, H. A., Albert, S., *et al.* (1974): Familial association of carcinoma of the breast and ovary. *Surg. Gynec, and Obst.,* **138,** 717.

MacDonald, I. (1966): The natural history of mammary carcinoma. *Am. J. Surg.,* **111,** 435.

MacKenzie, I. (1965): Breast cancer following multiple fluoroscopies. *Br. J. Cancer,* **19,** 1.

Macklin, M. T. (1959): Comparison of the number of breast cancer deaths observed in relatives of breast cancer patients and the number expected on the basis of mortality rates. *J. Natl. Cancer Inst.,* **22,** 927.

MacMahon, B. and Austin, J. H. (1969): Association of carcinomas of the breast and corpus uteri. *Cancer,* **23,** 275.

MacMahon, B., Cole, P., Brown, J. B. (1971): Oestrogen profiles of Asian and North American women. *Lancet,* **2,** 900.

MacMahon, B., Cole, P., Lin, T. M. *et al.* (1970): Age at first birth and breast cancer risk. *Bull. WHO,* **43,** 209.

MacMahon, B., Lin, T. M., Lowe, C. R. *et al.* (1970): Lactation and cancer of the breast. A summary of an international study. *Bull. WHO,* **42,** 185.

McWhirter, R. (1955): Simple mastectomy and radiotherapy in the treatment of breast cancer. *Brit. J. Radiol.,* **28,** 128.

Memorial Hospital for Cancer and Allied Diseases (1973): Epidemiology of Breast Carcinoma: A Review of Risk Factors. Breast Carcinoma Monograph, p. 17.

Mettler, F. A., Jr., Hempelmann, L. H. and Dutton, A. M. (1969): Breast neoplasms in women treated with x-rays for acute postpartum mastitis. *J. Natl. Cancer Inst.,* **43,** 803.

Meyer, K. K. (1970): Radiation induced lymphocyte immune deficiency. *Arch. Surg.,* **101,** 114.

Moore, D. H. (1965): Mammary tumor virus in mice. *Science,* **147,** 1158.

Moore, D. H., Charney, J. and Kramarky, B. (1971): Search for a human breast cancer virus. *Nature,* **229,** 611.

Moore, D. H., Sarkar, N. H. and Kelly, C. E. (1969): Type B particles in human milk. *Tex. Rep. Biol. Med.,* **27,** 1027.

Moss, N. H. (1965): Cancer of the Male Breast. In: Progress in Clinical Cancer (I. Ariel Ed.) Grune and Stratton, Inc., New York, p. 515.

Myrden, J. A. and Hiltz, J. E. (1969): Breast cancer following multiple fluoroscopies during artificial pneumothorax treatment of pulmonary tuberculosis. *Can. Med. Assoc. J.,* **100,** 1032.

Nohrmann, B. A. (1949): Cancer of the Breast. *Acta. Radio.* Suppl. 77.

O'Donnell, W. E., Day, E. and Venet, L. (1962): Early Detection and Diagnosis of Cancer. C. V. Mosby Co., St. Louis.

Okojie, X. G. (1974): Incidence of breast cancer among the Ishams of Nigeria. *Int. Surgery,* **59,** 209.

Papaioannou, A. N. (1974): Etiologic factors in cancer of the breast. *Surg. Gynec. and Obst.,* **138,** 257.

Peck, M. F. (1944): Malignant tumors of the male breast. *Surg. Clin. N. Amer.,* **24,** 1108.

Pelner, L. (1961): Host-tumor antagonism. XVII: Trauma and Cancer. *J. Amer. Ger. Soc.,* **9,** 58–76.

Petrakis, N. L. (1971): Cerumen genetics and human breast cancer. *Science,* **173,** 347.

Robbins, G. F. and Berg, J. W. (1964): Bilateral primary breast cancers. *Cancer,* **17,** 1501.

Schlom, J., Spiegelman, S. and Moore, D. H. (1972): Reverse transcriptase and high molecular weight RNA in particles from mouse and human milk. *J. Natl. Cancer Inst.,* **48,** 1197.

Schoenberg, B. S., Greenberg, R. A. and Eisenberg, A. (1969): Occurrence of certain multiple primary cancers in females. *J. Natl. Cancer Inst.,* **43,** 15.

Schottenfeld, D. and Berg, J. (1971): Incidence of multiple primary cancers – cancers of the female breast and genital organs. *J. Natl. Cancer Inst.,* **46,** 161.

Schottenfeld, D., Lilienfeld, A. M. and Diamond, H. (1963): Some observations on the epidemiology of breast cancer among males. *Am. J. Public Health,* **53,** 890.

Seidman, H. (1972): Statistical and Epidemiological Data on Cancer of the Breast. American Cancer Society, Inc., New York, New York.

Serrou, B., Dubois, J. B., Pourquier, H. and Romieu, C. (1974): Immunodepression in Multiple Primary Malignant Tumors (Ed. I. Severi) Perugia University Medical School Press, Monteluce, Itlay.

Shapiro, S., Strax, P., Venet, L. and Fink, R. (1968): The search for risk factors in breast cancer. *Amer. J. Public Health,* **58,** 820.

Shubik, P. and Hartwell, J. L. (1957): Survey of compounds which have been tested for carcinogenic activity. *National Cancer Institute,* Washington, D.C. *Monograph No. 6.*

Squartini, F. (1974): Multiple Cancers in the Mammary Gland System. In: Multiple Primary Malignant Tumors (Ed. I. Severi), Perugia University Medical School Press, Monteluce, Italy.

Stjernsward, J., Joundal, M. and Vasnsky, F. (1972): Lymphopenia and change in distribution of human B and T lymphocytes in peripheral blood, induced by irradiation for mammary carcinoma. *Lancet,* **1,** 1352.

Strax, P. (1974): Practical mass screening for earlier breast cancer detection. Post Graduate Course 045 # 15, Am. Coll. Obs. & Gyn. Meeting, Las Vegas.

Taylor, H. B. (1971): Oral Contraceptives and pathologic changes in the breast. *Cancer,* **28,** 1388.

Trichopoulos, D., MacMahon, B. and Cole, P. (1972): Menopause and breast cancer risk. *J. Natl. Cancer Inst.,* **48,** 605.

Turkington, R. W. (1970): Transfer RNA-methylating enzymes in mammary carcinoma cells. *Cancer Res.,* **30,** 650.

Urban, J. A. (1969): Bilateral breast cancer. *Cancer,* **24,** 826.

Wanebo, C. K., Johnson, K. G., Sato, K. and Thorslung, T. W. (1968): Breast cancer after exposure to the atomic bombings of Hiroshima and Nagasaki. *N. Engl. J. Med.,* **279,** 667.

Wynder, E. L. (1969): Identification of women at high risk for breast cancer. *Cancer,* **24,** 1235.

Wynder, E. L., Bross, I. J. and Hirayama, T. (1960): A study of the epidemiology of cancer of the breast. *Cancer,* **13,** 559.

14

Opportunities for Prevention

Robert W. Morgan and Damodar V. Vakil

In breast cancer, as in other diseases, we distinguish primary from secondary prevention. Our goal in primary prevention is to prevent the initial occurrence of disease. In secondary prevention, our goal is the earliest possible detection of disease, to be followed by prompt treatment aiming at cure. Unfortunately, most current preventive measures for breast cancer are based upon secondary prevention, which may already be too late for many patients.

Previous chapters have pointed out the epidemiologic and genetic factors associated with the development of breast cancer. Upon this knowledge we base our preventive program, knowing that there is no single magical factor, the control of which will eliminate breast cancer. Rather, it is a disease of complex etiology (Vakil and Morgan, 1973a; Vakil and Morgan, 1973b; Morgan, Vakil and Chipman, 1974) for which our method of control is based on the reduction of some, but not all of the risk factors (Morgan and Vakil, 1974). Thus each case of carcinoma probably represents an interaction of various environmental and genetic factors. Our control program cannot affect the genetic mechanism: we are unlikely to advocate a eugenic approach nor do we have available genetic engineering approaches to the susceptible genome. We therefore attempt to minimize the deleterious environmental influences in women known to bear a genetic predisposition to the disease.

PRIMARY PREVENTION

Ideally, we should aim at methods of primary prevention applicable to the entire population. For example, we should minimize the exposure of the breast to ionizing radiation, since there is evidence that such exposure contributes to later development of breast cancer (Myrden and Hiltz, 1969). Since it is not possible, as yet, to estimate the effect of low doses of radiation in the induction of breast carcinoma, we advocate caution to avoid unnecessary exposure. Unfortunately, this is the only protective measure which we are in a position to recommend for the entire population.

Most of our control programs must be based on an individualistic approach to the high risk patient. This means that we must identify the woman with unfavourable genetic or environmental factors so that we may manipulate her environment to avoid cancer development later. If we prevent the disease from occurring, we have achieved primary prevention. In breast cancer, as in most other diseases, this is our ultimate goal, and should be the most cost-effective. Avoidance of x-ray exposure is an attempt at primary prevention in the general population but in a selected population we can go somewhat further.

Table 1 Major Risk Factors for Breast Cancer in Approximate Order of Importance.

Approximate Order of importance	*Major Risk Factors for Breast Cancer*
1	Family history of breast cancer, especially bilateral or of premenopausal onset.
2	Late age at first pregnancy, or nulliparity.
3	Early age at menarche.
4	Late age of menopause.
5	Fibrocystic breast disease.
6	Radiation exposure (multiple fluoroscopies).
7	Family history of benign breast disease.
8	Upper middle-class or higher socio-economic status.
9	Above average height and weight.

Table I summarizes the major known risk factors, in approximate order of importance (Vakil and Morgan, 1973a; Vakil and Morgan, 1973b; Morgan, Vakil and Chipman, 1974). Obviously, we cannot change family history nor age at menarche. In women with family histories of breast cancer however, we might advise them to plan for children early in the childbearing years, rather than later. For many women, now, the timing of children is a matter of considerable choice and flexibility. If the patients were aware that they might reduce their cancer risk by earlier pregnancy, it could conceivably outweigh some of the socio-economic considerations which often delay childbearing.

A surgical menopause can greatly reduced breast cancer risk (Neel, 1955; Lilienfeld, 1956; Bucalossi and Veronesi, 1957; Hirayama and Wynder, 1962; Kaplan and Acheson, 1966; Feinleib, 1968; MacMahon and Cole, 1969; Trichopoulos, MacMahon and Cole, 1972). Although this is a drastic step, there may be surgeons who feel it is justified if there is a family history involving numerous premenopausal breast cancers, especially if it is associated with sterility and fibrocystic breast disease. Likewise, a case can be made for prophylactic bilateral mastectomy with silicone implantation for the person at very high risk and suffering from fibrocystic breast disease. Certainly, these women are a source of great concern to their surgeons and their family when they develop recurring breast masses. Again, surgery seems a drastic step but it is an available solution to the problem.

Another method of primary prevention which although not yet available is on the horizon, is endocrine modification on a long-term basis. Perhaps in the near future, we will identify teen-age women with an unfavourable estrogen profile. Recent work in this respect has been encouraging (Lemon *et al.*, 1966; MacMahon and Cole, 1969; Lemon, 1969; Cole and MacMahon, 1969; MacMahon *et al.*, 1971; Briggs, 1972), and if substantiated, leads us to the question of what to do about the women so identified.

One possible solution is the initiation of treatment with an oral contraceptive containing relatively large amount of estriol and low amounts of estrone or estradiol. This medication would provide the contraceptive effect desired by most women, while suppressing their natural ovarian function and supplanting it with a pattern of estrogens which is possibly less carcinogenic than their natural one. Naturally, there are numerous questions to be answered concerning the availability or efficacy of such treatment but, it is not unreasonable to anticipate a controlled clinical trial of such a method should current work on estrogen profiles continue to show promise. The role of exogenous hormones on the incidence of breast cancer is discussed also in Chapter 4.

Some authors report abnormally low androgen levels in some breast cancer cases and it is claimed that such an abnormality may predict a greater risk of developing the disease (Jull, Shucksmith and Bonser, 1963; Bulbrook, and Hayward, 1967; Adlercreutz, Luukkainen and Svanborg, 1967; Bulbrook, 1970; Bulbrook, Hayward and Spicer, 1971). While this may be of some etiologic importance, it has not yet provided a useful application in the primary prevention of cancer.

SECONDARY PREVENTION

Secondary prevention of breast cancer implies reduction in mortality or morbidity through early diagnosis and treatment, especially of asymptomatic disease (Shapiro *et al.*, 1968; Hutchison and Shapiro, 1968; Strax, Venet and Shapiro, 1969; Davey, Greening and McKinna, 1970; Shapiro, Strax and Venet, 1971; Venet *et al.*, 1971; Lynch *et al.*, 1972; Fink, Shapiro and Roester, 1972). Closely associated with early diagnosis is the question of screening. Screening does not diagnose breast cancer; it indicates women who probably have breast cancer. Actually, screening is even less specific, since it usually detects breast lumps rather than clearly distinguishing the benign from the malignant. In considering the usefulness of breast cancer screening, it is necessary to evaluate benefits against cost

Table 2 Annual Reduction in Mortality with Screening for Breast Cancer in Canada (from Morgan and Vakil, 1974)

Age Group	*Annual Deaths Without Screening*[1]	*Lives Saved Per Year With Screening*[2]	*Per cent Reduction in Deaths Through Screening*	*Years of Life Saved (per person)*[3]	*Person-Years Saved*
40–49	467	14	2.99	33.51	469
50–59	751	240	31.95	24.70	7668
60–69	760	69	9.07	16.71	1153
Total	1978	323	16.33	24.70	9290

[1]Statistics Canada (1972a).
[2]Calculated from data in Shapiro, *et al.* (1971).
[3]Calculated from data at midpoint of age 45, 55 and 65. Statistics Canada (1972b).

(Hutchison and Shapiro, 1968; Sackett, 1970), selective screening of the high-risk group as against the whole population (Dunn, 1969; Zippen and Petrakis, 1971) and the screening methods available (Furnival *et al.*, 1970).

There is not yet sufficient evidence to justify unselected mass screening for breast cancer. Table 2 indicates some of the potential benefits of early detection by mammography and physicians' examination. The projected savings of life are probably optimistic, given the variability in the quality of these examinations. Table 2 is based on the assumption that 65% (1,700,000) of Canadian women age 40–49 would participate (Shapiro, *et al.*, 1971; Statistics Canada, 1972a and b). Such a program would be unrealistic for Canada, especially in rural areas.

Although we cannot yet justify unselected mass screening, there may be a strong argument for provision of facilities for two types of women – high-risk individuals or study populations. We have sufficient knowledge of breast cancer risk factors to permit identification of many women destined to develop breast cancer (Morgan, 1974). For these women, primary prevention is not yet available. Are we justified in withholding from these women the probable, although unproven, benefits of screening? Already many such women are being screened by physician examination and mammography but unfortunately, there is no way to measure the extent or efficacy of the practice. An organized program might provide uniform screening standards as well as data for evaluation. There is also need for a series of controlled clinical trials of various screening methods, in order to determine whether or not screening will reduce mortality and morbidity, and among which age groups.

For each method of screening, one must assess sensitivity, specificity, yield, risk, acceptability, and cost of the test. Sensitivity is the ability to identify correctly the diseased person. Specificity is the ability to identify correctly the healthy person. Sensitivity, specificity, and disease frequency affect test yield. Risk from the procedure should not exceed the benefit produced. Cost is a function of capital outlay, frequency of testing, and cost of procedure. The procedural cost is closely related to the lowest level of skilled personnel required.

Table 3 illustrates some available screening methods and their evaluation derived from the literature (Lawson, 1956, Holleb *et al.*, 1960; Day and Venet, 1961; Gershon-Cohen *et al.*, 1964; Shapiro *et al.*, 1966; Connell and Ruzicka, 1966; Strax *et al.*, 1967; Shapiro *et al.*, 1968; Strax, Venet and Shapiro, 1969; Dodd *et al.*, 1969; Gray, 1969; Davey, Greening and McKinna, 1970; Furnival *et al.*, 1970; Thomas, 1970; Hodes, Wallace and Dodd, 1970; Shapiro, Strax and Venet, 1971; Venet *et al.*, 1971; Thiessen, 1971; Gilbertsen and Kjelsberg, 1971; Strax, 1971; Egan, 1971; Dowdy *et al.*, 1971; Wolfe, Dooley and Harkins, 1971; Lynch *et al.*, 1972; Nathan, Burn and MacErlean, 1971; Isard *et al.*, 1972).

Table 3 Comparison of Current Methods of Screening for Breast Cancer (from Morgan and Vakil, 1974).

Procedure	*Sensitivity*	*Specificity*	*Risk*	*Cost*
Self-examination	Good for large masses, not for smaller lesions	Poor.	None, except where false negative findings delay other screening.	Some moderate cost for individual teaching, but then very low continuing cost.
Physician examination	Not highly sensitive. Influenced by breast and physician characteristics, tumor size.	Poor.	None, except as above.	High, especially when done as separate procedure.
Nurse or technician examination	As above.	Poor.	As above.	Less costly.
Mammography and xeroradiography	Fair, especially over age 40. Will still miss some palpable tumours.	Not known, but likely poor.	Slight, but cumulative radiation effect.	High capital cost plus expensive technicians and radiologist interpretation.
Thermography	Poorer than above but perhaps better at younger age.	Not known, but likely poor.	No risk, except false reassurance.	Moderate-high capital cost, can often be operated and interpreted by technicians.

The varying sensitivity and low specificity of these methods is unlikely to improve and no method is ever likely to distinguish between a normal breast and one containing a microscopic tumour. A combination of methods will increase both cost and sensitivity. While mammography in conjunction with palpation by a physician is well documented (Shapiro *et al.*, 1966; Strax *et al.*, 1967; Strax, Venet and Shapiro, 1969; Davey, Greening and McKinna, 1970; Furnival *et al.*, 1970; Venet *et al.*, 1971; Strax, 1971), other combinations lack evaluation so far.

SELECTIVE SCREENING

Selective screening implies indentification and referral of women likely to benefit from screening programs (Morgan and Vakil, 1974, National Conference on Cancer Prevention and Detection, 1974). This approach reduces the need for facilities and personnel, while increasing the yield of the screening program. The selection may be through physician referral and it should be stressed that this means a program to educate physicians concerning risk factors (referral criteria), as well as the establishment of adequate screening facilities.

Table 4 suggests the screening procedures appropriate for women of various risk categories. We assume that referral for screening might also be modified by other factors such as the degree of patient anxiety, availability of services, transportation, and the presence of co-existing disease. Table 4 is not meant to be a rigid prescription for screening but rather, it represents a program based upon known risk factors (Vakil and Morgan, 1973 a, b). In applying the table, the appropriate category is the first column found applicable to that patient. Thus, for a person with no previous breast malignancy, but a positive family history of bilateral breast cancer, the recommendation in column (2) would be appropriate. The recommendations apply only to the specific age group. Since family and personal history change with time, periodic re-evaluation of the patient's category is suggested.

All categories given assume that there are *no breast symptoms.* The presence of a mass, pain, swelling, discharge or bleeding demand a full diagnostic sequence, not screening. The reader will note that the recommended screening activity decreases markedly for patients over the age of 80. The potential gains by early diagnosis in this age group are so small as to make expensive programs not worthwhile.

As an alternative or supplement to physician referral, one could implement a program of screening based on public education, individual self-assessment and self-referral for screening. There is no doubt that every woman should be a partner in her own health care. It is debatable, however, whether scarce screening facilities should be open to all (including those at low risk) or available only for physician referral. Until

Table 4 Selection of Appropriate Screening Procedures for Women with Variable Risks of Breast Cancer (From Moran and Vakil, 1974).

	Risk Factors					
Age	*Previous breast carcinoma* (1)	*Family history of premenopausal or bilateral breast malignancy* (2)	*Nulliparous or first pregnancy after age 30* (3)	*Previous cystic mastitis* (4)	*Menarche before age 12* (5)	*No known adverse risk factors* (6)
20–29	A,E,G,J,	A	A	A	A	A
30–39	A,E,G,J	A,B,H,L	A,C	A,C,H	A	A
40–49	A,E,G,J,	A,B,H,K	A,B,G,K	A,C,H,K	A,C,H,L	A,C,H
50–69	A,E,G,J	A,B,H,K	A,B,G,K	A,C,H,K	A,C,H,K	A,C,H,K
70–80	A,E,G,J until 10 yr. survival then F,H	A,F,H	A,C	A,C	A,C	A
80+	A	A	A	A	A	A

Breast self-examination monthly = A			
Clinical examination (M.D. or other)	Every 6 months = B	Yearly = C	Every 2 years = D
M.D. examination	Every 6 months = E	Yearly = F	
Thermography	Every 6 months = G	Yearly = H	Every 2 years = I
Mammography or xeroradiography	Every 6 months = J	Yearly = K	Every 2 years = L

facilities are widely available, the best compromise probably involves provision of facilities for physician referrals, with programs of professional and public education to encourage appropriate use of the physician as a counsellor in this matter.

It is not our intention to advocate, at this time, massive screening programs for detection of breast cancer. Rather, we see the use of existing or future screening facilities moderated by an intelligent pattern of referral based upon assessment of risk (Morgan and Vakil, 1974, National Conference on Cancer Prevention and Detection, 1974). Large-scale programs should be either designed as or preceded by major clinical trials of:

1. Breast self-examination, taught by various means (Day, 1960; Thiessen, 1971; Lynch *et al.*, 1972).
2. Thermography (Lawson, 1956; Gershon-Cohen *et al.*, 1964; Connell and Ruzicka, 1966; Freundlich *et al.*, 1969; Dodd *et al.*, 1969; Hodes *et al.*, 1970; Strax, 1971; Nathan *et al.*, 1972; Isard *et al.*, 1972).
3. Mammography (Shapiro *et al.*, 1966; Strax *et al.*, 1967; Shapiro *et al.*, 1968; Strax, Venet and Shapiro, 1969; Furnival *et al.*, 1970; Thomas, 1970; Shapiro *et al.*, 1971; Venet *et al.*, 1971; Strax, 1971; Egan, 1971; Dowdy *et al.*, 1971; Lynch *et al.*, 1972).
4. Breast examination by various health professionals (Gray, 1969; Lynch *et al.*, 1972).
5. Combinations of the above (Shapiro *et al.*, 1966; Strax *et al.*, 1967; Shapiro *et al.*, 1968; Strax, Venet and Shapiro, 1969; Davey, Greening and McKinna, 1970; Furnival *et al.*, 1970; Shapiro *et al.*, 1971; Venet *et al.*, 1971; Strax, 1971).

CONCLUSION

Breast cancer or its effects may be preventable. Childbearing at an early age will confer some protection. Until there are other methods of primary prevention, the physician must concentrate on secondary prevention including screening. In presenting risk factors as criteria for screening, we have attempted to make rational use of screening technology. While we have insufficient evidence to recommend mass screening, we do see a place for a vigorous approach to the high-risk patient. To develop more evidence for or against mass screening, we would encourage clinical trials of various screening methods. In the meantime, while we engage in a moderate amount of screening, we do so under the Scottish verdict of "Not Proven".

REFERENCES

Adlercreutz, H., Luukkainen, T. and Svanborg, A. (1967): Simultaneous determination of urinary estrogens, individual 11-deoxy-17-ketosteroids, total 17-ketosteroids, total 17 ketogenic steroids, pregnanediol and plasma cortisol during the menstrual cycle and in early pregnancy. *Ann. Med. Exp. Biol. Fenn.,* **45,** 277.

Briggs, M. (1972): Ethnic differences in Urinary Oestrogens (letter). *Lancet,* **I,** 324.

Bucalossi, P. and Veronesi, U. (1957): Some observations on breast cancer in mothers and daughters. *Br. J. Cancer,* **II,** 337.

Bulbrook, R. D. (1970): Prognostic value of steroid assays in human breast cancer, in Briggs, M. H. (Editor), Advances in steroid biochemistry, p. 387, Academic Press, New York.

Bulbrook, R. D. and Hayward, J. L. (1967): Abnormal urinary steroid excretion and subsequent breast cancer. *Lancet,* **I,** 519.

Bulbrook, R. D., Hayward, J. L. and Spicer, C. C. (1971): Relation between urinary androgen and corticoid excretion and subsequent breast cancer. *Lancet,* **II,** 395.

Cole, P. and MacMahon, B. (1969): Oestrogen fractions during early reproductive life in the aetiology of breast cancer. *Lancet* **I,** 604.

Connell, J. F. and Ruzicka, F. F. (1966): Thermography in the detection of breast cancer. *Cancer,* **19,** 83.

Davey, J. B., Greening, W. P. and McKinna, J. A. (1970): Is screening for cancer worthwile? Results from a well-known clinic for cancer detection. *Brit. Med. J.,* **3,** 696.

Day, E. (1960): What is an adequate "cancer checkup"? *Postgrad. Med.,* **27,** 274.

Day, E. and Venet, L. (1961): Periodic cancer detection examinations as a cancer control. In Fourth National Cancer Conference Proceedings, p. 705. J. B. Lippincott Co., Philadelphia.

Dodd, G. D., Wallace, J. D., Freundlich, I. M., *et al.* (1969): Thermography and cancer of the breast, *Cancer,* **23,** 797.

Dowdy, A. H., Barker, W. F., Lagasse, L. D. *et al.* (1971): Mammography as a screening method for the examination of large populations. *Cancer,* **28,** 1558.

Dunn, J. E. Jr. (1969): Epidemiology and possible identification of high-risk groups that could develop cancer of the breast. *Cancer,* **23,** 775.

Egan, R. L. (1971): Contributions of mammography in the detection of early breast cancer. *Cancer,* **28,** 1555.

Feinleib, M. (1968): Breast cancer and artificial menopause: A cohort study. *J. Natl. Cancer Inst.,* **41,** 315.

Fink, R., Shapiro, S. and Roester, R. (1972): Impact of efforts to increase participation in repetitive screenings for early breast cancer detection. *A.J.P.H.*, **62,** 328.

Freundlich, I. M., Wallace, J. D. and Dodd, G. D. (1969): Thermography and the venous diameter ratio in the detection of non-palpable breast carcinoma. *Amer. J. Roentgenol.,* **102,** 927.

Furnival, I. G., Stewart, H. J., Weddell, J. M. *et al.* (1970): Accuracy of screening methods for the diagnosis of breast disease. *Brit. Med. J.,* **4,** 461.

Gershon-Cohen, J., Berger, S. M., Haberman, J. D. *et al.* (1964): Thermography of the breast. *Amer. J. Roentgenol,* **91,** 919.

Gilbertsen, V. A. and Kjelsberg, M. (1971): Detection of breast cancer by periodic utilization of methods of physical diagnosis. *Cancer,* **28,** 1552.

Gray, L. A. (1969): Role of physician in the diagnosis of breast cancer. *Cancer,* **24,** 1183.

Hirayama, T. and Wynder, E. L. (1962): A study of the epidemiology of cancer of the breast. II. The influence of hysterectomy. *Cancer,* **15,** 28.

Hodes, P. J., Wallace, J. D. and Dodd, G. D. (1970): Thermography. *Med. Clin. North Am.,* **54,** 603.

Holleb, A. I., Venet, L., Day, E. *et al.* (1960): Breast cancer detected by routine physical examination. *N.Y.J. Med.,* **60,** 823.

Hutchison, G. and Shapiro, S. (1968): Lead time gained by diagnostic screening for breast cancer. *J. Natl. Cancer Inst.,* **41,** 665.

Isard, H. J., Becker, W., Shilo, R. *et al.* (1972): Breast thermography after four years and 10,000 studies. *Am. J. Roentgenol,* **115,** 811.

Jull, L. W., Shucksmith, H. S., and Bonser, G. M. (1963): A study of urinary estrogen excretion in relation to breast cancer. *J. Clin. Endocrinol. Metab.,* **23,** 433.

Kaplan, S. D. and Acheson, R. M. (1966): A single etiological hypothesis for breast cancer? *J. Chron. Dis.,* **19,** 1221.

Lawson, R. N. (1956): Implications of surface temperatures in the diagnosis of breast cancer. *Canad. Med. Assoc. J.,* **75,** 309.

Lemon, H. M. (1969): Endocrine influences on human mammary cancer formation. A critique. *Cancer,* **23,** 781.

Lemon, H. M., Wotiz, H. H., Parsons, L. *et al.* (1966): Reduced estriol excretion in patients with breast cancer prior to endocrine therapy. *JAMA,* **196,** 1128.

Lilienfeld, A. M. (1956): The relationship of the cancer of the female breast to artificial menopause and marital status. *Cancer,* **9,** 927.

Lynch, H. T., Harlan, W., Swartz, M. *et al.* (1972): Multiphasic mobile cancer screening: a positive approach to early cancer detection and control. *Cancer,* **30,** 774.

MacMahon, B. and Cole, P. (1969): Endocrinology and epidemiology of breast cancer. *Cancer,* **24,** 1146.

MacMahon, B., Cole, P., Brown, J. B. *et al.* (1971): Oestrogen profiles of Asian and North American women. *Lancet,* **II,** 900.

Morgan, R. W. (1974). In *Biochemistry of women: Clinical concepts,* p. 137; Curry, A. S. and Hewitt, J. R. (Ed.), CRC Press, Cleveland.

Morgan, R. W. and Vakil, D. V. (1973): Endocrine profiles and breast cancer. *Lancet,* **I,** 546, (letter).

Morgan, R. W. and Vakil, D. V. (1974): Etiology of breast cancer. III. Opportunities for prevention. *Can. Med. Assoc. J.,* **111,** 1105.

Morgan, R. W., Vakil, D. V. and Chipman, M. L. (1974): Breast feeding, family history, and breast disease. *Am. J. Epidemiol.,* **99,** 117.

Myrden, J. A. and Hiltz, J. E. (1969): Breast cancer following multiple fluoroscopies during artificial pneumothorax treatment of pulmonary tuberculosis. *Can. Med. Assoc. J.,* **100,** 1032.

Nathan, B. E., Burn, I. and MacErlean, J. (1972): Value of mammary thermography in differential diagnosos. *Brit. Med. J.,* **59,** 316.

National Conference on Cancer Prevention and Detection (1974): Summary of recommendations for early detection. *Cancer (suppl.),* **33,** 1759.

Neel, J. V. (1955): On some pitfalls in developing an adequate genetic hypothesis. *Am. J. Hum. Genet.,* **7,** 1.

Sackett, D. L. (1970): Can screening programs for serious disease really improve health? *Science Forum* **15,** 9.

Salber, E. J., Trichopoulos, D. and MacMahon, B. (1969): Lactation and reproductive histories of breast cancer patients in Boston, 1965-66. *J. Natl. Cancer Inst.,* **43,** 1013.

Shapiro, S., Strax, P., Venet, L. *et al.* (1966): Evaluation of periodic breast cancer screening with mammography. Methodology and observations. *JAMA,* **195,** 731.

Shapiro, S., Strax, P., Venet, L. *et al.* (1968): The search for risk factors in breast cancer. *A.J.P.H.,* **58,** 820.

Shapiro, S., Strax, P. and Venet, L. (1971): Periodic breast cancer screening in reducing mortality from breast cancer. *JAMA,* **215,** ,1777.

Stark, A. M. and Way, S. (1970): Screening for breast cancer. *Lancet,* **II,** 407.

Statistics Canada. (1972a): Causes of death. 84–203 Annual, Ottawa.

Statistics Canada. (1972b): Vital statistics. Canada Year Book, Ottawa.

Strax, P. (1971): New techniques in mass screening for breast cancer. *Cancer,* **28,** 1563.

Strax, P., Venet, L., Shapiro, S. *et al.* (1967): Mammography and clinical examination in mass screening for cancer of the breast. *Cancer,* **12,** 2184.

Strax, P., Venet, L. and Shapiro, S. (1969): Mass screening in mammary cancer. *Cancer,* **23,** 875.

Thiessen, E. U. (1971): Breast self-examination in proper perspective. *Cancer,* **28,** 1537.

Thomas, B. A. (1970): Screening for breast and gynaecological lesions. *Lancet,* **II,** 409.

Trichopoulos, D., MacMahon, B. and Cole, P. (1972): Menopause and breast cancer risk. *J. Natl. Cancer Inst.,* **48,** 605.

Vakil, D. V. and Morgan, R. W. (1973a): Etiology of breast cancer. I. Genetic aspects. *Can. Med. Assoc. J.,* **109,** 29.

Vakil, D. V. and Morgan, R. W. (1973b): Etiology of breast cancer. II. Epigemiologic aspects. *Can. Med. Assoc. J.,* **109,** 201.

Venet, L., Strax, P., Venet, W. *et al.*, (1971): Adequacies and Inadequacies of breast examinations by physicians in mass screening. *Cancer,* **28,** 1546.

Wolfe, J. M., Dooley, R. P. and Harkins, L. E. (1971): Xeroradiography of the breast: a comparative study with conventional film mammography. *Cancer,* **28,** 1569.

Zippen, C. and Petrakis. N. L. (1971): Identification of high risk groups in breast cancer. *Cancer,* **28,** 1381.

15

Role of the Breast Cancer Detection Centre

Philip Strax

INTRODUCTION

Preclinical breast cancer is defined as cancer detected before it would be presented in the usual course of clinical practice. It usually means cancer found before a woman presents it to her physician and mainly refers to minimal breast cancer which in some cases may be impalpable. It may also refer to advanced cancer which has been ignored by the patient, either deliberately or not.

Preclinical breast cancer may be found by the physician in the course of examination for some other condition, but more commonly is detected in a mass screening program. The breast cancer detection center which a woman can attend for regular and thorough breast examination even in the absence of symptoms, can play a key role in the earlier detection of breast cancer.

The detection of breast cancer by women themselves seems to offer no possibilities of any further reduction in mortality rates. However, the detection of preclinical cancer by mass screening has the potential to create a breakthrough in this respect. This concept has received its greatest impetus from a study by the Health Insurance Plan of Greater New York, in which mass screening has resulted in a one-third reduction in the death rate from breast cancer in an observed group even after 7 years of follow up.

Mass screening for earlier detection of breast cancer has been actively developed by the Guttman Institute of New York City and has culminated at a national level in the establishment of 27 demonstration programs involving 29 institutions throughout the United States for the purpose of evaluating feasibility and results. To date the results at the Guttman Institute, and in those centres in operation long enough to have gathered data, have produced a higher proportion of earlier breast cancer with substantially reduced axillary node involvement than would be expected in the usual course of clinical practice.

The greatest need for the future of screening lies in the delineation of the high risk group. This may come about on the basis of high risk markers in the history or in the hormonal milieu of a woman, or findings by clinical breast examination, mammography or thermography. Such selective screening on the basis of high risk factors would make periodic screening for the earlier detection of breast cancer both practical and widely acceptable.

THE PROBLEM

The breast is the site of 28% of all cancers and breast cancer is the most common cause of death in women between the ages of 40 and 44. It increases in incidence with age, so that the risk of developing the disease at the age of 70 is ten times greater than that at the age of 40.

Despite advances in surgical, radiotherapeutic and chemotherapeutic techniques, the mortality from breast cancer has not changed significantly in the past 40 years, although during that period, deaths from all causes in women have been declining. In the absence of any development in curative or preventive measures in the immediate future, our only hope of improving the prognosis from breast cancer is to aim at early detection—at a stage when we hope that tumour is still localized to the breast.

The question then arises, will the detection of more breast cancers at a stage when regional nodes are still uninvolved result in a lowering of a mortality curve that has remained stationary for 35 years? If the answer is yes, is there a practical method available today to implement such a concept. The following facts suggest that earlier detection properly carried out, might provide at least a partial answer to the problem:

It is well established that the detection of breast cancer at a stage when the axillary nodes are not involved, carries with it an 85% likelihood of 5 year survival. Yet, overall, one-third of women with breast cancer are incurable by surgical means when first seen, and of the remaining two-thirds, only about one-third are alive and well 10 years after diagnosis. Thus, only about 25% of breast cancers can be said to be curable at the present time.

The vast majority of breast cancers seen by clinicians are therefore late cancers for which we cannot offer a cure. Perhaps an important reason for this is that 9 out of 10 cancers detected today are found by the patient herself and not by the physician. Perhaps what is needed is to have physicians take over breast cancer detection—to have them examine a woman before she is aware of a problem—and possibly find cancer at an earlier, more curable stage.

Because we have been relying on women to detect their own cancers, breast self examination has been stressed in the past. Of the diagnostic procedures, this is the simplest to apply, the least expensive, the most readily available and it increases in value with regular repetition. It has been advocated by the American Cancer Society and health authorities for many years, yet this method, possibly the most effective of all, seems to have failed to affect the breast cancer death rate.

Why then have we not been more successful in saving more women affected by breast cancer. The answer must be that *our present treatment is not effective in the majority of cases discovered by our clinical methods.* We must consider two possibilities:

Firstly, are our weapons too weak to manage breast cancer? There seems no doubt that the surgical and radiotherapeutic approach used today can be successful when we are faced with a truly localized cancer, a single growth that is well confined to a small portion of the breast. On the other hand, when regional nodes show signs of involvement, removal of these nodes does not necessarily mean removal of all the cancer. Our weapons are therefore adequate for the early localized case.

Secondly, will it make any difference if we detect cancer earlier? Will earlier detection save lives, or by finding cancer earlier in its evolution, will it merely prolong life and not really increase the likelihood of cure.

In 1951 MacDonald enunciated his principle of "biologic determinism" in cancer of the breast, suggesting that the length of survival of a woman with the disease depended on the virulence of the cancer and the defensive mechanism of the host and not on the stage of the disease when presented to the physician. This concept was reinforced by a paper presented at the James Ewing Society meeting in Maui in 1974 by Gardner which indicated that patient delay of up to a year and physician delay of up to a month had no influence on survival.

Such statements would *a priori* dismiss mass screening for earlier breast-cancer detection as useless. It is the purpose of this chapter to show that in the earlier stages of breast cancer, the odds are strongly in favor of the patient and survival can be markedly increased. Even curability can be mentioned. What has been needed is substantial proof that earlier detection of breast cancer can substantially reduce the death rate from this disease. Such data would then logically lead to the widespread use of mass screening, or the involvement of large populations in the detection of unsuspected preclinical breast cancer. This proof is provided by the following clinical trial.

THE RANDOMIZED TRIAL

In December 1963, the Health Insurance Plan of Greater New York, a prepaid, group-practice plan, began a long-term randomized trial (under contract with the National Institute of Health) of mass screening for breast-cancer detection. The aim of the project was to find answers to two questions:

(1) Would mass screening using clinical examination and mammography result in a lowering of the death rate from breast cancer and not merely a longer survival?

(2) What would be the contribution of mammography in such mass screening – was it enough to make it a worthwhile addition to a screening program?

Of the 31 medical groups in the Health Insurance Plan, 23 participated in the study. Of their 500,000 members, 85,000 were women aged 40 to 64 years, reflecting a broad spectrum of ethnic and socioeconomic groups. They all received comprehensive medical care on a prepaid basis at their group centers. Within each of the participating groups, two systematic random samples of women aged 40 to 64 years were selected. Every "study" group woman was matched in the "control" group. The total number of women in each sample was 31,000, each medical group contributing a share proportionate to its size.

Study-group women were offered a screening examination in their medical-group centers. All women receiving the initial examination were invited for three follow-up studies at annual intervals, unless they were found to have conditions warranting earlier follow-up. Control-group women continued to receive their usual medical care at their group centers.

Each screening examination consisted of an interview to collect demographic information and a health history. The clinical examination, usually conducted by a surgeon of the group, was done without knowledge of mammographic findings. He recorded his clinical findings on a special form which included data on breast structure as well as on the masses found. He also included recommendations for follow-up care.

Mammography involved the use of industrial fine grain film (Eastman M type), low kilovoltage (under 30 kv) and variable target-film distance with close coning. Cephalo-cauded and medio-lateral views of each breast were taken by technicians specially trained for the procedure. Mammograms were read independently without knowledge of clinical findings by the group radiologist and then by two radiologists on the study staff. Differences of opinion were resolved by the chief radiologist on the study team. Radiological data were placed on special forms and included information on breast structural detail as well as abnormal masses and calcifications. Recommendations for follow-up were either for routine examination one year later, early recall because of suspicious findings, or for biopsy or aspiration.

Differences of opinion as to follow-up between clinician and radiologist were resolved by the staff clinical coordinator, who presented final recommendations for further care to the medical group responsible for the woman's follow-up.

Surgical and pathological findings in breast-cancer cases were obtained from hospital charts. The project's coordinating pathologist reviewed slides and conducted special studies of tissue blocks when available. All carcinoma cases were investigated for type of surgery performed, histological type, nodal involvement, and size of lesion. Records of post-operative radiation or chemotherapy were obtained.

About 65% (20,200 women) of the study group received their initial examinations. Of these, 80% appeared for their first annual re-examination, 74% for their second annual re-examination, and 69% for their third annual re-examination. About 60% of the participants in the screening program had all four examinations, 28% had two or three examinations, and 12% only the first examination.

Two important results are apparent after a 7 year period of follow-up:

1. There has been a one-third reduction in mortality from breast cancer in the study group as compared with the control group. There have been 108 deaths from breast cancer in the control group, compared with 70 in the study group, only two-thirds of whom had actually been examined. The remaining one-third has been carried in the study group for statistical purposes.

2. One-third of the cancers detected in the study group were found on mammography only and were not palpable by the clinician. In a group of 44 such cancers only 1 woman has died (Venet *et al.*, 1971; Strax, Venet and Shapiro, 1973).

It was particularly interesting that nodal involvement in the study group differed considerably from that in the control. The proportion with negative axillary nodes in the control group was 48%, which corresponds to the usual findings in medical practice. In the mammography-only cases, 79% were free of axillary nodal involvement. In the clinical-only cases, 75% were node-free. In cancers found by both modalities, 46% were free of nodal involvement.

In over 85% of breast cancer seen in normal medical practice, it is found that both x-ray and the clinician agree on a positive diagnosis. In the study, 33% of the cancers were found by mammography alone, 44% were found by clinical examination alone, and 23% were found by the combined use of the two modalities. It is therefore apparent that under screening conditions, the earlier cancers may be detected by only one modality and under these circumstances there is a high proportion with negative axillary nodes.

In the histologically confirmed cases of intraductal carcinoma (a group which would be expected to have a more favourable prognosis), 38% were detected by mammography alone, in contrast to the 11% found by clinical examination alone. Moreover the radiologist seemed to be more successful in diagnosing cancer in the larger fatty breast in women over 50 years of age, because, of those women whose cancers were found by mammography alone, 86% were over 50, and in 88% the breasts measured more than 5 inches in size. This compares with those cancers detected by clinical examination alone, where 66% were over 50 years of age and 70% had breasts measuring over 5 inches in size. In the case of cancer found by mammography alone 68% of the breasts were of the fatty type compared with 44% of those where the cancer was found by clinical examination alone.

A significant observation relates to the decreased death rate from breast cancer in the study group, in relation to the age of the patient. A lower death rate is evident among the study group women in the age groups 50–54, 55–59 and those 60 years and over. However, the death rates are almost identical in study and control groups at ages under 50 years. The screening programme appears to have resulted in a reduction of breast cancer mortality at the age of 50 and over, but not between 40 and 49 years.

Another important issue relates to the breast cancers detected in the study group. About 15% of them were detected within a year of a negative examination having occurred during the normal course of receiving medical care.

This quotation from an article on "Changes in 5-year Breast Cancer Mortality in a Breast Cancer Screening Program" (Shapiro *et al.*, 1973), sums up the conclusions: "In any event, the 5-year results of this investigation project the development of practical programs to screen for breast cancer as a high priority issue. In view of the costs, manpower and technical requirements, it would be unrealistic to expect a rapid spread of screening programs to cover major segments of the female population. But one might hope for two types of activities to be carried out simultaneously over the next few years:

(1) expansion of the availability of breast-cancer screening, either in conjunction with multiphasic examinations or in the form of single-purpose examinations; and

(2) further research that would lead to more efficient modalities, increased use of paramedical personnel and identification of women at high risk for breast cancer who would become special targets for screening programs."

The value of mass screening as a means of reducing the mortality of breast cancer had been demonstrated. It remained to determine a practical method for widespread application.

MANAGEMENT OF A SCREENING PROGRAM

Mass screening for breast cancer is not new. Many far sighted authorities like Holleb (1960) in New York, and Gilbertsen (1966) in Minneapolis believed that screening of apparently well women could lead to earlier detection of breast cancer and thus result in improved survival statistics. A series of reports by these authors showed that periodic examination could detect a higher proportion of breast cancers with negative axillary nodes. Gilbertsen especially found remarkable improvement in 5 and 10 year survival results in a group of women followed annually by palpation and inspection. Excellent studies by Holleb *et al.* (1960), Day and Venet (1961) and by Shahon, Santoro and Wangensteen (1961) were presented at a time when mammography was not in common usage.

In the early 1960s, Gershon-Cohen, Hermel and Berger (1961), Witten and Thurber (1964), Wolfe (1965), Sevens and Weigen (1966) and Friedman *et al.* (1966) discussed the use of mammography as a screening procedure in breast cancer. All reported the detection of occult, non palpable cancers, especially by periodic examination, but their conclusions varied from enthusiastic acceptance of the procedure to mild approval of its use in women over the age of 50 years. Most felt that the cost and effort of mass screening was too great in relation to the benefit ensuing.

These studies suffered by not using both clinical examination and mammography, and by the absence of a control group which was essential for evaluating the true potential of mass screening in reducing the mortality from breast cancer. Only a randomized controlled study as developed by the Health Insurance Plan, involving large numbers of women and containing a built-in matched control group, could provide the data necessary for a significant conclusion.

It must be emphasised that the mass screening of apparently well women for breast cancer differs in approach and methodology from the examination of obviously symptomatic women. As physicians we have been trained to diagnose and treat existing disease. We are in general so busy caring for the sick that there is simply not enough time available to hunt for unsuspected disease in the general population, and for this purpose we usually turn to paramedical personnel or to devices for help.

Moreover, early in the screening process, the cost factor is introduced. Should this particular screening program – let us say for breast cancer – have priority over some other health program? Is the cost of finding an unsuspected breast cancer (possibly saving a life) too great to make it worthwhile? In the symptomatic woman questions of expense, and questions as to radiation dosage received, duration of examination or even the proportion of benign to malignant findings at operation, are of little importance. Yet they seem to loom large when we begin to discuss the screening process. It may be useful to answer some questions that often arise.

(1) Whom should we screen? Only 7 out of every 100 women will develop breast cancer in their lifetime and if we knew which they were we could concentrate on them. High risk factors are being looked for, but in

my opinion, we are not certain enough of any one factor or practical combination of factors, to justify our turning women away from screening. It is to be hoped that reliable high risk markers will eventually be found, such as hormone ratios in urine or blood which can delineate the really high risk group.

(2) How frequently should women be screened for breast cancer? More data on many more women will be needed in order to decide which women should be examined and how often. Most investigators feel that at the present time a one year interval is most practical. Special provision must be made for those obviously at greater risk, such as those with previous mastectomy or those with a marked family history. Should a suspicious thermogram as the sole positive finding turn out to be a high risk marker, then certainly this should call for more frequent examinations. Provision must also be made for he clinician who may be specifically interested in breasts of special consistency or texture. At present there are no definite data on how frequently screening examinations should be done.

(3) Where should we screen? Screening should be available in the place appropriate to the woman being examined. Some segments of the population, especially the upper and middle income groups, prefer a medical institution and sometimes a prestigious one. For low-income groups, a hospital setting may be anathema. Such women should be examined in housing projects or churches or community rooms on a mobile basis. We must make the screening process available and accessible to those we seek.

THE GUTTMAN INSTITUTE

The success of the Health Insurance Plan screening program in reducing mortality from breast cancer in an observed group stimulated the formation of the Guttman Breast Diagnostic Institute in New York City (Strax, 1971). Its purpose was to determine the feasibility of periodic mass screening for breast cancer, to continue to improve its practicality, and to evaluate the roles of clinical examination, mammography and thermography in such screening (Strax, 1973).

Because mortality reduction had apparently been limited in the H.I.P. study to women over the age of 50 and because of the substantial numbers of "interval cancers" (i.e. cancers developing within a year of negative examination) three important modifications of the screening process were made:

(1) Since premenopausal women had breasts which were denser and more difficult to interpret in a mammogram, and since younger women might be subjected to more radiation exposure in periodic screening, the mammographic technique was modified to provide improved mammograms with greater resolution and enhanced contrast, yet with substantial reduction in radiation dose.

(2) Since thermography had come to the fore as a new method with potential for the detection of breast cancer and since it was effective in premenopausal women, it was added to the screening process.

(3) Since detection of an "interval cancer" depended on the woman herself, teaching of breast self-examination was included. Younger women are more easily motivated in this regard, and since they early demonstrated a demand for the examination, the screening study was offered to women over the age of 35.

The program has involved two projects – creation of a practical, accurate and economical examination and a program to motivate women to accept the examination. The value of the volunteer organization and staff of the American Cancer Society with its numerous divisions and units was recognized, and close association with this group has been most helpful in developing motivation of women at risk. The Institute now examines over 50,000 women per year at its centre in mid-Manhattan and at least another 15,000 women on an out-reach basis, usually directed to low-income communities.

The success of the Guttman Institute has stimulated the American Cancer Society and the National Cancer Institute to act jointly in establishing 26 other programs involving 28 other institutions to demonstrate the feasibility of mass screening for breast cancer throughout the United States. These additional projects are each being funded to screen 10,000 women for a total of 5 years. A data-collecting period of 5 years' follow-up will then ensue. All the programs offer a comprehensive interview for collection of demographic and health data, clinical examination performed by physicians or trained allied health personnel, mammography with film using a molybdenum-anode tube and compression, or with xerography and thermography. The Guttman Institute is being funded for examination of 20,000 women under the same auspices. Thus, data from a group of almost 300,000 women will be collected and should offer much insight into the potential of mass screening for breast cancer.

Examinations at the Guttman Institute are made available through the New York City Division of the American Cancer Society, which uses the press, radio, and television to make women aware of the problem and offers to provide them with further information, including an opportunity for examination at the Institute.

All studies are done independently so that the contribution of each modality may be assessed. Data are collected on special forms for easy compilation and retrieval. Details of the four-part technique offered at the Guttman Institute are as follows:

a. *Interview:* Demographic data, including ethnic background, education, menstrual, parity, breast and family history, are obtained, usually by volunteers specially trained for this task. Such information on a large scale may offer clues to detection of women at higher risk to breast cancer than others, and help delineate the group that needs more frequent watching.

b. *Clinical examination*: This phase is under the supervision of an experienced physician. It also is done by paramedical personnel, after training and under the guidance of the clinician. General breast characteristics are recorded on a special card and an impression of non-malignant no mass, non-malignant mass, or suspicion of maligancy is noted. Recommendation is made for one-year recall, early recall, or for biopsy or aspiration of masses. At this stage, emphasis is placed on breast self-examination. Women are taught the technique personally by paramedical personnel and are strongly urged to follow through on a regular monthly basis.

c. *Mammography*: Soft-tissue x-ray examination of the breast is performed with the Senograph, which is equipped with a molybdenum-anode tube to produce improved resolution and enhanced contrast. About 8 women per hour are examined with a radiation does of 2 to 2.5 rads per exposure, by using non-screen film, or 1 to 1.5 rads per exposure using a screen in a vacuum cassette. Two views, cranio-caudad and medio-lateral, are made of each breast.

A recent innovation has been the reintroduction of xerography by Wolfe (1969) as a display medium for mammography, instead of film. A charged selenium plate is exposed to the x-ray and a paper image produced which has considerably improved edge enhancement. This type of mammogram has found favor with many radiologists who consider it easier to interpret and many of the screening centers have opted for xeromammography. At the Guttman Institute the large number of patients makes the use of this display medium impractical at this time.

A xeromammogram needs an x-ray machine and ionizing radiation to produce the image, just as is the case with film but the technical factors are different. In general, the tungsten anode tube is more efficient with xerography and the molybdenum anode tube produces better quality mammograms on film. Both methods can produce excellent mammography and both have their strong points.

d. *Thermography*: A graphic representation of the infrared emanation from the breast is made with AGA Thermovision. This device produces an instantaneous photographic image on Polaroid film or on 70 mm photographic film. The examination takes only a few minutes if the patient is previously cooled. Although its complete role in screening has not yet been evaluated, most authorities agree that it should be part of the examination process because it is harmless, and because of its potential in alerting the clinician to the possibility of cancer in a breast with doubtful findings by the other modalities (Isard, Ostrum and Shilo, 1969; Isard and Ostrum, 1974).

Special forms are used to record impression of normal, symmetrical venous pattern or abnormal, asymmetrical patterns due to isolated hot vein, group of hot veins, or areas of increased heat or the edge sign. Recomendations are made for one-year recall, earlier recall for abnormal findings, or immediate recall for technical reasons. Inasmuch as areas of increased heat do not necessarily correspond to the location of a cancer, biopsy recommendation is not made on thermographic findings.

None of these methods is 100% in its accuracy. All can miss cancers or lead to surgical investigation of a benign condition. The combination of methods, however, increases the accuracy substantially. It is as though finer and finer sieves were put in place to catch the smallest cancer. Unfortunately, some cancers still elude our present traps, and some 10% of cancers become apparent within a year of a negative examination. Reliance is placed on breast self-examination to find these and every woman is taught this procedure at the time of clinical examination.

Training of paramedical personnel, supported in part by the American Cancer Society, is directed to several areas. Several of the Institute's personnel have been trained as pre-screeners in clinical examination of the breast. Several non-technicians have developed considerable skill in reading mammograms as pre-screeners. Non-technical personnel have been trained as health aides to canvass the community, spreading knowledge of the availability and value of the screening procedure.

With efficient logistics and concentration of examinations so that all are done under cooling conditions, the entire examination can be performed in less than 20 minutes. With at least 10,000 women examined per year, the cost for the complete examination can be reduced to less than $25.00.

Mobile screening:

The four-part technique used is the same as that described above. However, mammography may be performed with a 70 mm device that uses ordinary house current, is transportable, and is capable of examining up to 20 women per hour with a radiation dose of 1–1.5 rads per exposure (Strax and Oppenheim, 1968). Another unit for mammography is also transportable and has a stationary molybdenum-anode tube. It uses 110 v current and produces mammograms on 8 × 10 film.

A recent development is a 26-foot mobile unit that incorporates all of the four techniques (Strax, 1972). This makes the entire screening process completely mobile, and moreover, promotes widespread acceptance of the procedures on a community level. The equipment used on the van is the same as that used at the Center but all suspicious cases found in mobile screening are brought into the Center for definitive studies and follow-up.

THE RESULTS

In England, Agnes Stark and Stanley Way have been conducting a Breast Screening Clinic in Gateshead since 1968 (Stark and Way, 1974). At first, only clinical examination and thermography were used as the initial studies, with mammography being performed on women with positive thermograms. Because of the significant number of women turning up with cancer within a year of a negative study, it was felt that mammography should be added on a routine basis. Among 4,627 women screened, the cancer detection rate was 5.8 per 1,000 women examined. A high risk group which included 62% of the women, was screened by the three modalities of clinical examination, mammography and thermography in the period January 1970 to July 1972. In 2,684 of these "high risk" women a diagnosis rate of 19.3 breast cancers per 1,000 examined, was shown.

Table 1 Age distribution of women screened and of those proved to have cancer.

	Age Groups				
	35	*36–40*	*41–50*	*51–60*	*60+*
% of women examined	16%	15%	31%	24%	14%
% of women with cancer	1%	2%	29%	34%	34%

The more extensive program of the Guttman Breast Cancer Diagnostic Institute which has been in operation since 1968 carried out 49,450 examinations in the 3 year period 1971 to 1973. Of these, 24,246 examinations were initial and 25,204 were subsequent examinations. Of 2,071 cases recommended for biopsy or aspiration, 1,215 were carried out and 326 cancers found. The age distribution of the women and the cancers found is shown in table 1.

Table 2 Incidence of cancer and of node involvement according to whether examination was initial or subsequent.

	Number of examinations	*Number of ca. found*	*Rate per 1000*	*Negative axillary nodes*	
				no. of ca.	*% of ca.*
Initial examination	24,246	262	10.8	132	50%
Subsequent examination	25,204	64	2.5	40	63%

On initial examination, the number of cancers found was high because of the factors of self selection and the age of the women attending. Because these cancers had been present for varying lengths of time, only half of the women were free of axillary node involvement (Table 2). On subsequent examination, the number of cancers which have become detectable since the previous examination is much less, and the majority have no axillary node involvement.

The tandem technique, using clinical examination, mammography, and thermography gives the highest yield of positives because some cancers are detectable by only one of the modalities. It is interesting to note that those found by one modality alone, have a higher percentage of negative nodes (Table 3). Of the 326 cancers found, 300 were detected by the screening modalities while 26 were "interval" cancers found by the women themselves within a year of a negative examination. They are not included in Table 3. Since a positive thermogram alone is never the basis for biopsy, it also is not represented in the data. It should be noted that the absence of noted involvement is included in the data only when proven histologically. The surgical procedure in 12% of the cases did not include axillary dissection, so that the true percentage of negative nodes may be higher.

Table 3 Incidence of axillary node involvement according to method of diagnosis.

	All Cancers		*Negative Axillary Nodes*	
Cancers detected by:	*Number of Ca.*	*% of Ca.*	*Number of Ca.*	*% of Ca.*
Mammography only—not palpable	54	18%	35	65%
Clinical Examination only—not on X-ray	82	27%	50	61%
Both felt on palpation and seen on mammogram	164	55%	69	42%

Since 9 out of 10 breast cancers are detected by the women themselves, instruction in breast self examination is vital as a first step in screening. Women can be taught (and should be taught by the physician) to detect small lesions of 1 cm or less in their own breasts. Breast self examination is especially important to detect "interval" cancers and when practised as part of the screening process, "interval" cancers are detectable with a high frequency of negative axillary nodes. Of the 26 "interval" cancers in this series, 18 or 69% had no nodal involvement.

THE POTENTIAL

(1) Mass screening should result in earlier detection of minimal breast cancer and this should be reflected by a low percentage with axillary node involvement at the time of operation. Localized breast cancer with negative axillary nodes points the way to a reduction in the mortality rates.

In the mass screening programs now under way, self selection will be high at the initial examination and will account for a higher proportion of cancers being found on initial examination. After the initial examination, the majority of the cancers detected will be localized with negative axillary nodes. It should be noted that in the H.I.P. study, women were invited into the study on a random basis, so that self-selection was minimal. In that study, 70% of the cancers in the screened group had negative axillary nodes.

(2) Since all examinations in the screening programs will be done independently it will be possible to assess the contribution of the various modalities to the screening process.

(3) The educational value of the mass screening program for breast cancer is important. Not only is the female population alerted to the value of screening, but the physicians in the community also are educated in this regard. Every physician confronted with a non palpable cancer detected on mammography alone is likely to become converted to its value.

Motivation of middle and upper income women to accept breast cancer screening has been developed at the Guttman Institute to an increasing degree. In 1969, 6,500 women were examined. In 1974, over 40,000 were studied at the Center with an additional 15,000 examined on a mobile basis. However, even at the Gutmann Institute, where special efforts have been made to involve low-income women, less than 15% are black or Puerto-Rican. Mobile community screening is necessary to involve the low-income women.

Part of the examination involves instruction in breast self-examination. The potential of such education in breast self-examination is great and may become one of the most important benefits of the mass screening programs.

(4) Paramedical personnel are involved in the screening process in a major way – as interviewers, as clinical breast examiners, as technical personnel for mammography and as prescreeners of mammograms and thermograms. The Guttman Institute has had much success in this direction and many of the screening programs envisage the use of paramedical personnel, especially in the clinical examination of the breasts. Evaluation of their effectiveness in screening will be an important objective of the program.

(5) The extensive data being accumulated in the screening process will help to delineate higher risk groups and may shed light on the frequency at

which screening should be repeated. Information on mastopathy, menstrual, childbearing and demographic factors may provide further clues to high risk markers. Clinical examination will provide data on the breast structure of well women, and mammography, especially in repeated examinations, may help to delineate patterns more likely to be found associated with breast cancer.

Periodic examination presents the possibilities of restrospectively establishing earlier evidence of cancer than we are able to recognize at present. Additional information may be gathered on the value of thermography as an indicator of the woman requiring further investigation. Study of cancers found at a repeat examination may indicate the frequency of examinations needed in relation to age, and to the findings by the different modalities.

(6) "Interval" cancers, or cancers developing within a year of negative examination, were detected in about 15% of cases in the H.I.P. study. Large scale screenings will shed further light on such cases and may help us to detect some early signs which we do not recognize at present. There will also be a chance of evaluating the potential of breast self-examination in finding "interval" cancers at a localized stage.

(7) Much expertise in the modalities of clinical examination, mammography and thermography is present in the 29 institutions involved in the screening programs. It can be expected that improvements in technique will be generated – in the direction of economy, efficiency and safety. The centers will act as foci for the dissemination of knowledge on screening modalities to the medical profession.

(8) There are already indications that the concept of mass screening has been accepted by other groups – both public health authorities and the private medical sector. For early detection of breast cancer to become widespread in our society, many groups will have to become involved. There is here the potential that the 29 institutions involved in mass screening will produce the ripples that will extend far beyond them. The greatest possible gain of the breast cancer screening centers would be to produce on a national level, the one-third mortality reduction achieved in the Health Insurance Plan study.

REFERENCES

Clark, R. L., Copeland, M. M., Egan, R. L. *et al.* (1965): Reproducibility of the technic of mammography (Egan) for cancer of the breast. *Amer. J. Surg.*, **109**, 127.

Day, E. and Venet, L. (1961): Periodic breast cancer detection examinations as a cancer control measure, in *Fourth Natl Cancer Conf. Proceedings*, p. 705, Lippincott Co., Phila.

Egan, R. L. (1960): Experience with mammography in a tumor institution. *Radiology,* **75,** 894.

Friedman, A. K., Askovitz, S. I., Berger, S. M. *et al.* (1966): A co-operative evaluation of mammography in seven teaching hospitals. *Radiology,* **86,** 886.

Gershon-Cohen, J., Hermel, M. B., Berger, S. M. (1961): Detection of breast cancer by periodic x-ray examination: A five year survey. *JAMA.,* **176,** 1114.

Gilbertsen, V. A. (1966): Survival of asymptomatic breast cancer patients. *Surg. Gynec. Obstet.,* **122,** 81.

Holleb., A. I., Venet, L., Day, E. and Hoyt, S. (1960): Breast cancer detected by routine physical examination. *New York J. Med.,* **60,** 823.

Isard, H. J., Ostrium, B. J. and Shilo, R. (1969): Thermography in breast carcinoma. *Surg. Gynec. Obstet.,* **128,** 1289.

Isard, H. J. and Ostrum, B. J. (1974): Breast thermography – the mammatherm. *Radiologic C1. of N. America,* **12,** 167.

Lawson, R. N. (1957): Thermography – a new tool in the investigation of breast lesions. *Canad. Serv. Med. J.,* **13,** 517.

MacDonald, I. (1951): Biological predeterminism in human cancer. *Surg. Gynec. Obstet.,* **92,** 443.

Shapiro, S., Strax, P. and Venet, L. (1968): Periodic breast cancer screening in pre-symptomatic detection and early diagnosis, p. 203, Sir Isaac Pitman & Sons, Ltd, London.

Shapiro, S. *et al.* (1971): Periodic breast cancer screening in reducing mortality from breast cancer. *JAMA,* **215,** 1777.

Shapiro, S., Strax, P., Venet, L. and Venet, W. (1973): Changes in 5-year breast cancer mortality in a breast cancer screening program, in *Seventh Natl Cancer Conf. Proceedings*, p. 663, Lippincott Co., Phila.

Shahon, D. B., Santoro, B. T. and Wangensteen, O. V. (1961): Periodic examinations of the breast, in *Fourth Natl Cancer Conf. Proceedings,* p. 225, Lippincott Co., Phila.

Stark, A. M. and Way, S. (1974): The screening of well women for the early detection of breast cancer using clinical examination with thermography and mammography. *Cancer,* **33,** 1671.

Stevens, G. M. and Weigen, J. F. (1966): Mammography survey for breast cancer detection: two-year study of 1,223 clinically negative asymptomatic women over 40. *Cancer,* **19,** 51.

Strax, P. and Oppenheim, A. (1968): New apparatus for mass screening in mammography. *Amer. J. Roentgen,* **102,** 941.

Strax, P. (1971): New techniques in mass screening for breast cancer. *Cancer,* **28,** 201.

Strax, P. (1972): Female cancer detection mobile unit. *Preventive Med.,* **1,** 422.

Strax, P., Venet, L. and Shapiro, S. (1973): Value of mammography in reduction of mortality from breast cancer in mass screening. *Amer. J. Roentgen,* **117**, 686.

Strax, P. (1973): Mass screening for breast cancer. *Rev. Franc. Gynec.,* **68,** 457.

Venet, L., Strax, P., Venet, W. and Shapiro, S. (1971): Adequacies and inadequacies of breast examination by physicians in mass screening. *Cancer,* **28,** 1546.

Witten, D. M. and Thurber, D. L. (1964): Mammography as routine examination for detecting breast cancer. *Amer. J. Roentgen.,* **92,** 14.

Wolfe, J. N. (1965): Mammography as screening examination in breast cancer. *Radiology,* **84,** 703.

Wolfe, J. N. (1969): Xeroradiography of the breast. *Oncology,* **23,** 113.

16

Screening for Occult Metastases

James L. Quinn, III

INTRODUCTION

The detection of occult metastases in patients with breast cancer is vital for treatment planning. Radiotracer scanning has been used in breast cancer since the 1940's when workers at the University of California (Low-Beer, 1946; McCorkle *et al.*, 1948), found a significant increase in the uptake of ^{32}P tagged sodium hypophosphate in 34 of 41 malignant breast lesions. Inflammatory diseases of the breast caused false positive findings, and false negative findings occurred with small cancers that were located deeply within large breasts.

Radiotracer scanning techniques have been used: (1) to screen for occult metastases; (2) to screen for occult breast cancers in patients with a high risk of developing this disease; (3) to confirm the presence of suspected metastases; and (4) to help distinguish benign from malignant breast masses.

A practical problem in screening for occult metastases is that it is rare for a patient to be sent for scanning pre-operatively. The usual course of events is that a breast mass is found by the patient or her physician; a mammogram is usually obtained; the patient is referred for surgery for a biopsy of the mass; and appropriate surgery is performed on the basis of the pathologist's frozen section diagnosis. It is then that the patient may be sent to the Nuclear Medicine department *post hoc*, for one of a variety of diagnostic procedures.

SCREENING FOR OCCULT BREAST CANCER

The characteristics of a disease which make it suitable for screening include: (1) it has serious consequences; (2) it has a relatively high prevalence in the pre-clinical state; (3) there should be an improved prognosis as a consequence of earlier detection; and (4) a good screening test is available. Characteristics of a good screening test include: (1)

relatively high sensitivity; (2) relatively high specificity; and (3) the test is low in cost and of little inconvenience or discomfort to the patient.

Using these criteria, no current radiotracer scanning procedure can claim to be a very good screen for occult breast cancer. Yet, although we don't have an "ideal" screening test there is little doubt that breast cancer satisfies the above criteria of a disease for which screening tests should be applied. Repetitive screening for breast cancer leads to a one-third reduction in the death rate in older women over a five year period (see Chapter 15).

The two common measures of the validity of a diagnostic test are *sensitivity* and *specificity*. Senstitivity is defined as the proportion of those with the disease who are found "positive" or detected by the test, and specificity is the proportion of the group without the disease who are found "negative" by the test (Lilienfeld, 1974). At the moment there are no generally accepted guidelines which determine what constitutes an adequate screening program in breast carcinoma. Several studies are under way comparing thermography, xeroradiography and radiotracer scanning, but so far no results are available. Furthermore, the varied usage of the term "early" breast cancer makes the comparison of various screening results difficult.

BREAST UPTAKE OF RADIOPHARMACEUTICALS

The breast concentrates and secretes a variety of radiopharmaceuticals in addition to the earlier mentioned sodium hypophosphate. These include Gallium-67 citrate, pertechnetate, radioiodides, Bismuth citrate as well as the various phosphate compounds used for bone scanning.

Pertechnetate Uptake

In a small series, pertechnetate uptake was found in four breast cancers (Cancroft and Goldsmith, 1973). There was no increased uptake in two patients with fibrocystic disease. This procedure has technical drawbacks, such as interference from the background extracellular and cardiac blood pool radioactivity, that will probably discourage its widespread use.

Bismuth Citrate

Because of the strikingly high concentration of Bismuth-206 compounds in brain tumors we investigated its potential in detecting breast cancers (Jacobstein and Quinn, 1973). The emission energies of Bismuth-206 preclude scanning, so sample counting was done after biopsy, using standard well-counting techniques. In four out of five cancers of the breast there was a significantly elevated tumor to blood ratio 12 hours after intravenous injection of the material. One well-differentiated tubular carcinoma had no elevated activity. This technique is unlikely to have any significant impact on the diagnosis of breast cancers.

Iodine

Eskin of Philadelphia recently reported (1973) a study of 50 women, suspected of having either thyroid or breast disease. They had breast uptake measurements using Iodine-123. There was a statistically significant elevation of the radioactive iodine in clinically abnormal breasts. He reported that if at 24 hours, either breast shows a radioiodine uptake of 9% or greater, it is probably abnormal. Again it is unlikely, in view of the physical problems of measuring absolute breast uptake, that *in vivo* studies of breast masses will offer significant diagnostic information.

Phosphates

There has been a scattering of reports concerning the uptake of bone scanning agents in the breast. The largest series (Siegel, Friedman and Wagner, 1974), reported that of 33 patients with carcinoma of the breast, 24 had increased diphosphonate uptake in the clinically "normal" breast as well as in the abnormal breast. Only 2 of 17 patients who had no carcinoma of the breast had bilateral uptake of diphosphonate. Both of these patients had fibrocystic disease. Of those patients who had uptake in the clinically normal breast, 93% (24 of 26) had carcinoma. The authors suggest that the diphosphonate uptake in the breast may be a sensitive indicator not merely of breast disease but of breast disease that predisposes to breast carcinoma.

It has been proposed by another group of workers (Schmitt *et al.*, 1974) that the mechanism of uptake of both polyphosphate and diphosphonate compounds is related to large concentrations of acid phosphatase in human breast cancers and that these compounds bind to this enzyme's receptor sites.

BONE SCANNING

No single radiotracer scanning technique has had more application in the detection of occult metastases from breast cancer than the bone scan. A great deal of the impetus for this stemmed from the report of Sklaroff and Charkes (1968) that 10 out of 64 patients (16%) with surgical Stage II carcinoma of the breast had positive Strontium-85 bone scans. This was confirmed by Galasko (1969) who reprted that 12 of 50 patients (24%) with "early" cancer of the breast had positive bone scans with negative x-rays.

Then the race was on to "find the metastasis the radiologist missed!"

Significant technologic advances have occurred in bone scanning. The properties of clinically useful bone radiotracers are shown in Table 1. Technetium-99m compounds are the agents most frequently used. Although the bone scan is quite sensitive it lacks specificity, being positive in a variety of metabolic and non-neoplastic conditions.

Table 1 Properties of Clinically Useful Bone-seekers

Nuclide	*Half-life*	*Gamma Emission (keV)*	*Avg Skeletal Dose in Rads*	*Usual administered Adult Dose*
^{85}Sr	65 days	514	3.1/100 μCi	100 μCi
^{87m}Sr	2.7 hours	388	0.13/1 mCi	1–4 mCi
^{18}F	1.85 hours	511 (annihilation)	0.18/1 mCi	1–5 mCi
^{99m}Tc	6 hours	140	0.05/1 mCi	10–20 mCi

The strontium compounds are calcium analogues and could penetrate into the hydroxyapatite crystal in the bone remodeling unit. Fluorine-18 is thought to localize in the shell of hydration around the hydorxyapatite crystal. The precise site of localization of Technetium-99m phospate is unsettled and is currently thought to be in immature osteoid tissue (Rosenthal and Kaye, 1975).

Fluorine-18, a very good bone scanning agent, is not readily adaptable to camera scintigraphy whereas Technetium-99m compounds are. Technetium-99m diphosphonates (ethane or methylene) are more stable and more resistant to enzymatic degradation compared to either the pyrophosphate or the polyphosphate compounds (McAffee, 1975).

False negative bone scans can occur with breast cancers that are anaplastic, or in bone metastases that are quite sclerotic and metabolically dormant. Bone scans may also be called falsely negative when the entire skeletal system is involved by disseminated disease (Thrupkaew, Henkin and Quinn, 1974). The absence of renal activity in a Technetium-99m phosphate bone scan should alert one to that possibility. Approximately 50% of the fluorine or technetium compounds localize in bone and the other 50% in the urinary tract. This urinary tract activity can occasionally be of considerable diagnostic usefulness.

In 17–26% of patients with proven breast carcinoma, bone scans have been found positive and the x-rays negative (Pistenma, McDougall and Kviss, 1975; Hopkins and Kristensen, 1973). In contradistinction, x-rays are positive and the bone scans negative in only 1–2% of patients with breast cancer metastases to bone.

Of those patients who are clinically asymptomatic with Stage I breast cancer, only 8–10% show bone scan evidence of occult and unsuspected bone metastases. Whether this constitutes a high enough yield to advise a bone scan preoperatively has been challenged in several quarters (Brand, 1972; Green *et al.*, 1973). Using the bone scan to confirm the suspicion of metastases in patients who have musculoskeletal pain the yield is much higher; in our experience 15 out of 18 patients. However, occasionally the bone scan can be discouragingly insensitive.

Of greater importance is the inter-relationship of roentgenographic skeletal surveys and bone scanning. The bone scan should not be used alone as a diagnostic procedure and an x-ray of the area of scan abnormality is necessary to confirm the findings or to make a more specific diagnosis (Desaulniers *et al.*, 1973).

If one decides to perform a bone scan it should be a total body bone scan. A recent review (Sharazi, Rayudu and Fordham, 1974) of 100 "solitary" bone lesions reported that 54 were metastatic. Eighteen of these were from breast cancers and one quarter of these were in the extremities. Of interest is the frequently observed phenomenon of extensive metastases to bone but none to the liver. The converse is also seen not infrequently (Sharma and Quinn, 1972).

The bone scan may be used to select patients suitable for radical surgery or radiotherapy. If the scan and the x-ray are normal, then the patient should be considered free of metastases. If the bone scan shows equivocal areas, but the patient's history, examination, x-rays and biopsy of that region are all normal, then an equivocal scan is not sufficient to alter a plan for radical therapy. If the bone scan shows multiple areas of abnormal uptake, and the patient has pain in these regions, then even in the presence of a normal x-ray, the scan finding is sufficient to lead to serious consideration of less radical therapy (Butler and Brucer, 1974).

LIVER SCANNING

A variety of radiopharmaceuticals have been used to image the liver. The major ones are Iodine-131 tagged Rose Bengal which is selectively secreted by the polygonal cells of the liver, and colloids of either Gold-198 or Technetium-99m which are concentrated in hepatic reticulo-endothelial cells. The reported accuracy of liver imaging in searching for metastases varies from 77–84% (Lunia *et al.*, 1974). With the gamma camera and Technetium-99m compounds, it is generally felt that a metastasis must be at least 2 cm in size and located at or near the hepatic surface, to be detected by liver scanning. Both Rose Bengal and the radiocolloids show decreased or absent activity in hepatic metastases.

Gallium-67 citrate is of limited usefulness. This radio-pharmaceutical is taken up by many liver metastases but the tumor shows the same or slightly greater activity than the surrounding normal liver, making it extremely difficult to see. This is in contradistinction to hepatomas where gallium uptake is intense.

In a recent report of 1,424 liver scans used in the detection of metastases, an overall accuracy of 77.3% was reported. With regard to cancer of the breast there were 44 patients of whom 34 were correctly diagnosed by liver scanning (Lunia *et al.*, 1974; Fee *et al.*, 1974).

BRAIN SCANNING

In reviewing 550 patients with proved brain tumors on whom Technetium-99m pertechnetate brain scans were performed, 32 of 34 patients with proved intracranial breast cancer metastases showed abnormal brain scans (Quinn, 1971). It is most common to see breast cancer metastases as single or multiple areas of abnormal uptake which cross vascular boundaries and 50% are located deep to the surface of the cerebral cortex. However, metastases from breast cancer can occasionally mimic the findings seen in subdural hematoma when the tumor is implanted in a plaque like fashion in the dura.

Using radiopharmaceuticals, it is still difficult to distinguish a metastasis in the skull from one that is located on the surface of the cerebral cortex. Pertechnetate concentrates in both lesions and the bone scanning agents may also concentrate in metastatic intracranial tumors, as well as in the area of bone destruction from a metastasis in the cranial table.

LYMPH NODE SCANNING

The probability of metastases in the internal mammary lymph node chain is approximately 50% when the primary breast cancer is in the central or medial aspect of the breast and the axillary lymph nodes are histologically positive (Nelson and Montague, 1975). The preoperative determination of internal mammary involvement would be extremely useful in designing appropriate post-operative irradiation to one or both internal mammary chains.

Despite the fact that scattered reports continue to appear in the literature concerning lymph node scanning, the technique has not gained widespread acceptance in the evaluation of patients with breast carcinoma. At first, radioactive Gold-198 particles were used in these studies (Kazen *et al.*, 1968). These colloidal particles range in size from 9–15 millimicrons, and over a period of 24–48 hours are clearly identifiable in the lymph nodes. Abnormal or involved nodes will show either no uptake or filling defects in the uptake. The spatial resolution for the Gold-198 energy is inferior to that of the Technetium-99m energy, and this has discouraged its widespread use.

Technetium-99m labelled sulfur colloid prepared with the hydrogen sulfide method was described as being useful for lymph node scanning (Hauser, Atkins and Richards, 1969). These particles are from 10–50 millimicrons in size. Technetium sulfur colloid prepared by the thiosulfate method produces too large a particle to be picked up readily by the lymph system. An alternative method was reported using antimony sulfide for preparing suitable Technetium-99m colloidal particles that could be used for lymph node scanning (Garzon, 1965). The size range of these particles is from 4–12 millimicrons, and is thus comparable to colloidal Gold-198.

Ege (1975) at the Princess Margaret Hospital in Toronto, Canada has used this preparation in the evaluation of over 600 patients. He has found it valuable for assessing the integrity of parasternal lymphatics, and perhaps more important, in establishing a baseline pattern for each patient. There is considerable anatomic variation in parasternal lymph drainage and this technique has been dramatic in the demonstration of disparity between parasternal nodal uptake and the conventional borders of classic radiation therapy portals. This procedure is able to detect cross drainage between potentially involved nodes and contralateral lymphatics. Because of the ease of its performance, and the reproducibility of the test using the patient as her own initial control, it may have a considerable impact on future treatment planning of breast cancer.

Both sides are studied approximately 3 hours after a subcostal injection. Obvious disparity in the pattern of uptake between the two sides is thought to be reliable evidence of involvement of one parasternal internal mammary chain. As Dr. Ege says "this simple and reproducible technique offers a unique means for bridging the disparity between concepts rooted in anatomic dogma and the dynamic situation which pertains to each patient during life" (Ege, 1975).

CONCLUSION

Although no ideal screening test for occult metastases in breast concer exists today, several radiotracer techniques are useful in patient diagnosis and management if judiciously applied.

The bone scan may be the most sensitive of these and should replace routine total body x-ray surveys in screening for occult metastases, or during follow up, to confirm suspected osseous metastases.

The brain scan, also quite sensitive, has its greatest application in confirming suspected metastases. Its yield in an asymptomatic patient is almost *nil.*

Current liver scanning techniques have a low false positive but a significantly high false negative rate (about 25%). This makes a "positive" liver scan more meaningful in the confirmation of suspected metastases than is a "negative" liver scan in excluding metastases.

We are in the second generation of lymph node scanning with the use of the scintillation camera and colloidal Technetium-99m. It is possible that investigation of internal mammary node drainage will have a dramatic effect on field planning in radiotheraphy.

REFERENCES

Brand, W. N. (1972): AEC Symposium 27 "Clinical Uses of Radionuclides: Critical Comparison with Other Techniques", p. 156.

Butler, D. E. and Brucer, N. (1974): Interpretations of Bone Scans, Editorial. *JAMA,* **229,** 1783.

Cancroft, E. T. and Goldsmith, F. J. (1973): Technetium-99m Pertechnetate Scintigraphy as an Aid in the Diagnosis of Breast Masses. *Radiology,* **106,** 441.

Desaulniers, N., LaCourciere, Yves, Lisbona, R. N. and Rosenthall, L. (1973): A Detailed Comparison of Bone Scanning with Technetium-99m Polyphosphate and Radiographic Skeletal Surveys for Neoplasm. *Journal De L'Association Canadienne des Radiologists,* **24,** 340.

Ege, G. N. (1975): Personal Communication.

Eskin, B. A Parker, J. A., Bassett, J. G. and George, D. L. (1974): Human Breast Uptake of Radioactive Iodine. *Obstet. Gynec,* **44,** 398.

Fee, H. J., Jr., Prokop, E. K., Cameron, J. L. and Wagner, H. N., Jr. (1974): Liver Scanning in Patients with Suspected Abdominal Tumor. *JAMA,* **230,** 1675.

Galasko, C. S. B. (1969): The Detection of Skeletal Metastases From Mammary Cancer by Gamma Camera Scintigraphy. *Brit. J. Surg.,* **56,** 757.

Garzon, O. L. (1965): A Technetium Labelled Colloid. *Int. J. Applied Rad. Isotopes,* **16,** 613.

Green, D., Jeremy, R., Towson, J. and Morris, J. (1973): The Role of Fluorine-18 in the Detection of Skeletal Metastases in Early Breast Cancer. *Aust. New Zeal. J. Surg.,* **43,** 251.

Hauser, W., Atkins, H. L. and Richards, P. (1969): Lymph Node Scanning with Technetium-99m Sulfur Colloid. *Radiology,* **93,** 1369.

Hopkins, G. B. and Kristensen, K. A. B. (1973): Whole Body Skeletal Scintiphotography in the Detection of Occult Metastatic Breast Carcinoma. *Calif. Med.,* **119,** 10.

Jacobstein, J. G. and Quinn III, J. L. (1973): Uptake of ^{206}Bi Citrate in Carcinoma of the Breast. *Radiology,* **107,** 677.

Kazem, I., Antonaides, J., Brady, L. W., Foust, D. S., Croll, M. N. and Lightfoot, David. (1968): Clinical Evaluation of Lymph Node Scanning Utilizing Colloidal Gold-198. *Radiology,* **90,** 905.

Lilienfield Abraham, M. (1974): Some Limitations and Problems of Screening for Cancer. *Cancer,* **33,** Number 6.

Low-Beer, B. V. A. (1946): Surface Measurements of Radioactive Phosphorus in Breast Tumors as a Possible Diagnostic Method. (Letters to the Editor). *Science,* **104,** 399.

Lunia, Shantilal, Parthasarathy, K. L., Bakshi, S. and Bender, Merrill, A. (1975): An Evaluation of ^{99m} Tc-Sulfur Colloid Liver Scintiscans and Their Usefulness in Metastatic Workup: A Review of 1,424 Studies. *J. Nucl. Med.,* **16,** 62.

McAffee, J. G. (1975): Personal Communication.

McCorkle, H. J., Low-Beer, B. V. A., Bell, H. G. and Stone, R. S. (1948): Clinical and Laboratory Studies on the Uptake of Radioactive Phosphorus by Lesions of the Breast. *Surgery,* **24,** 409.

Nelson III, Alvah J. and Montague, Eleanor D. (1975): Resectable Localized Breast Cancer. *JAMA,* **231,** 189.

Pistenma, D. A., McDougall, I. R. and Kriss, J. P. (1975): Screening for Bone Metastases – Are Only Scans Necessary? *JAMA,* **231,** 46.

Quinn III, J. L. (1971): Use of Diagnostic Nuclear Medicine Procedures in Breast Cancer. *Cancer,* **28,** 1695.

Rosenthal, L. and Kaye, M. (1975): Technetium-99m Pyrophosphhate Kinetics and Imaging in Metabolic Bone Disease. *J. Nucl. Med.,* **16,** 33.

Schmitt, G. H., Holmes, R. A., Isitman, A. T., Hensley, G. T. and Lewis, J. D. (1974): A Proposed Mechanism of Technetium-99m Labelled Polyphosphate and Diphosphonate Uptake by Human Breast Tissue. *Radiology,* **112,** 733.

Sharazi, P. H., Rayudu, G. V. S. and Fordham, E. W. (1974): Review of Solitary Fluorine-18 Bone Scan Lesions, *Radiology,* **112,** 369.

Sharma, S. M. and Quinn III, J. L. (1972): Sensitivity of ^{18}F-Bone Scans in the Search for Metastases. *Surg. Gynec. Obstet.,* **135,** 536.

Siegel, M. E., Friedman, B. H. and Wagner, H. N., Jr. (1974): A New Approach to Breast Cancer, Breast Uptake of Technetium-99m-Hedspa. *JAMA,* **229,** 1769.

Sklaroff, D. M. and Charkes, N. D. (1968): Bone Metastases from Breast Cancer at the Time of Radical Mastectomy. *Surg. Gynec, Obstet.,* **127,** 763.

Thrupkaew, A. K., Henkin, R. E. and Quinn III, J. L. (1974): False Negative Bone Scans in Disseminated Metastatic Disease. *Radiology,* **113,** 383.

Index